THE PHARMACY LEADERSHIP FIELD GUIDE

Cases and advice for everyday situations

D1616690

Michael A. DeCoske, PharmD, BCPS
Associate Chief Pharmacy Officer,
    Ambulatory Services
Department of Pharmacy
Duke University Hospital
Durham, North Carolina

Jennifer E. Tryon, MS, PharmD
Assistant Director of Inpatient Pharmacy
PeaceHealth Southwest Medical Center
Vancouver, Washington

Sara J. White, MS, FASHP
(Ret.) Director of Pharmacy
Stanford Hospital and Clinics
Mountain View, California

American Society of Health-System Pharmacists®
Bethesda, Maryland

Any correspondence regarding this publication should be sent to the publisher, American Society of Health-System Pharmacists, 7272 Wisconsin Avenue, Bethesda, MD 20814, attention: Special Publishing.

The information presented herein reflects the opinions of the contributors and advisors. It should not be interpreted as an official policy of ASHP or as an endorsement of any product.

Because of ongoing research and improvements in technology, the information and its applications contained in this text are constantly evolving and are subject to the professional judgment and interpretation of the practitioner due to the uniqueness of a clinical situation. The editors, contributors, and ASHP have made reasonable efforts to ensure the accuracy and appropriateness of the information presented in this document. However, any user of this information is advised that the editors, contributors, advisors, and ASHP are not responsible for the continued currency of the information, for any errors or omissions, and/or for any consequences arising from the use of the information in the document in any and all practice settings. Any reader of this document is cautioned that ASHP makes no representation, guarantee, or warranty, express or implied, as to the accuracy and appropriateness of the information contained in this document and specifically disclaims any liability to any party for the accuracy and/or completeness of the material or for any damages arising out of the use or non-use of any of the information contained in this document.

Director, Special Publishing: Jack Bruggeman
Acquisitions Editor: Rebecca Olson
Senior Editorial Project Manager: Dana Battaglia
Production Editor: Kristin Eckles
Cover Design: Carol Barrer
Page Design: DeVall Advertising

ISBN 978-1-58528-249-4

Dedications

I dedicate this book to my loving mom and dad for their years of sacrifice and support; to my Grandma Gladys for giving all that you have without ever asking anything in return; to my Aunt Donna for helping our family to flourish from the start; to my sister Madison for being such a great friend; and to my pharmacy mentors who daily help me navigate through and triumph over leadership challenges.

—*Michael A. DeCoske*

I dedicate this book to my mom and dad, Joyce and Robert (Sam) Tryon, who inspired my passion for leadership, to my husband and best friend Rene Mandrones for loving and supporting me, and to my mentor Sara White for unconditional support as I face the successes and challenges of my leadership journey.

—*Jennifer E. Tryon*

I want to dedicate this book to all of the staff, students, and residents I have had the pleasure to work with in over 40 years. They have been instrumental in teaching me what a good leader needs to do to be successful, and I will be forever grateful. My leadership philosophy began with Clifton J. Latiolais as my role model at Ohio State during my MS-Residency and was enhanced by working with Harold N. Godwin at the University of Kansas for 20 years. I also want to dedicate this book to current young leaders, such as Jennifer and Mike, who encourage me to continue contributing professionally even in retirement.

—*Sara J. White*

Acknowledgments

We would like to thank our case content reviewers for their valuable contributions. New practitioners Drs. Vicki Tkacz Brown, Jennifer Devos, Brent Reed, and Tim Ulbrich, as well as veteran mentors Drs. Marialice Bennett, Rebecca Chater, Kelly Goode, and Janelle Ruisinger, helped us to ensure that our pharmacy leadership cases are applicable to a broad range of pharmacy practice settings. We would like to thank our case content reviewers for their valuable contributions.

The Editors

Contents

Foreword

It is gratifying to witness the evolution of the profession of pharmacy over the past 40 years. We take the existence of unit-dose drug distribution and intravenous admixture programs for granted and expect the delivery of the right drug to the right patient at the right time. Many health systems such as Ohio State University Medical Center Department of Pharmacy also offer comprehensive patient care services in various specialties including internal medicine, pediatrics, and surgery as well as subspecialties such as cardiology, infectious diseases, and transplantation. ASHP surveys of health-system pharmacies, however, have reported marked variability in the types of pharmacy services offered and in the use of technology to achieve the best health outcomes for our patients.

The public expects community pharmacists to fill prescriptions accurately, efficiently and safely at the lowest cost. Medication therapy management or disease management programs are being offered in an increasing number of pharmacies; however, wide variability exists in the availability of these services in the community setting. Why are some health-system or community pharmacies able to offer more comprehensive and patient-focused services than others? One among many distinguishing features is the quality of leadership provided by the directors, managers, supervisors, pharmacists and technicians working in some practice settings as change agents or change leaders versus others.

Most of us have learned about leadership unconsciously and informally (e.g., through participation in student associations or attending a few lectures as a part of other courses). I do not recall ever learning specifically about leadership during my college years. In fact, I thought knowledge and training of leadership were needed by only those pursuing administrative or managerial positions. Several years after graduation I realized the importance of learning about leadership for all pharmacists for both professional and personal development. Most of my learning about leadership came from reading books, observing leaders, good mentoring, and active involvement in local, state, and national organizations. Since 2006, I have enjoyed teaching a course on leadership at Ohio State University to our pharmacy students, and it has been a tremendous learning experience for me and for our students based on the evaluation of this course.

Although there is a vast amount of literature including books and articles written on leadership, no specific book exists with direct applications for pharmacy students. This book, edited by DeCoske, Tryon, and White, is a welcome addition to the available resources and is particularly timely as we identify our unique roles in the healthcare reform to achieve the desired cost-effective health outcomes. I believe leadership education and training must begin in the college of pharmacy. This work would, of course, need to continue throughout one's career as is true for the continuous development of our professional competence.

This book has nine chapters from various authors on topics related to leadership. An excellent feature of the book is a series of case studies on pharmacy-related leadership challenges. Completion of these exercises should teach students how to address practical issues in effective ways.

The book discusses leadership versus management principles, attributes of effective leaders and managers, and the importance of passion, vision, integrity, trust, and calculated risk taking. It emphasizes that everyone is a leader ("little L") even though only some will become positional leaders ("big L"). The roles of professional organizations, mentoring, strategic planning, and effective communications in developing leadership are well described. One must also know how to work efficiently, negotiate, prioritize, delegate, and engage in difficult conversations and manage conflicts. The book discusses the importance of using people skills in developing positive relationships with individuals and inspiring them to become a part of the team to achieve collective goals. Finally, leaders must enthusiastically embrace change and know how to continue leading and marketing ideas. The key concepts and case studies in this book are an excellent substrate for developing leadership among pharmacy students. The editors are to be congratulated for conceiving and completing this important and much needed book.

Milap C. Nahata, MS, PharmD
Professor and Division Chair
College of Pharmacy
Professor of Pediatrics and Internal Medicine
College of Medicine
Ohio State University (OSU)
Associate Director of Pharmacy
OSU Medical Center
Columbus, Ohio

Preface

Every pharmacist faces leadership challenges every day, whether they realize it or not. The manner in which these challenges are handled can promote a positive image for the pharmacy profession or result in catastrophic outcomes for everyone involved. While pharmacists receive exceptional didactic clinical training, leadership skills are another crucial, often underdeveloped, skill set necessary for the success of a pharmacist. As leadership skills are studied, practiced, and mentored, pharmacists will enjoy greater career success in any setting they choose to work.

Some pharmacists may choose to be a "big L" leader, pursuing a career with a formal leadership title (manager, director, lead pharmacist). All other pharmacists, however, must be a "little L" leader on their shift, in their practice, or as an informal influencer of people and pharmacy practice.

The purpose of *The Pharmacy Leadership Field Guide: Cases and Advice for Everyday Situations* is to present pertinent leadership concepts using real-life cases that apply to pharmacy students, residents, and new practitioners. The authors of each chapter consist of a veteran mentor—chosen because of a proven leadership track record in pharmacy— and a new practitioner—selected for their strong leadership abilities and diverse practice settings. Each chapter contains profiles of its authors, which include their pharmacy experience and leadership career advice. Each case focuses on a different leadership topic specifically chosen for the early part of a pharmacy career. Because each chapter is written by a different veteran mentor/new practitioner team, the writing styles and perspectives vary in consistency, which adds to the richness of the book's content; the reader can benefit from the diverse practice experience brought by the author teams.

The concepts presented in the book are case based and apply to general leadership topics that are pertinent to every pharmacist irrespective of your career choice. The cases and skills in the book are ones that every pharmacist will encounter throughout the rest of your personal and professional life. You will find that some of the topics transcend the content of this book and are at times repeated, which will assist in your learning and ability to apply the concepts in multiple, real-life situations. To optimize your use of the book's content, refer to the book as an "in-print mentor," where you identify a leadership skill to work on from one of the chapters, read the advice from the veteran mentor and new practitioner, and try to apply your learning to a real-life situation or to the exercises at the end of the chapter. This book demonstrates in print how to utilize mentors. The more you practice, the more you'll optimize your learning opportunities.

CHAPTER FORMAT

Each chapter begins by introducing the overall leadership concept being presented. The introductory section is not meant to be a comprehensive coverage of the leadership topic, as many books have been written covering each concept in detail. Instead, the brief content overview at the beginning of each chapter is meant to set the stage for the main points presented in the chapter and to introduce the cases that will be covered.

Each chapter covers a contemporary leadership topic, broken into component parts. Each subtopic is introduced by a pharmacy practice leadership case written by the chapter's new practitioner from his or her personal experience. The protagonist of the case finds himself in the midst of a particularly challenging dilemma. Much as a pharmacy school module might be introduced by a patient case, the leadership cases are similarly structured. At the end of each case, the protagonist either makes some difficult decisions or leaves matters unresolved in their decision-making process. The ambiguity in case resolution closely mirrors the reality of leadership. While therapeutic modalities are often based on evidence and science, the resolution to leadership dilemmas is often less clear because in the leadership world there is rarely one right answer.

Following the cases, we probe into the mindset of the main character. As you read, you may find yourself asking or thinking the same questions as the protagonist. The recurring "may be thinking" or "might reason" feature is designed to assure readers that their raw emotions to the case presented are natural and common. The point-counterpoint nature of the internal dialogue seeks to span the spectrum of first reactions.

Next, we hear sound advice from our veteran mentors. In the Mentor Advice section, our experts respond to the character in the case as though they were a personal mentor. The mentors give practical guidance on how to handle the specific dilemma presented within the case. In the What I Have Found to Be Successful section, the mentors broaden the scope of their advice to offer valuable pearls to the reader on success strategies for handling similar leadership dilemmas to those outlined in the case. These tips are based on the leadership acumen and experience of our veteran mentors.

Following the veteran advice, we engage new leaders to offer their experiences. Each new leader has, in one shape or another, found him- or herself struggling with a challenge similar to that presented in the case. Thus, the New Leader Advice section gives practical advice, which is specific to the dilemma faced by the character. Expect to learn what has worked and, conversely, what to avoid (what our new leaders have learned the hard way). This "in the trenches" learning technique will guide the reader to form the correct thought process (though not necessarily to the perfect solution) when attacking a similar leadership problem. The What I Have Found to Be Successful section will again offer broad tips and techniques for similar challenges.

Subsequent cases are presented in a similar fashion to comprise the core content of each chapter. Each chapter closes with a Leadership Pearls section. Review this list often for an overview of the content and some quick tips that are necessary before diving into a real-life issue. Have some time to practice? Each chapter contains a Leadership Exercises section that offers practical ways to refine your leadership skill set. Take a few minutes and try out one of the suggestions after reviewing the chapter. These proven strategies will build your confidence as a leader.

Chapters conclude in varying ways. Depending on the concept explored, a unique assessment or chapter review has been prepared. Take a moment to review key terms and material before finishing your study of the chapter. These tools will help to reinforce a leadership competency and vocabulary that is otherwise scarcely present in the pharmacy curricula.

How to Use This Book

The cases in this reference are a valuable way to be introduced to leadership concepts. In-depth, chapter-by-chapter study may be an effective way to cover the material. However, in the busy lives of pharmacy students, residents, and new practitioners, it may be more practical to think of this book as a reference to use when you find yourself in a jam. Consult the table of contents or index whenever you find yourself in the middle of a messy situation. Odds are, you are not alone. In some way, shape, or form, another colleague has likely been in your shoes. Reviewing the most appropriate case or concept will offer a real-time refresher to help guide you in making the best decision possible.

ASSOCIATED WEBSITES

You can find additional and supplemental material for *The Pharmacy Leadership Field Guide: Cases and Advice for Everyday Situations* at www.ashp.org/fieldguide. This site contains all of the "Success Skills for Pharmacists" articles that have been published in the *American Journal of Health-System Pharmacy* over the past several years. Some titles include "Working Efficiently," "Building and Maintaining a Professional Network," "Public Speaking Revisited: Delivery, Structure, and Style," and "Maximizing Your Pharmacy Brand." As more articles are published they will be added to the website. Based on the "Success Skills" series, there are additional posted tips, checklists, and pearls that have not been published.

Mike A. DeCoske, Editor

Jennifer E. Tryon, Editor

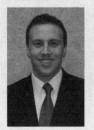

Michael A. DeCoske, PharmD, BCPS
Associate Chief Pharmacy Officer, Ambulatory Services
Department of Pharmacy
Duke University Hospital
Durham, North Carolina

Why pharmacy: While in high school I was looking for a profession that allowed me to pursue my strengths in math and science—one that also allowed me to satisfy my strong desire to help improve people's lives. I attended a career fair and realized there were two schools of pharmacy within commuting distance of home and, thus, pharmacy it was!

Advice to readers: In school, be serious about classes and seek out opportunities to get involved in professional organizations, which provide great travel opportunities, allow you to meet other leaders, develop a professional network, build lasting friendships, and have high-level intellectual interchanges. Set aside the payday for 1 or 2 more years and do a residency. The doors it will open for you are numerous. Residencies will also help you learn how to deal with people, best practices in medication use, and key elements of a high performance pharmacy. In launching your career, utilize mentors who understand where you want to go in your career and who are willing to listen to your thoughts. Carefully select mentors who do not put their own agenda ahead of yours. It is best to have several mentors; one a year or two ahead of you, one 5–10 years ahead, and one toward the end of his or her career. Realize at graduation that you only have a basic skeleton of pharmacy knowledge and you will spend your career continuing to put the flesh on those bones. Look at your first job as only the first step toward your dream job, not the pinnacle of your career.

Tips for work-life balance: Have a nonpharmacy passion that gets you away from work. Every 1–2 months, rebalance yourself by stepping away from the day-to-day grind and remind yourself of your personal mission statement and what motivates you to be a pharmacist.

Personal career: I am most proud of having successfully completed two residencies. In my first position, I coordinated projects where I had the privilege to work with a talented pharmacy team on generating ideas, solving problems, implementing new processes, and following up on our efforts. Being part of a project on all levels feels great. My career goal is to be in a leadership position within the healthcare industry as I want to be able to affect issues and patients on a broad scale. My career success is having a measurable impact on safe and effective use of medications and a positive impact on the development of the staff I work with.

Why leadership: I became interested in leadership during my PGY1 residency during my practice management rotation. Thus, I highly encourage readers to go into each new learning experience with an open mind. My favorite leadership books are Patrick Lencioni's *Death by Meeting: A Leadership Fable. . .About Solving the Most Painful Problems in Business*, Mark Walton's *Generating Buy-In: Mastering the Language of Leadership*, and Jim Collins' *Good to Great: Why Some Companies Make the Leap. . .and Others Don't*.

Recommended change for pharmacy: We need to continue to reinforce the value of our profession to other healthcare professionals and to the public. A key to this is ensuring that every pharmacist views our profession as a 24/7/365 commitment.

Why willing to coordinate this book: I have enjoyed the significant professional satisfaction of learning from the experiences of the various contributors, each with a different background and perspective. It is also an honor to fill a gap in the pharmacy leadership literature by creating a resource that is practical and serves as an "in-print" mentor for real issues that new practitioners will face at some point and in some shape or fashion. I hope this reference will be used on a daily basis by new practitioners as they face challenges in their school or career.

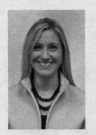

Jennifer E. Tryon, MS, PharmD
Assistant Director of Inpatient Pharmacy
PeaceHealth Southwest Medical Center
Vancouver, Washington

Why pharmacy: In high school I was intrigued with science and the complexity of biology and chemistry. My mother suggested pharmacy so I talked with a pharmacist and was impressed with the combination of science and patient care.

Advice to readers: As a student I wish I had been more curious and inquisitive in asking questions about the care delivery processes versus just trying to memorize and recite facts. Once in practice, I have learned there are no quick wins, and there rarely is a single right answer. It is also very apparent to me that I can't accomplish much alone and I can have a greater impact working collaboratively with a team of individuals. I also learned it is okay to fail as long as you learn from it. Consider doing a residency because it gives you the building blocks and tools to be successful, not just in your first job but throughout your career. A residency helps you develop and perfect your approach to practice. Get involved in professional organizations because they promote networking and provide you with new ideas, new approaches, and resources across the country. For your first job, try and find a good fit for you—perhaps a dynamic practice that improves care and provides opportunities to perfect your leadership skills. Your superior should be someone you can continue to learn from, that is committed to your continued growth, and who will set you up for success.

Tips for work-life balance: Use a mentor and invest in making the relationship useful for you by maintaining contact and sharing what you are experiencing. Prioritize your personal life with your career. Schedule your priorities, and don't let work issues stand in the way of your personal life priorities.

Personal career: My best career decision so far has been to seek a leadership track. I want to influence and improve care for our patients. My major successes so far have been developing a leadership team from individuals with a variety of ages and experiences that trust and care for each other. Our team has a shared vision, goals, and the satisfaction of actual accomplishments. My career goal is to advance in leadership responsibilities, love what I do, grow every day, and continue to learn. My measure of career success will be having made a difference in the care of patients and having helped my team grow and be successful.

Why leadership: In school I was asked by an upperclassman to run for president-elect of the ASHP student chapter, and I saw how we could have an impact and improve things for students via innovative ways such as community service projects, which intrigued me. My favorite leadership book is Stephen Covey's *The 7 Habits of Highly Effective People.*

Recommended change for pharmacy: I would like to see clarity of what it means to be a clinical pharmacist so the public, legislators, other healthcare providers, and patients know what to expect no matter where they encounter a pharmacist.

Why willing to coordinate this book: This book has been an exciting and helpful learning experience because of being able to create something totally new. It is enhancing and broadening my leadership skills. We are working with very successful writers, which enhances my network. I think it will be useful to readers because it combines the "little L" leadership realities of young pharmacists with the experience of seasoned mentors. I hope students, residents, and new practitioners will find it useful early in their careers as a basis of discussions with colleagues, small groups, meetings with deans, etc.

Publisher's Note

ANOTHER WAY TO ACCESS BONUS CONTENT FOR THIS BOOK

What is this? It's a QR Code, or two-dimensional bar code. Below and following each of the nine chapters in this book you will find a QR Code. Using a free application for your smartphone, these codes can be used to connect to bonus content to accompany *The Pharmacy Leadership Field Guide.*

By downloading a QR Code reader on your smartphone, you can quickly go to the online location of this bonus material. To get a free code reader for iPhone, Android, or Blackberry, search in your smartphone app store for a QR code reader and download the app. "Scanlife" is one such app.

Once you have downloaded the app, start it and you will see it access the camera on your phone. Point the camera over the QR Code at the end of each chapter and you will be taken to the webpage containing companion "Success Skills" articles from the *American Journal of Health-System Pharmacy.*

It is not necessary to use the codes and the app to access the articles—it just makes it a little quicker. The articles can also be found by clicking on the "Bonus Content" link found on the book's webpage at www.ashp.org/fieldguide.

For companion "Success Skills" articles related to the preface, scan the code above and read articles 1 and 3.

Editors

Michael A. DeCoske, PharmD, BCPS
Associate Chief Pharmacy Officer, Ambulatory
   Services
Department of Pharmacy
Duke University Hospital
Durham, North Carolina

Jennifer E. Tryon, MS, PharmD
Assistant Director of Inpatient Pharmacy
PeaceHealth Southwest Medical Center
Vancouver, Washington

Sara J. White, MS, FASHP
(Ret.) Director of Pharmacy
Stanford Hospital and Clinics
Mountain View, California

Contributors

Roberta M. Barber, PharmD, MPH
Assistant Vice President of Pharmacy Services
Virtua Health System
Marlton, New Jersey
Adjunct Associate Professor of Clinical
   Pharmacy
Philadelphia College of Pharmacy
University of the Sciences in Philadelphia
Philadelphia, Pennsylvania

Cindi Brennan, PharmD, MHA, FASHP
(Ret.) Director of Clinical Excellence
UW Medicine Pharmacy Services
Clinical Professor
University of Washington School of
   Pharmacy
Seattle, Washington

Philip W. Brummond, PharmD, MS
Pharmacy Manager
Department of Pharmacy Services
University of Michigan
Ann Arbor, Michigan

Toby Clark, RPh, MS, FASHP
(Ret.) Director of Pharmacy and Adjunct
   Professor of Pharmacy
University of Illinois at Chicago Medical Center
Chicago, Illinois
Lead Surveyor, Accreditation Services
American Society of Health-System
   Pharmacists
Bethesda, Maryland

Kyra Corbett, PharmD
Community Pharmacist
Liberty Pharmacy
North Liberty, Iowa

Jeanne R. Ezell, MS, FASHP
Director of Pharmacy and Residency Program
Blount Memorial Hospital
Maryville, Tennessee

Christopher R. Fortier, PharmD
Manager, Pharmacy Support & OR Services
Clinical Assistant Professor
Medical University of South Carolina
Charleston, South Carolina

Harold N. Godwin, MS, RPh, FASHP, FAPhA
Professor of Pharmacy Practice and Associate
  Dean
University of Kansas School of Pharmacy for
  Clinical and Medical Center Affairs
Overland Park, Kansas

Staci A. Hermann, MS, PharmD
Pharmacy Manager, Informatics and
  Automation
The University of Kansas Hospital
Kansas City, Kansas

Lindsey R. Kelley, PharmD, MS
Manager, Pharmacy Operations
Department of Pharmacy and Therapeutics
UPMC Shadyside Hospital
Pittsburgh, Pennsylvania

Paul R. Krogh, PharmD, MS
Pharmacy Manager
Abbott Northwestern Hospital
Minneapolis, Minnesota

Katherine A. Miller, PharmD
Pharmacy Operations Manager
United Hospital
St. Paul, Minnesota

Rafael Saenz, PharmD, MS
Director, Acute Care Pharmacy Services
University of Virginia Health System
Charlottesville, Virginia

Ross W. Thompson, MS, RPh
Director of Pharmacy Services
Tufts Medical Center
Boston, Massachusetts

Samaneh T. Wilkinson, MS, PharmD
Clinical Manager, Inpatient Clinical Services
PGY-1 Residency Director and HSPA PGY-2
  Residency Coordinator
Department of Pharmacy
The University of Kansas Hospital
Kansas City, Kansas

Karol Wollenburg, MS, RPh
Vice President and Apothecary-in-Chief
NewYork-Presbyterian Hospital
New York, New York

Reviewers

Lea S. Eiland, PharmD, BCPS
Associate Clinical Professor and Associate
  Department Head
Department of Pharmacy Practice
Auburn University, Harrison School of
  Pharmacy
Huntsville, Alabama

Charles Hartig, PharmD, JD Candidate 2012
Registered Pharmacist
Hartig Drug/MedOne Healthcare Systems
Dubuque, Iowa

Ashley M. Overy
PharmD Candidate, Class of 2012
Rudolph H. Raabe College of Pharmacy
Ohio Northern University
Ada, Ohio

Todd D. Sorensen, PharmD
Associate Professor and Associate Department
  Head
Department of Pharmaceutical Care and Health
  Systems
Director, Ambulatory Care Residency Program
University of Minnesota College of Pharmacy
Minneapolis, Minnesota

CHAPTER ONE

Professional Leadership

Christopher R. Fortier, PharmD; Sara J. White, MS, FASHP

Introduction

In July of 1960, John F. Kennedy said "It's time for a new generation of leadership…For there is a new world to be won." Many decades later these words are still significant and pose somewhat of a challenge to the current students, residents, and new practitioners within the pharmacy profession. Unfortunately, most pharmacists have not been exposed to any substantial formal training in leadership or management. Additionally, many pharmacists lack a well-established relationship with a mentor, such as a professor or preceptor, to provide career advice and guidance. Yet, it is mentoring and leadership skills that are truly essential to becoming a well-rounded practitioner, to achieving career success, and ultimately to advancing our profession.

Understanding the importance of professional leadership early in your career as a student or new practitioner will provide you with numerous advantages and opportunities. Professional leadership, however, must be actively worked on, developed, and enhanced. Having your own personal vision and strategies for what you want to achieve, developing a career plan, and creating a dialogue with multiple mentors is a great starting point. Another key element is understanding the "big picture" of how you and your peers can impact the pharmacy profession and also understanding the professional duty we each have to expand the pharmacists' role in patient care. It is you as the "everyday leader" who can leave your mark on enhancing the pharmacy practice model, optimizing the performance of medication-use technologies, improving medication safety, and impacting patient outcomes. If we don't seize these leadership opportunities that come our way, other clinicians and administrators will grab them up, leaving pharmacists and the profession behind.

In this chapter, we will introduce several core competencies you need to develop professional leadership skills. These following nine essential principles should serve as a foundation for your own personal leadership development.

- **Don't mistake a good manager for a leader.** All pharmacists are managers, since the focus in management is ensuring that specific predefined tasks are done correctly. Leadership, on the other hand, is defining what those tasks are and what direction they should take. It is, therefore, important to keep in mind that the precision, perfection, and fear of failure that ensures pharmacists protect patients from harm is almost 180 degrees different from the creative, visionary leadership skills outlined below. All pharmacists need to blend being a manager with also leading.

Managers	Leaders
Administer	Innovate
Ask how and when (processes)	Ask what and why (vision/mission)
Focuses on systems (drug distribution)	Focuses on people
Maintain current services	Develop new services
Rely on controls (checks and balances)	Inspire trust and engages people

Have a short-term perspective	Have a long-term perspective
Accepts the status quo	Challenges the status quo
Keep an eye on the bottom line	Keep an eye on the horizon
Are classic "good soldiers"	Are their own people
Are a copy	Are an original
Play it safe	Take calculated risks (not with drug therapy but with how work is organized and processed)
Schedule staff	Develop staff

- **Every pharmacist must be a change agent or "little L" leader.** Leadership is important—not just sometimes but *all* of the time. On every shift, in every practice setting, from clinical, patient-care rounds to the IV room, from the "In" window to the mail order room floor, leadership must pervade the way we think and act. It was not just the "big L" leaders (those with formal titles such as director, store manager, assistant director, clinical coordinator, supervisor, etc.) who are responsible for pharmacy services evolving from compounding to a drug therapy, patient-oriented service, but those "little L" leaders on the front lines exhibit the skills of a leader every day. For example, hospitals haven't always had pharmacy services to compound intravenous medications; this was traditionally the nurse's job. Community pharmacists were not always permitted to counsel patients on their medications; this was traditionally only the domain of the physician. Needless to say, the ability of pharmacists to use their drug expertise to improve patient's medication use has come about by both "little L" and "big L" leaders seeing a need and experimenting with creative ways to fill it, thus evolving the pharmacists' role.

- **Employ situational leadership.** Situational leadership means adjusting your approach by taking into account the various factors and context in each circumstance such as what specifically needs to be achieved, the individual people involved, the history surrounding the challenge and other applicable factors such as regulatory and legal challenges. This approach also involves facing issues head on, rather than putting off dealing with uncomfortable situations such as performance issues, failing to seek key peoples' input before decisions are made, not being clear about performance expectations, and not completely training and orienting new staff.

- **Never think "It's not my job."** Some of the most poisonous words in a pharmacy, of any setting, are "that's not my job." Leaders avoid, at all cost, the elitist mentality that it is below them to work in the trenches when required. Rather, leaders use those opportunities to develop good working relationships. All organizational workgroups—

whether between a pharmacist and a technician or the entire pharmacy department—function best when there are good trusting relationships between all members. To develop a good working relationship with another person, don't be afraid to rub elbows with them, getting to know them on a personal basis. Delegation is a key skill for a successful leader, yet one that is often lacking in new practitioners who prefer to "just do it myself." To maintain job satisfaction and avoid "burn-out," delegation must be mastered. It works best when the individual and delegated task are matched. Resistance to delegation can arise from insecurity about being successful, from lack of adequate communication about goals and expectations and from creating a feeling that the person delegating is taking advantage of their employee. A successful leader will thoroughly discuss the potential task, ask what resources might be needed to get it accomplished, get consensus, and express the willingness to assist and to ensure the person's success. Frequent "touching base" or personal contact with the person about their progress without micromanaging will often provide the person with the confidence they need. It's important to avoid insisting that a delegated project be completed exactly as you would have done it, especially if the outcome is acceptable.

- **Don't miss "the forest for the trees."** Understanding the "big picture" requires that we survey the whole forest and not just focus on an individual tree. This approach means considering all the available options, as well as what is going on in society, congress, healthcare, technology, and science (not just the current pharmacy or healthcare silos). Societal trends will ultimately affect pharmacy and each pharmacist, so it is better to proactively create a professional future instead of waiting and having others impose it on us. A wise tactic is to always have a fall-back plan for when the unexpected happens, as it undoubtedly will many times over the course of your career.

- **Always be accountable and take responsibility for the therapeutic care of the patient.** Society has entrusted pharmacists and physicians with the responsibility to safely dispense and steward lifesaving and sometimes extremely dangerous medications and thus expect that patients will be protected from harm. Society understands that using medications requires a unique knowledge of therapeutics and patient specifics that laypeople, even with the information available today via the internet, are unable to safely interpret by themselves. Professional leadership is to always living up to this societal obligation no matter the consequences. A pharmacist must ensure not only that patients are protected from harm but that they obtain their needed medication. This might mean staying late for a patient, stepping out of our comfort zone, or going above and beyond what is required to care for unique patient needs.

- **Be the CEO (chief executive officer) of your career.** Being a CEO means taking charge, being responsible and accountable for how a career and life will "play out." While schools and colleges of pharmacy provide practical exposure and experience in a variety of employment opportunities, leadership is exploring as many as possible because it is impossible to understand what each is really like without some actual experience. Leadership is also benefiting from the experience of individual faculty and preceptors by asking them about their career decisions, unique employment opportunities, employment competition in the marketplace, qualifications employers are looking for, and their strategies for achieving work-life balance. Another telling question is what, if they had their career to do over again, are the key decisions they would have made differently. Realize that everyone views things differently so collect as many "career stories" as possible. Document this "career research" so it can be compared/analyzed at different points in your career, as your perspective will invariably change. As your career progresses consider developing a career "board of directors" composed of several mentors each representing a possible direction that your career might go in the future as additional inputs.

- **Employ a career development plan.** A career development plan will require some work, but really, what could be more important than your greatest personal investment. Engaging in the planning process will allow you to take control of the direction of your career. It involves thinking through what is important to you and understanding exactly what it is you absolutely do not want to be doing, and then defining and documenting the goals needed to achieve the plan. For each goal, develop a list of steps that are needed, prioritize them in the order needed to achieve the goal, and create a realistic timeline for the accomplishment of the planned goal. Periodically review the plan to track your progress and make any needed revisions. Seek assistance and advice from trusted mentors or veteran pharmacists in the planning and revision process. The plan may not be a document you refer to daily or even monthly, but always be aware how the decisions you make on a daily basis will affect your career plan.

- **Perfect leadership skills through involvement in professional organizations.** Professional organizations allow pharmacists to pool their resources and hire staff that work on their behalf. Professional organizations can do things that it would be very difficult for individual pharmacists to achieve, such as lobbying for or against applicable legislation, testifying in congressional hearings, conducting continuing educational meetings, publishing journals, establishing best practices, and communicating with the public. Generally pharmacy organizations—whether local, state, national or international—all function with policy recommending committees/councils where members determine how the organization's monetary and staff resources are allocated. Active involvement in professional organizations is a fantastic way to stay informed and energized. For a leader, professional involvement is not just attending meetings but also a professional commitment to serve. Volunteering as a member on national committees and to enthusiastically give your time and energy working with a professional organization is one of the greatest ways leaders can give back.

CASE 1.1

Don't mistake a good manager for a good leader

PRINCIPLES ■ Leadership ■ Management

Sarah is a coordinator for 15 clinical pharmacists who are responsible for order-entry, drug information, and clinical pharmacy activities within their patient-care units. As a clinical pharmacist, Sarah has great relationships with her coworkers, covers extra shifts, and socializes with them outside of work. When a coordinator position opened up, all of her coworkers encouraged her to apply. Once she assumed the coordinator role, Sarah did a great job of keeping the operation running smoothly. She was extremely organized, made sure to send the staff schedule out 1 month ahead of time, and was diligent about replying to staff e-mails within a couple hours. Overall, she was great at keeping the daily responsibilities of her staff in order and under control.

About 8 months into her coordinator role, a couple of clinical pharmacists resigned from their positions. In their exit interviews, they stated that they were becoming "bored" with their position and wanted to participate in more innovative initiatives and to expand their clinical roles. Being down two pharmacists, the already stressed clinical pharmacy group was asked to work more shifts and went from working every 3rd weekend to every other weekend. In addition to dealing with staffing and recruitment issues, Sarah was also concerned about the upcoming implementation of computerized physician order entry (CPOE) and bar code medication administration (BCMA). Whether she knew it or not, these technologies would drastically change the way that the clinical pharmacists practiced and would position them as a front-line resource for nurses and physicians.

Even though Sarah was involved in the CPOE/BCMA roll-out team, she provided spotty staff pharmacist training and was not proactively communicating with her pharmacists about upcoming changes. Soon enough, the chaotic nature of the division became too much for her staff to bear. Sarah received two additional letters of resignation from her staff who had taken new jobs at another hospital in the city. Sarah needed to quickly regroup in order to deal with these additional vacancies, recruitment, technology implementation, and with a very dissatisfied staff.

WHAT SARAH MAY BE THINKING...

- Everything is going great and my staff does not need much direction.
- Why is my staff looking for and accepting other jobs?
- Why do people think that implementing these technologies is going to be difficult?

ON THE OTHER HAND, SARAH MIGHT REASON...

- Should I be considering new innovative clinical projects for my team to work on?
- How can we continue to promote pharmacy and expand our clinical pharmacy services in my area?
- It will be critical for me to set direction for my staff and prepare to lead the changes coming with this technology implementation.
- I really dropped the ball.

MENTOR ADVICE

Sarah is a great manager in keeping things running, getting the schedule completed in a timely manner, and quickly responding to e-mails; however, she needs to become the leader that the group deserves. This is a great opportunity for her to stretch herself and move toward her full potential. If having the time to lead is a challenge for her, she could consider delegating some things such as the schedule or day-to-day staff supervision to others. This delegation will help them grow and develop their own management skills.

While leading encompasses many aspects, Sarah's immediate priority is to engage and inspire her staff including the technicians to tap their potential and, thus, become the employer of choice for recruitment and retention. Sarah should begin by leading her staff in developing their practice vision in the new CPOE/BCMA world. In order to facilitate the staff, she needs to be clear about how the systems will work and understand the timelines and expected benefits of the new technology. If she isn't completely committed to the new vision, she will have trouble translating it to the staff and, thus, being a successful leader. Staff members are very conscious of her attitude and approach, not just what she says but what she does and believes. Obviously Sarah's technology vendor and technical personnel can provide her with some education, but if the system is implemented anywhere locally, she can plan a visit and see it in action. If nothing is available locally, then Sarah can ask the vendor for pharmacy contacts that have implemented the system around the country and talk with them. Many vendors would be willing to provide an on-site demonstration.

Sarah needs to prepare the staff to think about how practice needs to change. She could organize several educational sessions for the staff, being sure to include everyone that will be affected on the benefits of the new systems and how they are anticipated to work. As the leader, Sarah must be optimistic, enthusiastic, have a "can do, will do" attitude, and verbally express her faith in their ability to maximize this opportunity. Sarah should consider using visual aids or handouts that show the high level, pharmacy-related processes in the present system and the parallel anticipated workflow in the new system. She should include only as much detail as needed for them to contrast the systems so they aren't overwhelmed. Sarah needs to ask for questions and concerns and listen very carefully for kernels of things that need to be resolved (but she shouldn't justify or defend the system changes). Sarah could conclude the session by again discussing the benefits and the opportunity to enhance pharmacy's contribution to patient care. She can give them the assignment of thinking through what their ideal future or practice vision/mission should be in this computerized world, and then schedule another session to get feedback as to what this practice would look like, how it would feel, and what they would be doing. It may be helpful to facilitate their thinking to suspend, for the moment, any barriers, obstacles, feasibility, etc. Sarah should have a system to capture the terminology they use because their words are important as a window into how they are thinking, and then put together a draft vision/mission using their words. The staff should review and modify it so it is truly their practice vision/mission. At future staff meetings, Sarah should keep their vision/mission in front of them by periodically asking for examples of how they are moving toward it in their daily activities.

As Sarah is engaging them in this visioning exercise, she needs to work closely with her human resources department to fill vacant positions, being sure they are using a variety of recruitment options such as professional meetings, professional placement services, residency training programs, graduates, recruiters, etc. Sarah could also contact former staff to tell them about her current role as a leader, her pharmacy vision, and the exciting roles that are being created should they be able to return one day.

What I have found to be successful

It is so easy to be consumed by only the management tasks that you never get to lead. You must be a leader if your group is going to be successful even as a change agent or "little L" leader. Focusing on leadership will also help to ensure that you recruit and retain excellent staff. Scheduling leadership activities on your calendar before you put management activities on it will help. For me, this meant dedicating time talking with my team, asking the staff to routinely update their practice vision, engaging in strategic planning, and reading outside of pharmacy and healthcare. Try and do some leadership activities each day so you focus on the long term and leverage your peoples' talents. Don't focus on e-mail, voice mail, or meetings at the expense of leadership. Don't be afraid to delegate tasks to provide yourself the time to lead. Remember, leadership is focused on being sure the right things are done, not just doing things correctly.

NEW LEADER ADVICE

Unfortunately, many pharmacists never receive formal education on management and leadership in pharmacy school and are left on their own to learn these essential skills. Most pharmacists learn these skills as they go, read on the topics, and are provided advice from their mentors. New leaders need to have a blend of both management and leadership skills within their professional toolkit with the appropriate understanding of how to use the skills in a variety of situations.

Sarah was more of a friend than a leader for her staff, which made her well liked but not able to execute; in the end, her staff began to look for other positions. An old adage is "You don't quit your job, you quit your boss." In order to avoid these pitfalls, Sarah should meet with her staff or round on them regularly to communicate the status of the project and to seek their feedback, which will help them gain trust in her as a leader. Sarah may think that this all seems like a lot of work for one project, but gaining the trust of her staff is essential. These basic components of having open communication, setting a vision, and developing staff are three major pieces of being a leader.

To retain her staff, Sarah must work to develop her personal leadership skills and invest time in her staff. Delegating, coaching, and communicating are the areas she needs to focus on. Her staff wants to be further developed, to have more clinical responsibilities, and to progress in their careers. She needs to put herself back into their position and think about when she was a clinical pharmacist and what she enjoyed and disliked about it.

This is a good example of the major difference between a manager and a leader. Yes, when things were calm with Sarah's staff and project work was minimal, she was a successful coordinator. However, when staff was down and when implementing large-scale technology projects, Sarah's leadership skills needed to kick in. Even though Sarah thought she had good relationships with her staff, having recently been in a similar role with them, she was not aware of what their needs and future development were. Surveying or frequently rounding on her staff could have avoided this. Additionally, these strategies could have assisted her to better inform her staff of the impending changes with CPOE and BCMA. Not working closely enough with her supervisor and delegating tasks to her staff when things started to become overwhelming was another mistake.

What I have found to be successful

I have found success in being honest with my staff about new projects and helping them to see that I am dedicated to improving their work environment as well as improving my skills as their manager. I routinely meet with them as a group to make sure we have the opportunity for open communication and to address any staff concerns. When dealing with staff shortages, it is important to communicate what you are doing to fill the vacant positions with your current staff, so that they know what is going on. Finally, when implementing new technology, such as CPOE/BCMA, I have found frequent meetings with staff to discuss updates and implications to their workflow to be important. This may mean delegating some of the education and training to high-performing staff members.

CASE 1.2

Being a "little L" everyday leader

PRINCIPLE ■ The importance of every pharmacist being a leader

Having worked in a large hospital pharmacy during college, Harry decided to move back to his hometown and accepted a position at Pine Hill Community Hospital. Pine Hill Hospital is a 200-bed facility with only an inpatient pharmacy and no decentralized clinical pharmacy services. Harry has been working at Pine Hill for the past 3 months and has worked to establish relationships with the pharmacy director, five pharmacists, and 10 technicians. He continually offers suggestions for improvement within the department and even started a suggestion box for staff to submit their own ideas or concerns. Additionally, he has gained a good rapport with the hospital nursing and physician staff using his clinical knowledge and through his effort to offer improved clinical pharmacy services to Pine Hill's patients. Overall, Harry has the reputation within and outside of the department of consistently going the extra mile.

On one Monday afternoon the lead hospitalist, Dr. Lewis, meets with Harry and his director to discuss his plan for pharmacy to lead a new hospital-wide initiative. Dr. Lewis describes that anticoagulation management is a Joint Commission National Patient Safety Goal and that he would like Harry to lead the implementation of the hospital's program. Dr. Lewis tells Harry that he considers him an "everyday leader" and is confident that Harry can work collaboratively with the hospital staff in optimizing anticoagulation therapy for their patients. Harry's director agrees to allow him to lead this effort and pledges to provide Harry with the time and resources necessary to get the job done.

Even though he did not have a formal leadership title and was continuing to work in the central pharmacy, Harry was excited to begin to lead the anticoagulation initiative across the institution, but he feels slightly overwhelmed. He doesn't really know where to start and was nervous about getting a group of pharmacists, nurses, and physicians to look at him as the leader and decision maker on the project. After getting some advice from his director, Harry decides to crack open his notes from a leadership course he took in college and re-read some essential strategies and potential pitfalls to lead a successful project.

WHAT HARRY MAY BE THINKING...

- I am just a staff pharmacist.
- I am concerned about having the time to work and implement this project in addition to my other job duties.
- Am I going to upset any of my pharmacy colleagues because I was asked to lead this project and they were not?
- How can I get nurses and physicians to work with me as a team on this project?

ON THE OTHER HAND, HARRY MIGHT REASON...

- This is a great opportunity to promote the pharmacy department across the organization.
- This project should help to continue to reinforce the relationship between pharmacy and the other disciplines within the organization.
- This will allow pharmacy to be at the table and have our perspective represented instead of other departments making decisions regarding the medication-use process.
- I need to work with my director to guide me in leading this project.
- The opportunity could help me with a future promotion to a clinical pharmacist position.

MENTOR ADVICE

This is a great opportunity for Harry to be a "little L" leader and implement innovative pharmacy services at Pine Hill Hospital. He shouldn't squander this leadership opportunity as he now has the chance to make a significant impact and improve patient care. He should keep in mind that he can do anything he puts his mind to and be aware that he will encounter some challenges and obstacles but use them to stretch himself and move toward his potential while improving pharmacy services. When others raise concerns and obstacles, he must listen carefully and be willing to make any needed changes. The key is to keep moving the process forward and learn from experiences. Harry is wise in seeking out guidance from his "big L" pharmacy director on how to approach this project.

Harry needs to educate himself on how others conduct pharmacy anticoagulation services. Sources for this education would be searching the medical literature, resources on professional organizations' websites, best practice guidelines, archived listserves, meeting abstracts, slides and recorded presentations, upcoming programs, anticoagulation program speakers, and asking the director and veteran pharmacists if they know any local or state places that provide the service that he could visit. Given Harry's education, he can think through the decisions that need to be made by the group and commit to a finite number of meetings, allocating the decisions among them per formal agendas. People quickly lose interest if there are too many meetings and decisions aren't being made. Harry must keep concise minutes of who attends and the decisions made and be sure to keep the other pharmacy staff informed and seek their input during the development process. Harry needs to be aware that some pharmacists are not going to be comfortable taking on this additional responsibility without significant training and "hand holding" or individual attention, but with time they will adapt.

Harry should look at this experience as a journey of leadership learning and persevere through the "bumps in the road" that will undoubtedly occur. He needs to keep his eye on the desired outcome of helping patients and keep track of the daily successes/victories without giving up when the challenges seem a bit overwhelming. Harry must remember to constantly evaluate and re-evaluate the clinical program to make sure it is reaching its full potential.

What I have found to be successful

I have enhanced my leadership skills by being willing to take on new challenges, many of which required that I get myself "up to speed" quickly. Never fear the unknown as you will only figure it out by getting experience in the area. Don't be afraid to ask others to assist you since you will never have all the answers. Remember that leading the implementation of a new service is not a science where you can be assured of the exact result of each change, nor can you look to a textbook for all the right answers. Implementing new services is a process that develops with time, proper evaluation, and reassessment. Leadership is an art where you take calculated risks and are willing to make changes once you get some experience with change. Involving others in the design assists in making the best decisions possible during the planning, and it also allows for multiple points of view that make for a better evaluation of a service. Anticipate that it is human nature to be resistant to change so don't let concerns expressed by others delay starting. Be sure to take into account any valid concerns by carefully listening to the feedback of your colleagues. In my experience, always keeping in mind the desired outcome of the new service has gotten me through the "bumps in the road."

NEW LEADER ADVICE

Everyone should have a 100-day plan when starting a new position—a strong plan of integrating and establishing oneself. Harry's plan was to strategically establish strong relationships with his peers and other clinicians as well as making recommendations for improvements within the department. Harry is an "everyday leader." We all need to be "everyday leaders"—whether students, residents, or new practitioners. We must seize all opportunities to be innovative and evolve our profession during situations such as team rounds, group meetings, or implementing new medication-use technology.

As the project leader, Harry needs to review resources and spend time learning about the topic to be knowledgeable from all angles. Additionally, he should read about project management to understand the formal components of leading a team (initiating, planning, executing, controlling, and closing), and he should acquire basic management knowledge of how to successfully run a meeting (putting together an agenda, setting expectations, and dealing with conflict).

As Harry takes on these new roles and responsibilities, he must work closely with his peers, supervisor, and mentors on time management and potential pitfalls and discuss his implementation goals and review his project structure/charter with his supervisor. Harry shouldn't forget about having a good communication plan for the task force members and for his supervisor and colleagues. He can ask his mentors about how to best celebrate project milestones and group successes throughout the life of the project and should remember to recognize task force members during meetings (departmental- and organizational-wide) that make significant contributions to the success of the project.

What I have found to be successful

When I was new to the hospital and fresh out of pharmacy school, I worked hard to develop a strong reputation with my colleagues. Using my clinical skills, not being afraid to provide feedback, and developing relationships, I was able to integrate into the department.

These positive interactions will allow others to view you as a leader within the pharmacy department. Having a good reputation with physician and nursing colleagues is also essential to get things done within a hospital. Having the confidence and support of your boss can also be very reassuring. I have found that asking my director to mentor me through challenging assignments and particularly in the initial planning phases of the project has been a fantastic way to learn how to set expectations, implement change management strategies, and create an environment that supports teamwork.

CASE 1.3

Employ situational leadership

PRINCIPLE ■ Assessing the context and adapting leadership

Joanne recently became the manager of a new community pharmacy scheduled to open in 2 months. Just after pharmacy school, Joanne starting working for a community pharmacy and after 1 year, she was hired to open this new pharmacy. Her previous experience is minimal in leading people and managing a pharmacy operation. As the president of an active pharmacy student organization, she learned the importance of dealing with issues based on the situation and that one type of strategy does not work for every case. She was confident that this community pharmacy position would have its issues and unexpected setbacks but also its successes. Over the next 2 months Joanne hired staff, prepared the pharmacy, promoted the new pharmacy within the community, and was anxious for the grand opening.

Joanne's pharmacy team consisted of a pharmacist just out of pharmacy school and three technicians, with only one having previous community pharmacy experience. Within the first week of the store opening, Joanne began to realize that one of her technicians was not adequately trained and that her pharmacist partner was not following up on things he was asked to complete. It soon became clear that these were issues she needed to be immediately addressed. Joanne recognized that she would have to deal with each staff member in very different ways. Ron, a new pharmacy technician, seemed to be making a lot of mistakes that were affecting patient safety. Joanne also realized she needed to focus her efforts on improving her working relationship with her pharmacist partner, Doug. Since the store opened, Doug, a new graduate, had been very defensive when asked to complete certain tasks. Joanne met one-on-one with Doug to explain her concern and to seek out Doug's feedback. Doug stated, "I feel like you give me all the jobs that you don't want to do" and "I am not a student anymore."

WHAT JOANNE MAY BE THINKING...

- I have only been out of school for a year and I am already a store manager and responsible for the successful opening of a new store.
- I am nervous of being in charge of four staff members.
- How do I know the people I recruited are going to listen to me?
- Do I address the issues with Doug now or just give him a negative annual evaluation?
- I am just going to let Ron figure things out by himself. He obviously was not paying attention during his training.

ON THE OTHER HAND, JOANNE MIGHT REASON...

- This is a great opportunity for me in the early part of my career.
- I am going to make some mistakes, but I vow to learn from them.

- I need to learn how to hire, evaluate, and develop relationships with my new staff.
- It is important for me to address things head on instead of letting them linger.
- My staff is going to appreciate me more for meeting with them, listening to their feedback, and continually communicating with them about how things are going.

MENTOR ADVICE

Joanne needs to sit down with Ron, explain her concerns, and ask him how she can help him do a better job. She should think through if some more training would be helpful and who would be appropriate to do the training and arrange it. When Joanne meets with Ron, she must clarify her goal to have him working independently by the end of the month. She should provide appropriate coaching points from her observation of him working, telling him that she will support him in any way she can and indicate that she will follow up every couple days. If Ron does improve, Joanne can recognize his efforts in front of his coworkers.

Working with Doug requires a different approach, because, while Joanne is the store manager, Doug is her professional colleague. To focus on improving the working relationship, Joanne needs to ask him about his defensive comments and find out what he would like his role to be. Understanding how he is thinking will enable Joanne to engage him. There are probably some aspects that Doug views as growth for him that he can be responsible for, so Joanne should jointly agree on potential new duties for him and indicate her trust in Doug by continuing to have an open dialogue with him to improve the relationship and the overall success of the new pharmacy. Furthermore, Joanne can take on some of the duties Doug finds to be tedious so he will see her as "pulling her own weight."

What I have found to be successful

Using situational leadership—often based on the background, education, and level of experience of my staff—has been a key to my success. Treating each person as a unique and special person has never failed me. When it comes to performance, I have learned that people often just do what makes sense to them and, unless you intervene, will continue their current behavior. It is critical to closely observe new employees as they begin their work and to let them know any concerns you have the first time you observe inappropriate behavior. If you overlook it hoping it will correct itself, you are condoning it. If you delay, when you are eventually forced to have the discussion, they will be confused because you hadn't brought up the concern until now and they might not be motivated to change. Even in the beginning, before you have the conversation, ask yourself if the job expectations were clear and whether their training was complete. It is always wise to give the employee the benefit of doubt and clarify expectations or redo training if you have any concerns before you attempt to discipline them. When it comes to patient safety issues, however, be careful how many chances you give the staff, as you want to be sure to avoid harming the patient. It's not the most glamorous part of the job, but to be an effective leader you are going to have to deal with performance issues sooner rather than later. Your staff deserves to work in an environment where everyone is held accountable for doing their jobs well. Leaders can avoid being unfair to their staff by "biting" the bullet and having the difficult conversations necessary to improve performance.

NEW LEADER ADVICE

Joanne is dealing with two separate issues that require completely different approaches. Situational leadership means no single "best" style of leadership. Instead, she must adapt the style to not only the person or group that is being influenced, but also to the task or job that needs to be fulfilled. In this situation, Joanne did a great job of addressing the issues head on and using the "best" style of leadership as it relates individually to Doug and Ron.

With Ron's situation, Joanne quickly learned the importance of staff training, feedback, and performance evaluation. She needs to focus on continuing to follow up with Ron and to recognize his improvements or to correct his missteps. Addressing the interactions with Doug is more difficult because Doug is her peer. She wants to improve her communication with Doug and use conflict management skills during the one-on-one meeting. She may need to help him realize the important role he plays in the pharmacy and discuss ways to improve their professional relationship.

What I have found to be successful

It is possible that you could be in a formal leadership role very early in your career, whether it be the pharmacist-in-charge or as a supervisor. Accepting and excelling in a position like this can be intimidating but also rewarding if you work at improving your skills as a leader. To succeed you first must understand and use various leadership styles for the many and varied situations you encounter. Adding multiple styles into your professional toolkit and working to improve those skills will be important to handle difficult situations.

I have learned that addressing issues quickly and head-on prevent future problems from developing. Scheduling a private face-to-face meeting will allow your staff to open up. Be sure to clearly explain your issue citing specific examples and use active listening skills to hear the other side of the story. To make this a win-win, work hard to show the other person that you want to partner with them to address and improve the issue. Make sure to set your expectations of the person and outline milestones over a projected time period. I would highly recommend documenting all of your interactions, so that you have a record of your conversations and the expectations you have set. Consistently follow up and during those encounters be sure to listen and set goals moving forward. If the situation is not improving after using this formalized method, take the necessary disciplinary steps based on the level of the situation. However, if the situation is being addressed, make sure to publicly and privately recognize your employee for their accomplishments.

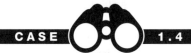

CASE 1.4

Never think "It's not my job"

PRINCIPLES ■ Responsibility ■ Accountability

Fresh out of his PGY-2 health-system pharmacy administration residency, Will has had his share of difficulties as the assistant director of inpatient operations at a 650-bed hospital. Prior to his arrival, the inpatient pharmacy was in disarray with medication errors, poor customer service, and minimal accountability for pharmacists or technicians. The board of pharmacy conducted a surprise inspection during Will's first week on the job and cited the pharmacy for numerous USP 797 violations. Within the medium-risk level IV room and a 24-hour inpatient pharmacy operation, Will oversees 45 staff members. During the first month in his new position, Will meets with each staff member in an effort to determine where the areas of opportunity in the pharmacy are and to determine performance improvement opportunities. Even though this is a time-consuming effort, he is able to learn more about each staff member, about their strengths and backgrounds, and about their life outside of work. After receiving this feedback and the results of the recent board of pharmacy inspection, it was clear to Will that some major changes to optimize their USP 797 process and procedures were in order.

Will worked quickly to develop a revised IV training, testing, and operation plan in order to comply with the USP 797 guidelines. He strived to get feedback from the staff pharmacists and technicians, knowing they have the most experience in this area and will be responsible for the daily, monthly, and quarterly tasks. Overall, the improvement project was going well as several pharmacy groups were working on different aspects of the project. Things took a bad turn, however, when Will asked one of his operations coordinators, Joe, to lead the ongoing compliance with the USP 797 project. Joe would be responsible for becoming the USP 797 expert for the department and the coordinator who would keep up with new standards, ensure staff training, monitor testing of products, and be accountable for the documentation of all associated tasks.

Joe was upset that he was being "told" to lead this program. He told Will that he did not appreciate the quick change in his job description and on repeated occasions stated that he "did not sign up for this" or "It's not my job." He went further to try to dissuade Will by asking him to assign the project to a staff pharmacist or technician. Will disagreed and stated that he wanted Joe to lead the project because he felt that Joe was the most knowledgeable about the topic. Will has the confidence that Joe would ensure the tasks would be completed and all board of pharmacy violations would be resolved.

WHAT WILL MAY BE THINKING...

- I am the boss and Joe needs to do what I ask.
- Should I have made this major change so soon?
- Do I not know Joe as well as I think I do?
- Does Joe know that he is the most knowledgeable and has the skills to do the job?

ON THE OTHER HAND, WILL MIGHT REASON...

- I should have included Joe more in the planning stages.
- Why did I not sit down with Joe earlier on to discuss my expectations and Joe's preferences about heading up this project?
- Should I just lead this project myself to ensure we continue to stay compliant?
- Do I need to ask someone else in the pharmacy to maintain this project?

MENTOR ADVICE

Will did an excellent job meeting with each person in his workgroup to view the pharmacy through their eyes and to get to know them on a personal basis. He should be applauded for seeking feedback from the staff as they are on the frontlines and truly understand the operational aspects of the pharmacy services. Once the improved processes are established, it is the staff that must comply and make them work. Thus, they are integral to resolving and maintaining the corrected board of pharmacy cited violations.

Needless to say, Will needs to back up with Joe and do some "high touch," which means asking his opinion, seeking his suggestions, and involving him in decisions. Will needs to find out what Joe perceives his role to be. Joe may be worried about what will be required and doesn't want to "look bad" in front of the staff, or Joe may not be that professionally interested in USP 797. Clearly defining expectations may help Joe better understand his new role. Will needs to offer himself as a resource to assist Joe if he has any problems with implementation and make sure to recognize the significant contribution that Joe is making to the department. Once Will "figures out" what Joe needs, he must assist him so he can be as productive as possible.

What I have found to be successful

Helping your team take ownership of their jobs is a key leadership skill. I found that being clear about what you as the leader value, such as taking care of the patient versus blaming others for not strictly following the procedures, is critical. As the leader you must "walk your talk." In other words, you must support people even when they make a different decision than you might have as long as the outcome is acceptable. If you undercut them or criticize their decision, the next time they will ask you what you want done versus making the decision themselves. If you feel their decision could have been better, then approach the situation as a training opportunity for them. Giving them permission to contact you anytime they are uncomfortable with the situation they encounter indicates your trust in their judgment, and I found it was rarely abused.

NEW LEADER ADVICE

Being a new leader with a large staff and a major issue of dealing with a board of pharmacy citation, Will needs to rely on his residency leadership training. He was smart to first meet with his staff to begin developing relationships with them and to learn more about the issues at hand. With the addition of the board of pharmacy citation to resolve, he knew he could not fix all the issues and needed additional assistance. Therefore, Will correctly delegated the oversight of the USP 797 improvements to Joe, knowing he was the best person for the task. However, Joe did not appreciate this new responsibility and voiced his dissatisfaction of the situation. Taking a step back and looking at how the situation was handled, Will should probably have included Joe regarding his initial thinking about this issue earlier in the process. With Joe already defensive, Will needs to pick his words carefully to "ask" instead of "tell" Joe that this is his responsibility as well as clearly setting his expectations. Moreover, after delegating this task, Will must continually show his support and assist Joe in being successful.

What I have found to be successful

In certain situations when I am asked to do a new task, I think to myself that "this is not my job." Maybe that is because it is a task I don't like doing, someone I don't like told me I had to do it, or the expectation of my position did not include this task. However, whether we like it or not, it is an opportunity to be a team player, gain respect from our colleagues, and improve things within the department. Conversely, vocalizing your discontent when given an assignment or uttering those poisonous four words—"It's not my job"—can alienate you from your colleagues or staff.

Delegation, for some, is often difficult because most like to be in control. However, you cannot take on everything and to be honest, there are likely people within your staff that can do the job just as well, if not better, than you. What I have learned to make delegation easier is to first develop relationships with your staff by getting to know their likes, dislikes, strengths, weaknesses. When you invest in your staff, they will look to you as the leader and be more likely to accept your request without pushback. Additionally, asking for feedback will confirm to staff that no matter their position in the department, they are looked on as a partner. In your daily interactions use words such as "team," "we," and "us" and work hard not to leave anyone out when recognizing staff.

In delegating a certain project or task, you must approach your staff by fully explaining the project and the specific reasons why it is important. Your staff is in the trenches and knows the process and limitations better than anyone so rely on them to come up with recommendations. Calm fears through showing your confidence in them and explaining how you will support them in their new role. Finally, key to employee satisfaction and engagement is recognition, so work to recognize staff for their involvement and successes.

CASE 1.5

Don't miss "the forest for the trees"

PRINCIPLE ■ Understanding the "big picture"

Ben is a third-year pharmacy student gearing up for his clinical clerkships that will begin in 1 month. He is looking forward to the didactic portion of pharmacy school being over, not very concerned with his upcoming rotations, and already talking to his peers about what he is going to be doing once he graduates. Ben spent the past summer as an intern with a large pharmaceutical company. He tells some of his close pharmacy friends that after graduating he is going to be a medical science liaison (MSL) with a pharmaceutical company. He is interested in the position due to the salary, flexible work schedule, and the reputation that goes along with working for a large pharmaceutical company. He is confident that he can easily get a position because he will be graduating from a PharmD/MBA combined program, has interned at the company, and is scheduled for additional industry rotations in the fall.

Knowing that he wanted to be an MSL following graduation, Ben purposely selected less challenging clerkships and attempted to schedule as many pharmaceutical industry rotations as possible. He selected two retail pharmacy rotations even though he had previously worked in retail, because past P4 students told him that they were an easy "A." Ben was not looking to get experiences in different areas of pharmacy and never considered the possibility of waiting to see how his rotations panned out before making a final decision on his career options.

In January, prior to Ben's graduation, he began looking for MSL positions. He found few vacancies and began to contact the preceptors that he had worked with during his industry internship and rotations to see if they could point him in the right direction. Despite his efforts, Ben was told that he was not qualified for the MSL positions, even with his PharmD/MBA degrees. Companies were looking for a PharmD with residency training in a specialty area and additional years of hospital experience. His preceptors consistently told him "You need more clinical experience other than college rotations to gain more clinical knowledge. It's important for you to develop relationships with physicians and understand their prescribing patterns." When he tried to sell that he has skills in both the pharmacy and business areas through his MBA, he was told that having an MBA was great but that he has not been able to take those skills and use them in the "real world." Ben was very discouraged, concerned that a jobless graduation day was approaching, and the deadline to apply for a residency had already passed. Feeling pressured, Ben decided to accept a position with a home infusion until he figured out his next career steps.

WHAT BEN MAY BE THINKING...

- I feel discouraged and am not sure how I could have prevented this.
- I have my PharmD and MBA degrees. Shouldn't that experience give me the edge?
- I did an internship and clerkships at various pharmaceutical companies. Based on that shouldn't I have the inside track for a position?
- It was my goal to work in the pharmaceutical industry and that is what I focused on.

ON THE OTHER HAND, BEN MIGHT REASON...

- I still have a pharmacy position and also enjoy working in this setting.
- I can continue to look for a job within industry and always leave my current position if an opportunity develops.
- Should I consider the feedback I received due to my lack of qualifications and seek out residency training?

- -

MENTOR ADVICE

When Ben finds himself in a less than desirable situation, he shouldn't be quick to panic or beat himself up. He needs to take the opportunity to think through what lessons he has learned and document his thinking so he can review it later and thus prevent himself from encountering a similar situation. One of Ben's lessons would be to always keep more than one option open and actually play out several simultaneously. In the future, if his circumstances change, he may want to alter his practice track, and his interests may change overtime as well. Another leadership lesson for Ben is to do his homework. This would mean inquiring what the employment requirements are and what the competition is for the MSL positions.

In making the best use of this "gift of time" while working in the home infusion pharmacy, he could join and attend local, state, and national professional organization meetings using these opportunities to get to know as many different pharmacists as possible. Before the sessions begin, during the breaks, meal functions, and social events, he can seek people out that he don't know and introduce himself (ask them where they work, what their job responsibilities are, what they like/dislike, what opportunities or openings might exist, and what qualifications their employers look for in new employees). Before he concludes his conversation, he should ask if they have a business card and give them his. If they don't have a card, he can ask them to write their e-mail address on the back of one of his, add their name to it, and XX out the front so he doesn't give it to someone else. He should use some type of filing system to maintain these business cards because they become his professional network and he may want to contact them later.

Since Ben needs "real world" experience, he should consider using some of his days off to "shadow" pharmacists he has met or work part-time in other settings. In his home infusion job, Ben can volunteer for projects and committees as a way to broaden his experience. Since the future is always an unknown, he needs to consider the additional experience that a residency ensures such as "researching" residencies by talking with graduates, visiting various residency programs, and reviewing the descriptive material on the ASHP Accreditation Website (www.ASHP.org) to enhance his knowledge.

What I have found to be successful

Keeping my options open proved valuable to me. I always try to have a backup plan in mind for everything I do so if the unexpected happens I am not thrown off balance. I completed a master's degree and residency program because I was interested in clinical practice. I actually had a male assistant pharmacy director tell me he was glad I was interested in clinical because there was no place for women in leadership. There had been only eight women in my pharmacy graduating class. Despite his negativity, my whole career has been spent in leadership positions. If I hadn't learned everything I could during my advanced program and two years of practice experience, I wouldn't have been able to move into formal leadership positions nor been successful enough to move into positions with additional responsibilities. My residency program opened many doors for me, if for nothing else, just in the people I met and the network I developed. Clearly doing a residency was the best career decision that I ever made.

When I went through pharmacy school, we used a slide rule since personal computers, word processors, PowerPoint, calculators, and the internet were not yet around. I was forced to learn these new things by taking classes, reading books, listening to tapes and having colleagues show me how to use them. Pharmacists today are bright and graduate with a doctorate degree. By mastering pharmacy school, you prove to yourself and others that you can learn anything you put your mind to. Be curious about the new things you encounter and ask yourself how you can make use of them.

NEW LEADER ADVICE

Being overconfident with his skills and what it takes to compete for an MSL position, Ben's career plans took an unplanned direction. Issues with not selecting challenging rotations, not developing a well-rounded skill set, and not having a career plan early on impacted Ben's situation. Ben could have had a better idea of the requirements for an MSL by talking with mentors earlier in his career and then building his curriculum vitae (CV) by completing a pharmacy residency.

However, Ben needs to be commended for accepting a position that will allow him to continue to develop his clinical knowledge and skills by working in home infusion. In the meantime, Ben needs to continue to advance his career experiences instead of going through the motions of just working his 8 hours a day and going home. The real test for Ben will be what he does next in striving toward his goal, an MSL position. He needs to continue to consistently meet with his mentors, network with his contacts within the pharmaceutical industry, stay involved in state and national pharmacy organizations, and should consider applying for a residency in the year ahead.

What I have found to be successful

I too have been in this situation and have learned how important it is to first ensure you learn from your mistakes. Sometimes we become overconfident in our abilities or caught up in daily activities that we fail to step back to look at the big picture. It is critical to seize every opportunity early in your career, even if it may be something of minimal interest, to give you the most options. You should consider focusing on being as well-rounded as possible and open to different experiences and areas of the profession. Always be conscious and look for ways to separate yourself from your peers.

Additionally, you may quickly learn that at times you may second guess some of your decisions and will need different perspectives on maneuvering your initials career goals. In this case, Ben wanted to work as an MSL but did not receive the advice that a residency would be the next logical step. Creating relationships and working with your professors, preceptors, student chapter advisors, and even people outside of the profession is an essential component of career planning. You may not always take your mentors advice directly, but at least you are getting a new perspective from people who have experienced it.

CASE 1.6

The pharmacist's role in relation to the patient and caregivers

PRINCIPLE ■ Doing whatever it takes

Erin is a community pharmacist working on a busy Monday morning at Benz Drug, where she has been working for the last 4 years. Benz Drug is affiliated with the Front Street Family Medicine practice and fills about 400 prescriptions on a Monday with one pharmacist, two technicians, and one clerk. Sabrina, a long-time customer, comes in during the busiest part of the day with two prescriptions for her teenage handicapped son. The technician accepts the prescriptions from Sabrina and begins to enter them into the pharmacy system when an alert pops up. Erin reviews the alert and determines a dosing error for one of the prescriptions and a significant drug interaction with the other. She looks down at the script to find that Dr. Taber wrote for the medications and she immediately sighs. Dr. Taber, a local physician at the Front Street Family Medicine practice, has an aggressive reputation and has insulted Erin on numerous occasions in the past.

Erin calls over Sabrina to ask her a couple questions and states that she is going to have to call Dr. Taber letting her know it could take some time. Erin continues to ask Sabrina about the purpose of her doctor's visit and conducts a brief medication history to ensure she has the most updated information. Since Benz Drug is affiliated with the family medicine practice, Erin logs into the electronic medical record to review the physician notes and patient labs. Upon review she quickly determines that Dr. Taber prescribed the same combination of drugs about 1year ago, but it was filled by another pharmacy. The medical record also notes that that Sabrina brought her son back to Dr. Taber about 5 days later with the complaint that he was having lack of urine output, nausea, and had developed a rash.

Erin gathers her notes, takes a deep breath, and calls Dr. Taber. After waiting on hold for 10 minutes, Dr. Taber picks up, and Erin politely describes the situation. Dr. Taber is immediately defensive and asks Erin, "Who are you to tell me what to prescribe"? Erin continues to explain the situation, stating that the patient was prescribed these same two medications in the past and suffered an adverse outcome. Dr. Taber again rips into Erin stating "you are not a doctor" and "shouldn't be questioning me." Erin pauses for a moment trying to come up with another strategy to persuade Dr. Taber.

WHAT ERIN MAY BE THINKING...

- I don't need this frustration today.
- I need to make sure I have all the clinical information to justify my recommendation.
- It is going to take me some time to collect this information. I have patients waiting.
- Should I wait until the other pharmacist comes in for the afternoon shift and have him call Dr. Taber?

ON THE OTHER HAND, ERIN MIGHT REASON...

- It is important to use my training, clinical knowledge, and available resources to collect the relevant information before I call Dr. Taber.
- This is an opportunity for me to improve my relationship with Dr. Taber.
- It does not matter if Dr. Taber is too abrasive or not. This is the right thing to do for the patient.

- -

MENTOR ADVICE

Erin did an excellent job getting all the facts and utilizing the information available to her so she was prepared for how Dr. Taber might react. She should keep in mind that she is not trying to be liked, but respected by those she interacts with. Erin shouldn't let anyone intimidate her by throwing their "perceived power" around such as, "I am a doctor and I'll take the responsibility." No one can absolve her of her professional responsibilities. As a new practitioner, she may want to ask other veteran pharmacists or her store manager for suggestions in handling difficult people.

A tactic she might want to try is explaining that she is in no way trying to upstage him and truly wants to create a better partnership to provide the best care to his patients. She could confidently make the recommendation for an alternative medication and a reduced dosing regimen. If he accepts, she can ask for a verbal order. Before hanging up, Erin should thank him and tell him that she is available anytime to answer any questions he may have and that she would like to work on strengthening the relationship between him and Benz Drug. Erin should document on the computer or prescription these interactions with the date and brief specifics so she can recall the details at a later date.

When Sabrina and her son come back later asking what happened, Erin should politely explain the situation. Sabrina may thank Erin for her intervention to help her son, which is what pharmacy practice is all about.

What I have found to be successful

When dealing with difficult people, focus on what is right for the patient and what you would want done if you were the patient's family member. Remember it takes two to have an argument so if you don't argue back, the person '"loses steam" fairly quickly. Often the other person wants to "place blame" versus solving the problem at hand so again don't play the blame game. When you encounter a difficult person, you don't have to answer attacks or defend yourself or your actions. Stay calm and merely ask what needs to be done to take care of this patient and assure them you will do it. Follow up later if in fact there are system issues that need to be resolved to prevent a similar situation from occurring in the future. Keep in mind that when someone attacks you, they are upset with something you have done and not with you personally. Sometimes they are upset by their own mistake and can take it out on you. At all times, you have a responsibility to society to protect your patients from harm.

- -

NEW LEADER ADVICE

There are going to be numerous situations in our careers that are going to be intimidating and uncomfortable. As in this case, Erin knew Dr. Taber had a long history of being rude and intimidating. However, it is ultimately about our duty as pharmacists to the patient. The goal is about having the leadership skills to be your own person, supporting data for your inquiry, being able to pick your battles, and be willing to swallow your pride.

As a community pharmacist, Erin has worked hard to enhance the role of pharmacists in the community by balancing the prescription volume with clinical pharmacy interventions and improved patient care. But, it is inevitable that she is going to have situations in which she could just let go or decide to address head on. Erin is going to make some mistakes as she first takes on these difficult situations with nurses, physicians, insurance companies, and even other pharmacists. Having a set of conflict management skills to influence and negotiate are essential in these situations.

What I have found to be successful

This situation is one that can make a bad day worse. However, I always keep in mind the Oath of a Pharmacist and my professional responsibility to the patient, despite backlash from others. I try to always think about what I would do in this scenario if the patient was my family member. It is crucial, in this case, to keep the lines of communication open with the patient. Putting the patient at ease and proactively addressing any of their concerns will gain you immense respect. When working with physicians or other healthcare professionals, I always make sure to have all my ducks in a row. I take the time to do the necessary research and make sure I have the necessary facts before proceeding. Using leadership, communication, and negotiation skills are then imperative as you try to find a resolution to possible conflict. To improve my conflict management skills, I role play with my mentors and ask how they have been successful with handling these situations. At times, I call them just before having to deal with a difficult situation, to get their input on my planned approach. As a pharmacy student, strive to develop relationships with medical teams you work with and watch how your preceptors are successful or unsuccessful in getting pharmacy recommendations acted on.

CASE 1.7

Be the CEO (chief executive officer) of your own career

PRINCIPLE ■ Professional development

Meg is in the midst of her clinical clerkships and is unsure about what she wants to do following graduation. She currently works in a community pharmacy, has some interest in residency training, and enjoyed a long-term care rotation. During the past year, Meg has felt pressure about completing a residency as all of her preceptors are pushing her in this direction and her best friend has already begun contacting sites to schedule interviews at the ASHP Midyear meeting. Being unsure about her career path but not wanting to miss any opportunities, Meg takes a step back and begins to think about her pharmacy school experiences and previous rotations. She begins to jot down those experiences and possible career options. She then write outs the pros and cons to these opportunities. A week later she reflects on the career opportunities she had listed and determines that she is most interested in pursuing residency training.

One major concern of Meg's is that she does not know where to start in determining which residency programs to apply to. She reaches out to her current preceptor Marlene, an ambulatory care specialist, who completed PGY-1 and PGY-2 residency just 3 years ago. Marlene sits down with Meg one day following a journal club in order to learn more about her background and her goals moving forward. Meg states that she does have an interest in applying for an ambulatory care residency but is unsure how to go about it, whether she has the necessary qualifications, and whom to talk to for more information. Marlene provides Meg with some contacts of her colleagues that direct residency programs and encourages Meg to reach out to these program directors. Overwhelmed with completing her current rotation projects, finishing her grand rounds presentation, finding housing for her March rotation in Washington DC, and preparing for the ASHP Midyear meeting, Meg gets to work immediately.

During Meg's last day of rotation, Marlene asks Meg where things are with her residency search. Meg tells Marlene what she has done to shorten her list of programs and shows her the ones where she is hoping to apply. Meg asks Marlene if she would be willing to review her CV and possibly even write her a letter of recommendation.

WHAT MEG MAY BE THINKING...

■ I like so many different aspects of pharmacy and I am unsure what I should be focusing on.

■ Is residency training the right choice for me?

■ I need to make sure to cover all my bases and not close off any opportunities for either residency training or a full-time job.

■ I have so many other things going on right now, how am I ever going to get this done and done well?

ON THE OTHER HAND, MEG MIGHT REASON...

- I like ambulatory care, the patient interaction, and am doing well on this rotation.
- Marlene has provided insight for me and given me the contacts to learn more about residency programs.
- Marlene is willing to mentor me to be competitive for this opportunity and hopefully into the future as well.
- I have put a lot of effort into learning more about the various programs and feel that I can be very competitive as an applicant.

- -

MENTOR ADVICE

Meg is doing a great job in becoming the "CEO" of her career. She should ask Marlene to assist her in mapping out the steps she needs to complete over the next month prior to the ASHP Midyear meeting in order to determine the programs that she will apply to. You can find residency program information on the ASHP residency directory, which links to individual program websites. It is important to assess the individual program requirements and application dates. Meg should indeed call the people that Marlene suggests, having some standard questions to ask each program. If timid, asking Marlene to make the connection between her and the contacts would be appropriate. Marlene might consider making a virtual introduction via e-mail. Meg could consider visiting a couple other ambulatory care sites that her college has relationships with to learn more about their practice models. Concurrently, she should begin working on her CV, letter of intent, and select preceptors she will ask to write letters of reference. Once she has completed this preparation, she should have shortened her list to a reasonable number of sites that she would like to schedule an initial interview with and visit at the residency showcase at the ASHP Midyear meeting. This decision will have a major impact on her career and possibly life direction over the next few years, so she shouldn't short-change the time she devotes to it or wait until the last minute to do her "homework."

What I have found to be successful

I learned that I was the most important person I would ever lead. My mentors have been critical for me as they have set the expectation that I will be successful, which gave me the confidence to "rise to the occasion." Mentors guided me based on their experience and opened doors with their professional network.

While I was a pharmacy student just getting through the courses, graduating and getting licensed were my goals. Neither of my parents had the opportunity to go to college so I never considered any education or training beyond my undergraduate degree. However, I listened as a professor in my hospital pharmacy course described residencies and graduate programs. After working for 2 years and realizing I was bored with practice, I took charge of my career, contacted the professor for advice, and applied to MS residency programs. For me, being in charge of my career was the best decision I ever made. Never feel you are a victim of your circumstances as you always have choices and must take the responsibility for having a satisfying career.

NEW LEADER ADVICE

In this chapter there are numerous examples of finding mentors to guide you. It may have taken 3 years of pharmacy school to realize this, but Meg has begun to truly take charge of her career. She must first learn to manage herself as a young adult and professional before her mentors can help her to be successful. Meg is correct to be concerned if a residency is the right option for her as there are numerous opportunities for pharmacists. Once she decided this would be the right path, she worked with her mentor and preceptor, Marlene, to develop a short-term plan that she was able to execute even in a short time period. In an ideal situation, she may have started on this career planning earlier; however, she should know that is it never too late to start planning and take hold of her career.

What I have found to be successful

Even being a student, it is never too early to take charge of how your career evolves. Something as simple as goals and objectives on paper will suffice. However, you will need to get some insights from an array of mentors that have well-rounded perspectives. I began by putting down five goals that I wanted to achieve for both the short and long term. Have three to five objectives that will support achieving each individual goal helped me. Think big but be realistic with yourself. I recommend starting your CV early on and continually update it.

Understand that evolving your career is totally based on your desire to achieve your goals in the most effective way. Consider seeking out more than one or two mentors who could be your professors, preceptors, work supervisors, and even people outside of the pharmacy profession. Think of these mentors as your career "board of directors." In my short career I have focused on using mentors of different ages, who have worked in various areas of the profession that I am interested in. Stay in regular contact with these mentors, creating an ongoing dialogue in order for them to get to know you not just professionally but personally. Send your career planning document along with your CV out to your mentors and ask them to review it. Discuss with them their overall thoughts about your vision, what may be missing from your CV, and some ways to avoid potential pitfalls. Continually update and review your planning document throughout your career and celebrate your achievements. Always remember that your plan needs to remain flexible and that you may not succeed in every aspect. Be able to learn from those disappointments and remain persistent with your future goals and vision.

CASE 1.8

Employ a career development plan

PRINCIPLE ■ Professional development

Wendy is a pulmonary clinical specialist at a large, academic medical center. Her career goals over the last 6 years have taken her down different paths. As a first-year pharmacy student, Wendy sought out a clinical faculty member to provide professional guidance. Soon after developing this relationship with her professor, Wendy was encouraged to develop a written career plan. After a couple of drafts, Wendy and her mentor completed a flexible career plan that included objectives to work on over the next 4 years. The plan included participating in state and national professional organizations, attending state and national pharmacy meetings, conducting research, presenting a poster, developing her leadership skills, and of course keeping up with her coursework. Each year Wendy sat down with her mentor to review the plan, noting her accomplishments, and updating the plan into the year ahead.

Wendy continued to check off the accomplishments of her career plan throughout pharmacy school all the way into being selected for a PGY-1/PGY-2 pharmacotherapy residency. Again, as she started her residency she updated her career plan, still working with her original mentors and developing new relationship with others. This time her plan expanded to gaining clinical expertise, building relationships with physicians, writing a peer-reviewed publication, delivering a podium presentation, and expanding her professional network all while continuing with professional organizations involvement.

Again, as a new practitioner, Wendy continued to be successful in completing the objectives of her career plan that now helped her to be offered a full-time clinical pharmacy specialist position at the same organization where she completed her residency. After the first couple of months in her new position, she focused on updating her career goals by establishing relationships with her team, precepting students and residents, and looking to balance her work and family life. This time, her goals centered less around research, publications, and presentations and more on time with her husband, having kids, and outside activities. Many of Wendy's colleagues were surprised about her new career goals being that she had always been focused on being a well-rounded pharmacist both within the medical center and on the state and national level. However, Wendy was conscious of the commitment she still needed to make to perform at a high level in her daily job tasks.

Now that Wendy has been able to completely balance work and family, she has begun to update her career plan for her next stage. Her current plan still involves spending time with her family and on nonpharmacy activities, but it also includes a future goal of being a clinical coordinator and possible residency program director.

WHAT WENDY MAY BE THINKING...

- I am only a P1. Why do I need a career plan?
- Will I disappoint my mentors if I am not able to achieve the goals outlined in my plan?
- Will people think any less of me because I want to focus on family and nonpharmacy activities?
- Will focusing on family change people's perception of my commitment to my position?

ON THE OTHER HAND, WENDY MIGHT REASON...

- I have accomplished a lot in my early career because of my plan and mentor support.
- I plan to stay involved, just not to the level that I once was.
- I will need to be flexible as career goals can easily shift and change.
- Being able to balance these activities is important to me and keeps me happy.
- Having continually updated my career plan has allowed me to focus on areas of opportunity and then looking to the next opportunity based on my current situation.

MENTOR ADVICE

Wendy has done an excellent job so far in her career using mentors and a career plan. Now that she has established for herself the goal of being a clinical coordinator and possibly a residency director, in addition to having a balanced work-life career, she needs to think through and update her career plan. She should ask pharmacists who are currently clinical coordinators and residency program directors what knowledge, skills, and abilities they have found to be useful in these roles and how were they able to develop themselves professionally. Wendy shouldn't be afraid of deviating from the plan she first set, as priorities and circumstances will undoubtedly change over the course of her career. She needs to remember that her career is a marathon, not a sprint. There will be plenty of time to accomplish all of her career goals, but she just needs to be flexible.

What I have found to be successful

Leaders always keep themselves motivated by not only celebrating their success, but by quickly setting their next career goal. Success and satisfaction come from the journey toward a goal, not merely the achievement of the goal. I have found that always knowing what my next goal is engages me and provides personal satisfaction. I have found that this strategy is even needed in retirement, otherwise it is easy to become bored. Being successful as a leader requires challenging yourself in new areas and exploring new adventures.

NEW LEADER ADVICE

Wendy has remarkable consistency toward achieving and continually updating her goals from a student, to resident, to new practitioner. This case exemplifies Wendy's forward thinking for what she needed to compete for a residency and clinical specialist position. Additionally, Wendy prides herself in giving back to the profession through presentations, research, participation in professional organizations, and patient care. However, most will have some disappointments along the way, so Wendy needs to be able to adapt when situations may not go as planned.

Following her time as a new practitioner, Wendy began to step back from some of her involvement to start a family and participate in more things outside of the profession. She could have been criticized by some for stepping away from her career plans, but she was happy with her job and family life. The important part was that Wendy was at least involved and engaged in something more than just her clinical pharmacy role. Maybe it was not to the level of participation of working on multiple groups and giving various presentations as before. As pharmacists, we sometimes have the mentality that we have to do it all and now. However, Wendy will have plenty of opportunities to contribute to the profession in the years to come. A year or two hiatus might seem long now, but on the grand scheme of things, it might be the right thing to do to keep personal and job satisfaction and balance.

What I have found to be successful

Having learned the importance of a career plan during pharmacy school, I have been able to navigate the challenges and achieve my goals from school, through residency, and now in my current role. Overall, my successes have been due to some good advice from various mentors. Use your mentors to review, provide advice, and let you know what they think is missing from your plan. Reach out to high level leaders within the profession (i.e., Harvey AK Whitney and Remington Medal award winners) to get insight about what new skills you will need in the future with the upcoming changes in healthcare, pharmacy practice models, and with the implementation of medication-use technology and automation.

Most importantly, I've had to learn to *manage* myself in my career journey. My priorities have changed throughout time and will continue to change, so I am constantly updating my career plan. It's sometimes a letdown when I don't achieve all my goals, but I work hard to avoid feeling guilty or disappointed when this occurs. I am also always sure to include achieving goals outside of pharmacy in my plan, such as starting a family or having a new hobby, as you need to have a balanced life outside of the profession.

CASE 1.9

Perfecting leadership skills through involvement in professional organizations

PRINCIPLE ■ How professional organizations function and the leadership opportunities

During pharmacy school, Trevor attended his first national pharmacy meeting in San Francisco and quickly understood the importance of being involved in professional organizations. At that meeting, he was able to network with student pharmacists from across the country, talk with pharmacy leaders, and learn about the issues affecting the profession. Throughout pharmacy school, Trevor was an active member of multiple student organizations and even became the president of a large chapter during his 3rd year of school. His involvement and networking in professional organizations helped him to get an internship in the Washington, DC area and strengthened his application for his PGY-1 residency interviews.

Trevor began his PGY-1 residency with all intentions of continuing to be involved in professional organizations as a new practitioner. However, the workload and time associated with completing his PGY-1 requirements quickly became a reality and he decided to abandon his participation within these local, state, and national organizations. During his quarterly meetings with his residency program director, Trevor was continually encouraged to participate within these organizations, especially on the state level. Again, Trevor could not figure out how to balance his work and professional involvement. Then during his pharmacy administration rotation in spring of his residency year he had his "aha" moment after being assigned by the director of pharmacy to begin advocacy work on state pharmacy technician legislation that was being presented to the state legislature. Trevor dove into the program learning the background, talking to pharmacy staff, reading the legislation, and working with both the state society and national organization on talking points. Additionally, he organized and hosted a state legislator in order for him to see the role and impact that pharmacy technicians play within the hospital setting.

WHAT TREVOR MAY BE THINKING...
- I enjoyed participating in pharmacy school organizations when I was a student.
- I just do not have time to participate the way that I want to.

- My mentors are encouraging me to stay involved but don't understand how over-whelmed I am.

ON THE OTHER HAND, TREVOR MIGHT REASON...

- Now that I am a new practitioner, I have different opportunities to be involved than when I was a student.
- Learning how to advocate on the state level will be important to move pharmacy forward.
- I need to continue to be part of professional organizations to grow my professional network.

MENTOR ADVICE

In school Trevor was focused on short-term priorities: completing his classes and experiential rotations so he would graduate. Now he needs to change his focus to his long-term career. He may have 30–40 years that he will work so he needs to think of his career as a marathon, not a sprint. Including his personal life (spouse, children), he can chart out by decades what he would like his major accomplishments to be, such as president of a state professional organization, more job responsibility, or graduate school. By spreading things over decades, he can have the time to enjoy each aspect. In other words, he shouldn't try and be president, have a new job, and young children all at the same time. Even though he could get it all done at once, he will likely sacrifice quality and his own job satisfaction.

What I have found to be successful

Finding the time for the things that you determine are important is a matter of first think-ing through what they exactly are and documenting them. Be sure to include the important people in your life. Periodically take the time to plan your next 1–2 weeks (or months). Sched-ule time to focus on your list of priorities because you have defined them as critical. This includes spending time with those people important to you. Then after your take care of "first things first," fit in the other tasks that you must do, carefully avoiding interference of these items with your priorities.

I have found the time I devoted to professional organizations to be very valuable throughout my career, and the leadership skills I developed have assisted me in both my professional and personal life. The professional network I developed continues to be useful as I explore new professional opportunities in retirement. It is clear to me I would not be asked to speak or participate in programs without the reputation I developed in professional organizations. When it is all "said and done," it is the people who you have met throughout your career that mean the most, and many become your close personal friends.

NEW LEADER ADVICE

Trevor is a typical new practitioner who was highly involved during pharmacy school but became less involved when he became a new practitioner. It takes more effort when one does not have the college of pharmacy support system, and in many ways Trevor is now a "small fish in the big pond." However, there are numerous opportunities to continue to be involved in professional organizations and leadership. Many organizations now have specific new practitioner groups that focus on the needs of and provide resources for young practitioners. Additionally, there are numerous leadership positions within these groups that can be pursued. The myth of being involved—that it takes up too much time—is just a myth. Following his "aha" moment, Trevor should apply for nomination to a new practitioner committee that only requires a one-hour monthly call and some extra time working on projects. Most importantly, through this new role he will be able to network among his peers across the country, making new friends and sharing best practice resources from other sites.

What I have found to be successful

As a resident, I quickly learned the difficulty of balancing residency and involvement outside of work. However, even during a busy residency year there is an opportunity to stay involved professionally as some even might consider it a professional duty. Ultimately, this will grow your CV to compete for future job opportunities as well as allowing you to give back to the profession. It is critical for pharmacists to financially support these state and national organizations that work on our behalf to provide member resources, lead the development of professional policies, and spearhead legislative advocacy efforts.

Initially, you should look for opportunities to be a member of student or new practitioners' committee and if that is successful, consider pursuing additional leadership opportunities within the committee. Using the same method as developing your career plan, create a professional career timeline starting with student and new practitioner groups, specialty area sections, state delegates, and possibly board member or president positions of an organization.

The rewards for me have been plentiful as I have been able to travel across the country to attend various pharmacy meetings, give presentations, and meet both young and seasoned practitioners. I even met my wife from another college of pharmacy through participation in professional organizations.

Summary

The direction provided within this chapter from the perspective of a veteran mentor and new practitioner provides the foundation for exploring leadership opportunities and the importance of learning from your mistakes. Understanding and working toward developing your professional leadership skills will provide you with future job success, professional opportunities, and most importantly, the ability to advance the profession. Every young pharmacist needs to know that they can be an everyday "little L" leader even without a formal leadership title. Additionally, one must use the suggested strategies to begin to build their resume, to develop relationships with mentors, and to create a career plan. It is inevitable that sometime in your career you will encounter difficult scenarios. Being able to use a variety of leadership styles, delegating tasks, actively listening, and effective communication will help others to develop a trust in you and see you as a leader. Finally, consistent involvement within professional organizations, as a group leader, and through advocacy efforts is not only fun and rewarding, but your professional obligation.

Leadership Pearls

- Leadership is being in charge of your career and having a career plan that is reviewed and updated periodically.

- Leadership is being a "little L" everyday leader and continuing to evolve pharmacy services as a change agent.

- Leadership is consistently supporting your patients to optimize their therapy even in difficult situations.

- Leadership is adapting your style to the situation and learning from your mistakes.

- Leadership is belonging to and holding positions in professional organizations to advance the practice of pharmacy.

Leadership Exercises

- Seek out a high-level pharmacy leadership person and ask their vision for the profession over the next 10 years and what new skills you will need to be successful with these changes.

- Apply for student or new practitioner professional organization leadership opportunities and actively participate.

- Develop a career plan of both short- and long-term goals and have multiple mentors review it to see what is missing. Research and consider residency programs even if already in practice.

- Volunteer to lead a project or committee to improve your leadership and project management skills, using your mentors/supervisor for advice along the way.

- Read leadership books (i.e., *Good to Great: Why Some Companies Make the Leap. . .and Others Don't, The Five Dysfunctions of a Team: A Leadership Fable,* and *The 7 Habits of Highly Effective People*), journal articles, Harvey Whitney lectures, John Webb lectures; attend webinars; and review available pharmacy leadership videos and the leadership resource center at www.ASHPfoundation.org.

- Seek out opportunities to distinguish yourself from your peers, such as presenting, publishing, teaching, and volunteering for projects.

VETERAN MENTOR PROFILE

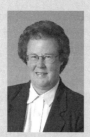

Sara J. White, MS, FASHP
(Ret.) Director of Pharmacy
Stanford Hospital and Clinics
Mountain View, California

Why did you decide on a career in leadership? I was exposed in my residency to improving pharmacy services and the challenge of fully utilizing our drug therapy knowledge. I chose a career in leadership because I liked the challenge and variety in experiences that I was exposed to. I also liked that no two days are alike.

Where do you turn for advice when you are stressed? I have a network of colleagues whom I turn to when I need advice. I also find that a walk in nature provides me with a good opportunity to reduce stress and contemplate problems and solutions.

What is your favorite leadership book? I have some favorite leadership authors, which include Peter Druker, John Maxwell, and Steven Covey. I find I can relate to and apply many of the leadership principles they write about.

From your perspective, what is the most important issue facing pharmacy leadership today? I think we are challenged with our reporting relationships in an organization. It's important that we are "at the table" when strategic decisions are made, which means we need a pharmacist at the senior leadership level. A chief pharmacy officer or some other title that reports to the COO or CEO would fill this need, where the CPO could have an impact on strategic decisions that impact not just the pharmacy but the whole organization such as the allocation of resources.

The other important issue we face is ensuring we have enough leaders in pharmacy for the future. In order to ensure that pharmacy departments continue to report to a pharmacy director, we need to develop leadership skills at all levels, starting with students and new practitioners.

Looking back over your vast experience in pharmacy, what one to two things do you know now that you wish you would have known as a student and new practitioner?

1. Leadership is all about helping others be successful at work. It is important to "pay it forward" and help others achieve their goals and stretch beyond their imagination. By doing so, new leaders will emerge in the pharmacy profession.
2. It is important to be a part of the solution and not the problem. Don't just complain about the current state of affairs; think about ways to improve them and volunteer to help.

What is your best advice for a new pharmacist today? Look for and seize opportunities to better utilize your expertise. Find a need and fill it. And don't wait to be discovered—look for opportunities to practice your leadership skills and to make a difference.

How do you envision this publication assisting student and new practitioner leaders? I hope the book stimulates young pharmacists to think of themselves as at least a "little L" leader on their shift or in their clinical practice and take the responsibility to apply this material and take their leadership skills to the next level. This will benefit patients and the profession and will result in a very fulfilling career.

NEW PRACTITIONER PROFILE

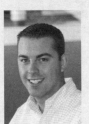

Christopher R. Fortier, PharmD
Manager, Pharmacy Support & OR Services
Clinical Assistant Professor
Medical University of South Carolina
Charleston, South Carolina

Why pharmacy: I had a mentor in high school who advised me to check out pharmacy. I shadowed a clinical pharmacist and was impressed with the role in patient care, relationships with the medical team, and the overall impact a pharmacist can make.

Advice to readers: As a student I wished I had worked in a hospital as an intern for a better knowledge of a variety of drugs and pharmacy operations. My biggest learning since graduation has been the importance of relationships with your healthcare peers and colleagues to ensure that we have a seat at the table where major decisions are made. My involvement in professional organizations has provided me with opportunities to network, travel, and the ability to meet people all over the country and to learn about their innovative pharmacy practices. It is critical when starting your career to have various mentors, a career plan on paper that you update periodically, and to proactively seek out career opportunities.

Tips for work-life balance: You need to prioritize, manage your time, and consciously say yes and no as appropriate. Based on the stage of your career and priorities at the time, you will need to modify ways to balance things and to be most efficient. For example, when my son was born I quickly switched to arriving early at work so that I could pick him up from day care and spend time together.

Personal career: My best career decision was to do a residency, which I hadn't planned on doing. My residency also provided me with how to manage myself, making the most of my strengths, providing opportunities, and fine-tuning my time management skills. I am most proud of being in a leadership role, my public speaking skills, and the ability to work with a great staff that understands teamwork. My career goal is being innovative in advancing the pharmacy practice model. Ultimately, I would like to be a director in the near future and additionally have a large interest in public health sector. Career success for me is first to be happy in my role and second working to advancing practice by trying new things to promote the role of the pharmacist on the local, state, and national levels.

Why leadership: My mother sparked my interest in leadership at an early age by encouraging me to seek out leadership roles. My favorite leadership book is Daniel Goleman's *Emotional Intelligence: Why It Can Matter More Than IQ*.

Recommended change for pharmacy: I would like to see a larger role for technicians to free up pharmacists' time. Rather than just talking about the needed changes, we must actually make them happen.

Using this book: I think this book provides useful quick tips and strategies as lessons learned can be taken and implemented immediately in order for each reader to become well rounded and successful.

Suggested Additional Readings

Blanchard K, Johnson S. *The One Minute Manager*. New York, NY: Berkley Trade Press; 1983.

Collins J. *Good to Great: Why Some Companies Make the Leap. . .and Others Don't*. New York, NY: Harper Business Press; 2001.

Covey S. *The 7 Habits of Highly Effective People*. New York, NY: Free Press; 2004.

Maxwell JC. *The 21 Indispensable Qualities of a Leader: Becoming the Person Others Will Want to Follow*. New York, NY: Nelson Business Press; 1999.

Pierpaoli P. Mentoring. *Am J Hosp Pharm*. 1992;49:2175-2178.

White SJ. Are you a manager or a leader? *Am J Health-Syst Pharm*. 2005;62:1206.

White SJ. Will there be a pharmacy leadership crisis? An ASHP Foundation Scholar-in-Residence report. *Am J Health-Syst Pharm*. 2005;62:845-855.

Zellmer W. Pharmacy vision and leadership: revisiting the fundamentals. *Pharmacotherapy*. 2008;28(12):1437-1442.

Zellmer W. Reason and history as guides for hospital pharmacy practice leaders. *Am J Health-Syst Pharm*. 2005;62:838-844.

Zilz DA, Woodward BW, Thielke TS, et al. Leadership skills for a high-performance pharmacy practice. *Am J Health-Syst Pharm*. 2004;61:2562-2574.

Additional Materials

Assessing Your Professional Leadership Skills

(Complete the following and be candid.)

Professional Leadership Skill	Always	Frequently	Occasionally	Never
I look for ways to improve pharmacy services and propose them in the form of solutions to my superior/preceptor	❏	❏	❏	❏
I keep various areas of professional practice open	❏	❏	❏	❏
I see myself as a "little L" everyday leader	❏	❏	❏	❏
I see myself as CEO of my career	❏	❏	❏	❏
I use mentors to help guide my decision making	❏	❏	❏	❏
I have a current documented career plan	❏	❏	❏	❏
I do what is right for the patient no matter the consequences to me personally	❏	❏	❏	❏
I communicate with and seek input from everyone in my workgroup before implementing changes	❏	❏	❏	❏
I do "what it takes" to get my job done even if it requires me to do things beyond my usual responsibilities	❏	❏	❏	❏
I seek leadership positions in professional organizations	❏	❏	❏	❏

Analysis: What do you need to do to move your assessments to the "always" column? Pick one and work on it using your mentor's and your career plan.

Read "Success Skills" articles 2, 6, and 11.

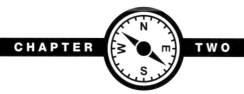

CHAPTER TWO

Becoming a Leader

Paul R. Krogh, PharmD, MS; Ross W. Thompson, MS, RPh

Introduction

Contrary to what many might believe, a title alone does not make someone a leader and those without a designated *leader* title can and do make a difference in the lives of others every day. Further, not all leaders reside at the top of an organizational structure. Many provide effective leadership from middle management and even front-line positions. The word *leader* usually calls to mind someone at the head of a pack, a group, or a company.

A leader is a person who influences a group of people toward the achievement of a goal. Leaders come in all sizes, shapes, and dispositions. What they share in common, however, are several characteristics and skills:

- A clear guiding vision

- Passion

- Integrity

- Trust

- Curiosity

- Calculated risk taking

With these skills, they serve as models for emulation and inspire others to follow them.

In our knowledge-intensive world of ceaseless innovation and change, every pharmacist must be attuned to the challenges of providing healthcare and actively communicating the important role pharmacists play in providing optimal patient care. Pharmacists must continually be working and studying to improve their skills in order to direct the future of the profession. It is imperative that every pharmacist be a leader in order to influence optimal medication therapy for patients by building a reputation of integrity and accountability, working on strong communication skills, and focusing on relationships with patients and healthcare providers.

Becoming a leader takes a good deal of dedication and time. It is not learned overnight; it is an ongoing process. As professionals, we must strive to learn something new every day, be successful in sharing our knowledge to promote quality patient care, and promote our value to the patient and organization in an ongoing manner. This includes expanding our horizons—internally by developing our leadership skills and externally by identifying leadership opportunities within our organization and community—and recognizing and taking advantage of the skills and talents of those around us.

Although there are numerous topics related to becoming a leader, we have chosen to discuss the following:

1. Varying your leadership style

2. Mentorship

3. Seizing growth opportunities

4. Negotiation

5. Prioritization

We chose these topics as they are perhaps the most important elements for emerging leaders to incorporate into their management skill set beyond the baseline tools that one typically acquires through routine work experience, which tends to focus on individual skills such as organization, time management, etc.

VARYING YOUR LEADERSHIP STYLE

Effective leadership requires awareness of multiple factors including your personal style, the skill and experience of your team members, the type of work to be completed, and the organizational environment. Through awareness of these factors, an effective leader will help determine the optimal leadership tactics to leverage for the initiative at hand.

Within the literature, it is common to see a total of eight leadership tactics described, which include direction, persuasion, negotiation, involvement, indirection, enlistment, redirection, and repudiation. Depending on the situation, a savvy leader will know which of these tactics to employ for maximal results and be able to smoothly transition between these approaches as the circumstances of the situation evolve.

There is simply no single leadership style or tactic that is universally ideal for all situations. Each of us has a "default" leadership style that we would naively apply to every situation until we gain an awareness of what leadership tactic is best suited for the immediate situation. Emerging leaders must invest time in understanding each of these tactics and gaining comfort and experience with each one, realizing not all eight will be intuitive or naturally based on individual style.

I found this concept most clearly illustrated by authors Paul Hersey and Ken Blanchard within the framework known as "Situational Leadership." Within this framework, any leadership scenario falls into one of four categories with each requiring a unique approach for optimal results. These leadership approaches consist of directing, coaching, supporting, or delegating. Depending on factors such as the team's competence and commitment, one of these four approaches should be leveraged. If the team has low competence and low commitment, the leader should utilize the "directing" approach where the leader is somewhat autocratic. A team with high competence and high commitment can be led using "delegation."

A skillful leader is able to identify these factors within any given scenario and realize which tactic to employ to maximize the performance of the team. The challenge is that this skill requires a significant effort to adopt into your leadership repertoire to the extent that you are able to fluidly move from one approach to another based on the situation at hand. This requires extensive practice, observation of others who possess this skill, and an awareness of your personal style.

Guiding and developing teams to function with a high degree of competence and commitment allows you to lead the team optimally through use of delegation. Leading through delegation is the most efficient of these scenarios, as this requires the least amount of time and intervention by the leader. Team members tend to enjoy this leadership approach over others as it allows them more autonomy and creativity and how the work is organized and completed.

Thus, delegation and empowerment are essential skills for a manager. Newer managers often face the reality that they must transition from completing the tasks at hand to delegating those tasks to their employees. This is not always an easy transition especially for those who are highly effective at "doing." The simple truth is that "doing" is much less productive than coordinating the efforts of several "doers" within the organization.

Successful delegation includes a series of steps. For larger projects, it is wise to formalize a project plan that entails far more detail than is typically necessary for delegating a simple task or activity within a larger project. Regardless, a few key steps occur in any form of effective delegation: define the task—provide as clear of a picture of the outcome as possible.

1. Select the individual(s) to complete the task with appreciation for the needed skills and current capacity to complete the activity.

2. Provide context such that the individual(s) understand how the task or project aligns with strategic direction of the organization—make it meaningful versus laborious. Personalize why you are asking that specific individual to contribute to inspire them and acknowledge their strength. Leaders inspire colleagues and promote a vision of the collective impact of individual efforts.

3. Evaluate availability of resources (time, equipment, subject matter expertise, etc.) that could be accessed over the course of the project and clarify how they can be accessed.

4. Agree on a timeline for completion and the need for any preliminary "check-in" activity prior to completion. In the instance of longer-term projects, establish criteria for how progress will be measured including a mechanism to proactively report progress to plan. This step is critically important to allow you to measure progress without being perceived as micro managing or interfering if things slip off track.

5. Provide encouragement, guidance, and support as the task or project is completed. By providing consistent feedback you will establish a rapport with the individual(s) that will make future collaboration more efficient and effective as you reconcile personal styles and techniques.

If executed properly, a manager can delegate tasks to individuals in such a way that the employee is more engaged than if the manager independently completed the task or project without any contribution from the employees.

Delegation can give way to empowerment as the manager gains trust in the employee and the employee gains confidence in interpreting needs and prioritizing, which allows a coordinator to enjoy even greater synergy from team members contributing to a common goal. This can be most clearly illustrated by describing a continuum of the levels of delegation. In the most basic level of delegation, the employee is truly being directed/instructed on what is to be completed. At this level, an employee has little room for interpretation and will likely find little to no satisfaction in the task at hand. As the level of delegation increases the employee is truly empowered, which allows creativity and interpretation by the employee and minimizes the need for the coordinator to implement a rigid system of managing oversight of delegated tasks.

The following is a simple illustration of the continuum of delegation giving way to empowerment:

1. Please take responsibility for completing this report. I have prepared instructions for how to generate the data, who should receive a copy of the report, and when it is due.

2. Please take a look at the information being requested of us. Provide me with your recommendations on what sources of data we should access so we can review it together to make sure we are in agreement before we generate the first report.

3. Please draft a template for this new report that also includes the source of data we will use to populate the template. Once prepared, please run it by me for my formal sign-off before you route this to the Quality of Care Committee.

4. Please formulate a response to this request on behalf of the Department of Pharmacy and let me know what feedback you receive after you present the report.

As you can see in these latter examples, the employee is being empowered to think and act more independently. It should be easy to see how empowerment is the most effective level of delegation. It is also the most enjoyable for the employee who senses a significant amount of flexibility and trust. However, this level of delegation is the most risky for the manager as the majority of control/oversight is relinquishing to the employee. This must be managed carefully especially in newer working relationships where you and the employee don't have as much working history. To effectively delegate a task, one must determine what level of delegation is appropriate for the specific task/project at hand while also accounting for the skill level of the employee being assigned the task.

MENTORSHIP

Access to a mentor is a success factor for emerging leaders. This resource is typically an individual who is older and more experienced. The mentor provides support and guidance in support of the personal and professional development of the protégé (AKA mentee). The mentor volunteers his or her time and knowledge for the sole purpose of supporting the protégé without any concern for personal gain.

Many larger employers offer formalized mentorship programs to be accessed by employees. It is also common for professional organizations to provide this type of program for members. However, the best place to look for a mentor might be within your department. Especially as a new practitioner, you are likely to find professional colleagues who possess valuable perspective and insight based on extensive experience within the organization and within pharmacy practice.

It is not uncommon to find mentorship outside of pharmacy practice but within a parallel industry or discipline within healthcare. This can afford you with unique perspectives that become increasingly valuable as you mature within the pharmacy profession and perhaps feel the need to expand your perspective beyond the traditional thinking within pharmacy practice.

Once you identify a potential mentor, you should carefully consider the goals you hope to achieve through the relationship. By thinking this through in advance, you will be able to share a clear set of expectations at the time you approach the individual and ask them to commit to your development by serving as your mentor. At a minimum, you should be prepared to describe what qualities you've observed in them that motivated you to seek their mentorship and a general sense of what you would hope to learn from them. You should also be prepared to discuss the amount of time you would like to spend and potentially even how your interactions would be structured. Recognize that this individual may counter with alternatives based on personal preference or constraints.

SEIZING GROWTH OPPORTUNITIES

As an emerging leader within an organization, you are expected to invest time understanding departmental and institutional goals. Committing to staying current on these agendas will require you to carefully review general communication that is shared with the employee population. Even after reviewing routine communication via staff meetings and hospital announcements, it may require additional effort to gain perspective of organizational goals/priorities depending on the exclusiveness of the organization's communication plan or if there are several management levels between you and senior leadership of the organization. Additionally it is important for you to demonstrate an active interest by asking clarifying questions as you solidify your understanding of these goals and priorities. This will impress your supervisor who might realize your potential role in participating in organizational planning and/or expanding your roles and responsibilities within the organization as opportunities arise.

Armed with this additional perspective on the goals of the organization, you may encounter opportunities to provide ideas for new initiatives or services that could support the organization's goals. If positioned as suggestions for consideration, this too will lead to your gaining additional insight and perspective as leadership provides feedback on the merits of your idea. By taking this patient and persistent approach, you will be in a great position to anticipate opportunities for growth and advancement within the organization. The opportunities could be involvement in the drafting of a business plan to start a new service or even an opportunity to lead a new program.

NEGOTIATION

A skilled negotiator will find an outcome that is mutually beneficial for the involved parties. This goal of finding a "win-win" scenario is critically important in maintaining satisfaction and engagement of all parties. A common misconception is that a negotiation ends in a "win-lose" or even a "lose-lose" scenario where both parties compromise on what they truly needed as an outcome.

There are a few keys to preparing for a successful negotiation:

1. Approach the negotiation objectively and with your emotions in check.

2. Differentiate between your wants and your needs as outcomes of the negotiation and focus your effort on addressing your needs. Recognize that a negotiation has nothing to do with being right or wrong. Instead, it is related to assigning a value to tangible and intangible outcomes.

3. Never assume you know the value the other party is placing on any given term within the negotiation. This is often subjective and you are best served by asking for clarification as to why certain terms are more important than others. This allows you to determine how each term is valued by the other party.

This background on negotiation principles is most relevant to business/contract negotiations but can also bring valuable insight into how to handle situations that arise in the workplace as well as other facets of your life. Unfortunately, pharmacists rarely have formal training in negotiation. As a result, this skill is most consistently learned "on the job" as a pharmacist. Thus, becoming familiar with books/articles on the topic is perhaps the best approach to gaining this skill.

Many conversations incorporate some level of negotiation perhaps without our even noticing. A simple example is a husband who agrees to take out the garbage if his wife is willing to pay the utility bills. A pharmacist offers to send an intern home early to study for an exam if she assists a nurse with a controlled substance discrepancy on her way out of the hospital.

Although many individuals shy away from negotiations, it is important that your needs be known in order for you to maintain a sense of control of your work environment. By avoiding negotiation you place yourself in a position where you could become overburdened and frustrated which will only compromise your productivity and job satisfaction.

On the other extreme, it is important to realize that not every request should result in a negotiation. We all should embrace the fact that our job responsibilities are subject to change and that our flexibility is an incredible benefit to our employer. By turning every request—large or small—into a negotiation you run the risk of compromising your reputation as a team player and alienating yourself. Simply stated, not every request of an employee's time should result in a negotiation, as this is likely to develop into a strained relationship.

PRIORITIZATION

Competing priorities are simply a reality of life and especially prevalent in an acute care environment where patient needs and so many other factors are constantly changing. To effectively navigate through competing priorities, it is critically important to raise awareness of the existing dilemma and explore options for reprioritizing in order to address the most critical needs at hand.

Saying no is rarely easy and is never enjoyable simply because of how we are programmed within our society. We would not have chosen a field in healthcare if we didn't have an underlying motivation to assist members of society. However, we must learn how to say no in order to fulfill our current commitments and maintain a balance between work, family, and community involvement.

Perhaps the only time it is easy to decline an offer is in the scenario where you are being asked to do something inconsistent with your morals or ethical values. In that situation you have no choice but to decline in order to remain true to yourself.

If being asked to volunteer time for an organization or event in which you are not invested, it is absolutely acceptable to say no. This should also be relatively easy since you are not likely to face any ramifications of declining based on your disinterest in the requesting organization.

These initial scenarios are clear-cut. It is far more difficult when you are approached with an opportunity that you are truly interested in pursuing but lack the capacity to accept the responsibility. In this scenario it is wise to carefully consider options/ramifications before making your decision. Ask for a description of the responsibilities and estimated time requirements associated with the role. As you gain an understanding of the expectations, consider the option of discontinuing other obligations that would free an offsetting amount of your time. If there is simply no option of freeing-up the time needed to fulfill the role being offered, you could consider a couple of options:

- It is not uncommon to say "Yes, with the following conditions..." and you shouldn't be shy about doing so.

  - I'm happy to assist with reserving the meeting room and preparing the agenda, but you will need to find someone else to coordinate the travel arrangements of the guest speaker and getting the program accredited.

  - This might result in your being passed over for the immediate opportunity but might demonstrate your willingness to contribute at some level as future needs arise.

- When you simply don't have the capacity and need to say no but would truly be interested, find a diplomatic way to say "not right now."

  - I appreciate the opportunity and I would say yes if given the opportunity next year [i.e., you want the individual asking to know you appreciated the offer and are interested in the opportunity (for example, serving on a committee), just not right now.]

  - Just be prepared to say yes when the offer comes back around next year.

  - Saying yes but not fulfilling the responsibility is clearly the most devastating to your reputation as well as to your future involvement in that organization.

Worst-case scenario is your acceptance of a new responsibility and subsequent failure to fulfill the expectations. This reflects poorly on you as an individual and may decrease your self-confidence.

The next to worst-case scenario is your acceptance of additional responsibility and subsequently compromising your quality of life by over committing and feeling overly burdened and stressed. It is a difficult balance, as you won't get more accomplished and efficient with managing multiple responsibilities without occasionally stretching yourself.

In the context of an employer's request of your time, it simply is not appropriate to say no. Rather, you should pursue a deeper understanding of the need and potentially help explore alternatives if it is a responsibility you are not interested in assuming. Take the opportunity to ask for clarification for why you are being asked. If it is not a responsibility you would prefer assuming, make sure you describe why it is not your "preference" while conceding that you understand there are no other options at least in the short-term. As a result of this process you might discover an option to assume a different responsibility in exchange.

Building your leadership skill repertoire and knowing your personal style

PRINCIPLES ■ Delegation ■ Empowerment ■ Developing and understanding your leadership style ■ Taking charge by letting go

Tara is an energetic, highly motivated new practitioner who is well-liked by the pharmacy team members, nurses, and providers alike at Lakes Area Community Hospital, a 200-bed community hospital. Since starting at Lakes Area Community Hospital 4 years ago, Tara has been a key group member in numerous projects including an analysis and redesign of the sterile products dispensing processes to reduce waste and improve turnaround time, development of a pharmacy staff practice council, and creation of a multidisciplinary, subgroup of the pharmacy and therapeutics committee charged with reviewing and reporting on all medication errors.

Tara's expertise, attention to detail, and willingness to do whatever it takes to get the job done has not gone unnoticed; as one of the managers put it, "Tara is our go-to person when you need a task completed ASAP, as she is always willing to come in early or stay late and takes personal responsibility for completing the task on time."

On a personal level, Tara is very committed to her family, which includes her husband Mark, 3-year-old daughter Candice, and 1-year-old son Scott. Although Tara has enjoyed working as a staff pharmacist, she has commented to other team members that the varied day and evening shifts and every other weekend staffing requirements make it difficult to balance work and family responsibilities, in particular since the birth of her second child.

Tara was therefore delighted when the department decided to create a new "department project coordinator" position to help lead the numerous quality, safety, and performance improvement projects going on in the department. Tara felt this position would be a perfect fit for her as she is passionate about medication safety and has helped lead some recent process improvement efforts for the department. In addition, the new position would be regular business hours and no weekends!

However, Tara soon found moving from a "doer" to an "overseer" was more difficult than she imagined. In previous projects, Tara often would take on much of the workload herself to ensure the project was moving forward as planned. At 5 months into her new position as project coordinator for the department, Tara felt overwhelmed. She was struggling to keep up with her numerous project lead responsibilities such as meeting minutes, scheduling, and project updates. Worst, she was working more hours than ever and was consistently bringing work home with her to catch up, which had a negative impact on her family life.

WHAT TARA MAY BE THINKING...

- I feel overwhelmed and unable to balance my work and personal life.
- If I don't continue to be involved in the details, I won't be able to successfully lead the projects.

- I'm concerned that the quality of the project will suffer if I don't manage each step of the way.
- Will my colleagues resent me if I simply make project assignments and monitor their progress?
- Am I cut out for this project coordinator position?

ON THE OTHER HAND, TARA MIGHT REASON...

- How can I take a step back from the details of the projects and still make sure they are proceeding as planned?
- What steps do I need to take to become comfortable with "overseeing" versus "doing?"
- What are some other leadership skills I could learn and use to be a better leader?

- -

MENTOR ADVICE

Transitioning from a staff member to a manager position is often a significant change in responsibilities. Tara is an exceptional employee who is known for getting things done, but she is struggling with how to accomplish tasks by working through others. Tara should study the concept of situational leadership and apply that approach to how she is leading others involved in the projects she is coordinating. Tara will likely need assistance in learning how to incorporate a variety of leadership styles into her repertoire, which will take time, experience, and self-awareness. To assist her in this process, she should find someone on the management team that models these styles and then reflect on how she can incorporate a wider variety of styles into her leadership approach. This should become part of a routine re-evaluation for the purpose of reflecting on overall leadership performance.

Tara should also consider completing formal training in project management methodology with the goal of recognizing methodology for truly managing projects versus owning each task within the projects. Project management training is offered by a host of training services and might even be provided by the hospital's human resources department. Understanding this methodology will allow her to draw on techniques for successful project management including aspects of delegating effectively. The intent would be to modify her approach so she is consistently focused on assuming responsibility for the outcome of the project while supporting and promoting the accomplishments of the team members completing the project.

Lastly, Tara needs to take full advantage of teams that are able to function at a high level by leading through delegation and essentially "getting out of the way." Recognizing when one has this luxury will significantly increase one's effectiveness and capacity to manage multiple projects.

What I have found to be successful

Observe capable and savvy leaders who utilize an array of tactics as different scenarios arise. Because an accomplished leader is able to fluidly transition between these tactics, this skill might not be easily detected and observed. In learning this skill, an observer might benefit from meeting with the leader in advance of an important committee meeting to understand what the leader expects to encounter and what tactics are likely to be leveraged during the interaction. This would allow insight into what tactics will likely be demonstrated. Through this type of observation you will quickly see how effective a leader becomes when the appropriate tactic is used for the specific situation at hand.

Recognize your personal style and instinct. I have gained a much greater appreciation for my personal leadership style by reflecting on how I navigated through various leadership scenarios over the years. Recognizing my style naturally trends a certain direction, and I sense the need to remain astute to the situation at hand in order to go away from my natural instinct when a different tactic would be more effective.

These perspectives can only develop through observations of others you work for and over the course of your career, as well as through a deliberate effort to monitor your own successes and failures while leading work groups over the years. Strike the right balance between providing adequate oversight without micromanaging. It is important to balance the need for clear direction setting without leaning too far toward micromanagement where you run the risk of stifling creativity.

Leaders inspire teams by illustrating how the project at hand supports a larger mission. You will want to connect the task you are assigning to the bigger picture in order to instill motivation and ownership of the project (Why is this project important? How does it help support the advancement of the department, organization, or profession?). I was struck by a story I was told of an administrator who was walking through an oncology ward of a hospital when he encountered an employee from housekeeping. When the administrator asked the man what he did for the hospital, the housekeeper stated that he was "part of a team who is trying to cure the world of cancer." Someone had clearly inspired this employee by illustrating the importance of his individual role that supported the larger mission. I can only imagine the level of performance that would come from an organization of employees who had such clear vision and inspiration.

NEW LEADER ADVICE

Tara appears to have found balancing her multiple new responsibilities in her new role difficult. It is not uncommon to fall back to "what has always worked" during times of stress, and it appears she may be reverting back to old habits as she attempts to manage the multiple responsibilities she has taken on as the new project coordinator for the department. For her to succeed in her new position, it is important for her to continually work on developing effective delegation skills, which allow her to fully maximize the performance of the project teams.

Tara should consider seeking out project management training and tools to assist her in more effectively leading the various projects she is involved in, while still maintaining a pulse on where each team member is regarding assigned project tasks. Developing a Gantt chart at the beginning of a project with the team members can be especially helpful and will help all those involved in the project better understand the project in its entirety. A Gantt chart outlines the desired outcome, project tasks, individuals assigned to each task, and deadlines for each task and the overall project. Tara may also benefit from establishing clear expectations on the level and frequency of checking in on each team member's progress, making incremental course corrections if necessary. With clear expectations, she should become more comfortable recognizing and modifying her leadership style to maximize the effectiveness of each team member.

Varying her leadership style based on each team member's individual skills and experience will also help increase her comfort level in stepping back from the details of the projects she is leading while still maintaining a pulse on the progress of the project to ensure things are progressing as planned. In addition, Tara's ability to "take charge by letting go" will empower group members to think and act more independently—improving the engagement of group members and, ultimately, the outcome of the project.

What I have found to be successful

- **Utilize project management tools to track the progression of complex projects.** I have found project management tools such as Gantt charts to be an excellent tool for planning and scheduling projects, setting out tasks and designating responsibility for those tasks, and defining time periods within which tasks should be completed. Outlining and sharing identified tasks and the timeline prior to beginning any work on the project will also allow other team members a chance to provide input on the tasks and the timeline you have developed, allowing for any issues and/or concerns with the project to be identified and addressed at the beginning of the project.

- **Consistently and frequently check in with team members to address any issues and/or concerns that have arisen.** It is important that you identify and assist team members in removing barriers to progress on the project by maintaining frequent and open lines of communication. Focusing the discussion on what issues, concerns, or barriers they are facing rather than simply asking for a status update will help ensure you are helping move the project forward without being seen as a micromanager.

- **After completion of the project, hold a review meeting with all those involved to obtain feedback on the management of the project and, in particular, your performance as the project lead.** Three questions I have found very helpful in obtaining feedback from team members on my performance as a lead on various projects:
  - What should I continue doing?
  - What should I stop doing?
  - What should I start doing?

Share this feedback with your immediate manager and mentor to identify areas to focus developmental efforts.

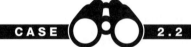

CASE 2.2

Finding and maximizing the mentor/mentee relationship

PRINCIPLE ■ Mentorship

Isaac recently completed a postgraduate year one (PGY1) residency and has been looking for a position in a small hospital where he can continue to grow his skills in both the outpatient and inpatient settings. After significant research, Isaac found what he thought was the perfect job with the one exception—the job is more than 2,000 miles away from home! Isaac has always been somewhat of a homebody, completing undergraduate and pharmacy school and his PGY1 residency 30 minutes from home and making frequent visits home on the weekends. In addition, he would be moving far away from one of the most influential individuals in his life—his uncle Gary, who is a pharmacist at the local community pharmacy where Isaac received his first exposure to the profession of pharmacy as a cashier and eventually a technician.

Isaac was immediately hooked and has continued to work at his uncle's store throughout undergraduate and pharmacy school and even occasionally during his PGY1 residency. Despite the distance, Isaac decided he would move forward with interviewing at Hobaken HealthCare, a 100-bed community hospital located just outside of San Diego, California. The interview went well and after significant discussion with his family and friends, Isaac decided to accept the position and move across the country to begin his professional career.

Two months after moving to San Diego, Isaac is becoming uncertain with his transition from resident to staff pharmacist as well as his move across the country for this position. That being said, he has connected well with a veteran pharmacist named Steve whom he has spent the most time with during his training. Steve reminds Isaac of his uncle Gary, which he thinks may be part of the reason he is so comfortable around Steve. Isaac feels Steve is a great role model and would like to continue to have regular contact with Steve as Isaac's career begins at Hobaken HealthCare. However, Isaac is unsure if Steve would be willing to be Isaac's mentor once his training is completed and hasn't formally discussed any mentorship relationship with Steve. In addition, Steve is the primary preceptor for all the interns at Hobaken—a responsibility that takes up a significant amount of his time.

WHAT ISAAC MAY BE THINKING...

- Steve likely is too busy to take me on as a mentee in addition to his mentor responsibilities with the interns.
- What if I make things uncomfortable between Steve and I by asking him to formally mentor me?
- Should I just look to my immediate manager as a mentor?

ON THE OTHER HAND, ISAAC MIGHT REASON...

- If I don't ask Steve if he would formally be my mentor, I will potentially miss a great mentor-mentee relationship.
- Steve's lead role as the interns' preceptor and as a trainer suggests he enjoys the role of mentor and thus may be willing to take me on as mentee as well.
- Steve may have other mentees who have recently made the transition from resident to staff pharmacist he could connect me with as well.

- -

MENTOR ADVICE

Isaac should ask Steve for his mentorship and gauge his interest in supporting him. Isaac might be pleasantly surprised with Steve's response. Even if Steve declines, Isaac will have made his interests known related to his personal and professional development goals. He will have flattered Steve by approaching him with this request. In reality it is rare for a colleague to decline if you approach them with a thoughtful request.

Once Isaac has a commitment from a mentor, he should consider formalizing a set of expectations that more clearly describes his commitment to the arrangement. This might include a meeting schedule as well as more detailed objectives or agendas for the time they spend together. Isaac needs to keep in mind that his mentor has priorities and that he should be respectful and deliberate with the time he requests from this resource.

Isaac should maintain regular communication with his uncle back home as he seems to provide him with a tremendous amount of comfort and perspective. Isaac might even consider bringing some formality to this relationship by establishing goals for what he wants those discussions to entail. That could influence those discussions more consciously in the direction consistent with a more formal mentor–mentee relationship. Those discussions can easily occur "remotely" by scheduling a standing meeting by telephone.

Isaac should also keep in mind that his direct supervisor may or may not have the ability to assist him in growing/developing his leadership capability. Managers aren't automatically mentors. The obvious candidates to become a mentor are often teachers/preceptors or managers. However, Isaac shouldn't forget to consider other, less obvious mentor relationships such as peers within his department or from different disciplines within his organization. Recognize that mentors might even emerge from outside of healthcare.

What I have found to be successful

- **Identify a mentor who will assist you as an emerging leader in pharmacy practice.** There is simply no substitute for this type of resource—especially earlier in your career. I personally found tremendous benefits through my experience with a mentor who supported me during my entrance into pharmacy practice.
- **Establish a network of colleagues who are aware of your personal and professional aspirations.** These individuals might represent a combination of former mentors, employers, subordinates, peers, and family. By maintaining this network you can gain a variety of perspectives as you contemplate a specific practice challenge or career dilemma. You can actively maintain this network. Although you must invest the time in maintaining this network, you will realize a great deal of benefit through being able to share your collective perspectives on real-time issues.

- -

NEW LEADER ADVICE

Mentorship is an essential component to continued growth and development throughout Isaac's career. Mentors can provide advice, professional growth opportunities, encouragement and feedback; all of which would be of benefit to Isaac as he makes the transition to staff pharmacist in an unfamiliar place.

Successful mentor–mentee relationships involve consistent communication between mentor and mentee and can occur via multiple venues, including e-mail or telephone, and thus relationships are not limited to geographic proximity of the mentor and mentee. Isaac has already developed a long-standing mentor relationship with his uncle and he would likely benefit from continuing to keep regular contact with his uncle during his transition.

Although Isaac may have some reservations in formally asking Steve if he would be a formal mentor due to Steve's other responsibilities, if Isaac doesn't ask he will never know! Multiple mentors can provide him with advice on different aspects of his life (perhaps one mentor on a professional level and another on a more personal level).

Finally, mentors can come from a variety of sources, including those outside of pharmacy and healthcare. Mentors from diverse backgrounds can help Isaac look at opportunities and challenges from a different perspective.

What I have found to be successful

- **Do not limit yourself to one mentor–mentee relationship.** You may find value in having more than one mentor; in particular, if the mentors exemplify different traits and skills you would like to emulate. As a new leader, I have found it valuable to have a couple mentors who provide me with a different perspective due to their distinct career paths.

- **Outline your personal and professional goals and share these with your mentors.** It is important to share your personal and professional goals with your mentors so they can best frame advice and provide examples of their experiences, which may assist you in reaching your goals. I've found regular review of my personal and professional goals assists me in taking a critical look at whether or not my recent activity and priority setting are enabling me to reach my goals. If yes, then share this progress with your mentors and if not, seek counsel from your mentors on potential strategies to take to get back on track.

CASE 2.3

How to recognize when an opportunity presents itself

PRINCIPLES ■ Goal setting and communication ■ Organizational awareness

Sara is a part-time staff pharmacist who has worked every Monday, Wednesday, and Friday the past 6 years in a pharmacy located within a geriatric medical clinic. Sara's interest in geriatrics began in pharmacy school and was reinforced after she completed a few of her advanced practice experiences at a local VA hospital.

Sara's boss, Kristi, shares her passion and has been instrumental in expanding the role of pharmacists in her clinic to include a diabetes medication therapy management (MTM) service, pharmacist consultations for all patients on eight or more medications, and they are in the beginning phase of development of hyperlipidemia MTM services as well. The diabetes MTM service is thriving and the pharmacy team members enjoy a great relationship with the physicians, nurses, and patients at the medical center. Sara feels extremely fortunate to have the opportunity over the past 6 years to participate in MTM service and continue to grow her clinical skills. In fact, she is considering increasing to a full-time position once her daughter, Erin, begins kindergarten this fall to help out with the additional workload the pharmacy team expects will be generated once the hyperlipidemia MTM service is implemented.

You can imagine how surprised Sara and the other team members were when Kristi informed them that she had accepted a promotion to oversee and lead the expansion of pharmacy services at the other four Heritage Medical clinic locations. Kristi also mentioned during her announcement that her plan is to spend the next few months hiring and training a new manager to take over her responsibilities at Sara's site and ensured everyone that she still will be working with the staff to take care of patients, just in a more distant role.

WHAT SARA MAY BE THINKING...

- Why did Kristi leave when we are in the midst of expanding our services to include a hyperlipidemia MTM service?
- Will our new manager be able to build the relationships with providers and nurses the way Kristi did?
- Do I still want to increase my hours to full-time if Kristi is no longer our manager?
- Am I or anyone else on our team able to lead our pharmacy team like Kristi did?
- Should I apply for this position or wait to be asked by the hiring manager?

ON THE OTHER HAND, SARA MIGHT REASON...

- I've learned a lot over the last 6 years and perhaps I'm ready to step into a formal leadership role.
- Kristi will still be around in the organization so if needed, I can still reach out to her.
- The strong team and collaboration with other providers Kristi has developed will provide a strong foundation to continue to advance pharmacy services, regardless of who is selected to fill the role Kristi is vacating.

MENTOR ADVICE

Sara owes it to herself to stay informed of the goals of the organization, how her role aligns and supports these organizational goals, and to fully appreciate the pressures her manager and the collective department feel toward achieving these goals.

One can appreciate Sara's surprise related to the news about Kristi. However, she should be well aware of the health system's plans to expand MTM services across all campuses. That insight should have helped prepare her for this organizational change associated with Kristi's promotion. Regardless, she is now in a position to look at the options for how to replace Kristi.

Sara needs to make her interests known if she wants to be considered as a candidate for Kristi's vacated position. It would be ideal if she had already laid this groundwork by communicating her short- and long-term career goals among the management team. There is no harm in voicing her interests as long as she is legitimately interested in the position's responsibilities.

In most instances it would be wise for Sara to approach Kristi to better understand the requirements of the position and determine if Kristi could provide insight on her potential candidacy if she decided she wanted to be considered for the promotion. If Sara chose to pursue the promotion opportunity, Kristi's advocacy would only enhance her chance of being considered.

If after a thoughtful review of the finer details of the expectations of the position she decides she is not interested in being considered, she could certainly offer to participate in the recruitment process as candidates are identified, screened, and interviewed. With 6 years of experience within this MTM clinic, her interests and opinions will be valued by the department's leadership team. Thus, Sara should have no hesitation in making her interests known.

What I have found to be successful

- **Approach a formal leader within your organization to express your leadership interests.** Leaders realize that individuals with interest in leadership are an incredible asset. These individuals are far more likely to support the accomplishments of the department and lead projects and new services as those opportunities arise.

If you have a sincere interest in expanding your role and responsibility in the direction of assuming a leadership position, your manager should recognize and appreciate the luxury of having you in the organization and look for ways to develop your leadership skills through activities such as committee and project involvement.

Be aware that demonstrating an interest with your supervisor (or even your supervisor's boss) will increase the organization's awareness of your goals and potentially lead to your gaining access to organizational plans and strategy. Volunteering for project involvement will also lead to a broader understanding of the organizational goals and direction and make you far more valuable as an employee.

- **Don't wait to be asked.** If you shy away from letting your interests be known, your supervisor may not even realize your potential capability for a larger role in the department. It is far too common for an employee to assume they are not a viable candidate for a promotion unless the supervisor solicits their interest. It is just as likely that the supervisor assumes the employee is not interested in the opportunity. This can obviously lead to disappointment and dissatisfaction that could have been avoided by simply letting your interests be known.

   The worst-case scenario is that you are passed-up for the promotion but will likely gain valuable perspective on what you will need to accomplish in order to be considered for promotion in the future. In addition, you are demonstrating your interest in supporting the organization.

- **If you are unsure of your interest, consider taking an interim assignment.** In this specific scenario, Sara might be well positioned to assume an interim role as a way to "test drive" the career opportunity if she is uncertain of the increased responsibilities. If presented properly, the management team would also see this as a way to ensure a smooth transition by not being solely dependent on recruiting an external candidate to replace Kristi.

   Demonstrate patience when seeking growth opportunities. Because people and priorities change within every organization, opportunities will arise. However, some opportunities may take longer than you would like. By giving your current employer an understanding of your interests, this type of opportunity is likely to materialize more quickly than if your interests remained unknown. If there simply is no growth opportunity, recognize that you need to choose to either be at peace in your current role or begin looking at other career opportunities that will enable your desired career growth.

NEW LEADER ADVICE

Kristi's strong relationship with staff and successful expansion of pharmacy services likely make her announcement a difficult and anxiety-provoking one for Sara and the staff. Her initial thoughts may include questions such as "Will the new manager be able to develop the same level of trust with the physicians, nurses, and patients at the medical center that Kristi has?" and "Will this person share the same passion for patient care that Kristi does?" For Sara in particular, "Do I have the necessary skills to step into the pharmacy manager position?"

After having some time to reflect on Kristi's announcement, Sara's thoughts appeal to change to take the leadership and clinical skills she has learned under Kristi's tutelage as the new pharmacy manager for the clinic. After all, she has a strong relationship with the pharmacy team, physicians, nurses, and patients at the clinic and has been considering moving to a full-time position.

The primary question Sara needs to ask herself is "Is moving into the pharmacy manager role in line with my career goals?" If yes, she should not let any reservations of not having "formal" management experience limit her from pursuing a new challenge or opportunity. On the other hand, if she is satisfied/fulfilled in her current role, she will want to participate and contribute in the selection process for her new boss. Either way, it is important for her to make her interest in the manager position or in being involved in the recruitment/hiring process of the new manager known to Kristi.

What I have found to be successful

- **Review your organization's goals and how your work supports attainment of these goals.** Understanding how your work supports the organization's goals allows for alignment of department goals with the organization and priority of work to support these goals. Sara's already established relationship with Kristi should provide her the opportunity to better understand the organization's MTM expansion initiative and what she can do—whether in her current role or as a new manager—to support this initiative.

- **Volunteer to be involved in an interdisciplinary project or committee.** Working with other disciplines on a project or as part of a committee is an excellent opportunity to expand your understanding of organizational goals and initiatives and what role the department and yourself can provide in supporting these. I have found interdisciplinary work valuable in gaining a greater understanding the role each discipline plays in setting and meeting organizational goals and where the expertise of pharmacists can support the organization's goals. It is also important you understand your department's current commitments and obligations to ensure you are able to speak on behalf of the department or defer to your leadership team for additional input when necessary.

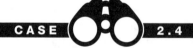

CASE 2.4

When and how to negotiate an outcome

PRINCIPLE ■ Priority setting

Khalid is a driven new practitioner who recently began a postgraduate year two (PGY2) specialty residency in infection disease at Java Medical Center, a 627-bed academic medical center. Khalid's major project for the year will be the development and cost justification of a pharmacist-managed, antibiotic stewardship program—an ambitious and likely time-consuming project to say the least!

Khalid is extremely excited about his major project and is confident that his discipline, work ethic, and time management skills will allow him to successfully balance the project workload, his rotations, and staffing requirements. Three months into his residency year, Khalid is keeping up with his residency rotations, staffing responsibilities, and project development timolinoo, although he is working long days and using his weekends to stay on track with his numerous responsibilities.

Khalid's primary preceptor has been very outspoken to other colleagues about how impressed she is with Khalid's ability to balance his residency requirements and his work developing an antibiotic stewardship program pilot, which will go live on two medical/surgical units in 2 weeks. In addition, development of an antibiotic stewardship program is a top priority for the organization and the progress of the antibiotic stewardship program pilot was even mentioned in a recent communication to all hospital staff from the CEO of the hospital. Khalid has been working feverishly to develop a formal communication plan outlining the pilot program for the pharmacy, medical and nursing staff, finalize note templates for the medical record, and tie up the format and content for the data collection forms. It's now Wednesday, 10 days before go-live, and Khalid is confident that if he stays focused he will meet the deadline of having the communication plan, templates, and collections forms completed by week's end for review by his primary preceptor.

On Thursday morning, Khalid gets an urgent page from his primary preceptor asking if he could do some research and communication on alternative options for a commonly used antibiotic that has suddenly become in short supply across the country. Khalid wants to help and doesn't want to let down his preceptor, but knows he won't be able to finish the communication plan, note templates, and data collection forms by the due date of this Friday if he shifts his focus to the drug shortage. On the other hand, he realizes the shortage will have a significant impact on care at the hospital and has been informed by the pharmacy buyer that the department does not have enough on hand to make it through the upcoming weekend.

WHAT KHALID MAY BE THINKING...

- I'll never be able to meet the established deadlines for my major project if I help out with the drug shortage.
- Why did my preceptor ask me to add the antibiotic shortage to my plate when she knows I have to have the communication plan, medical record templates, and data collection form templates completed by Friday?
- Does my preceptor recognize that what she is asking is not realistic based on everything else I have on my plate?

ON THE OTHER HAND, KHALID MIGHT REASON...

- It is important to our patients and department that I shift my focus to addressing the urgent situation of the drug shortage.
- Perhaps my preceptor will be willing to set my due date for the communication plan, medical record template notes, and data collection forms to early next week to allow me to work on the drug shortage and still meet the project deadlines.
- In the context of immediate needs for patient care and importance to the department, I should consider it a compliment that my primary preceptor came to me for assistance.

MENTOR ADVICE

Khalid is facing the unfortunate reality that he is not capable of meeting his project deadline if he redirects his focus to formulating a response to the drug shortage. As soon as he reaches this conclusion, he needs to immediately raise the concern with his preceptor to discuss options. Upon discussion, he might find that his preceptor didn't realize the scenario she created by delegating this drug shortage response to him.

As the discussion ensues with the preceptor, it would be important to understand if the Friday deadline for his stewardship program materials was an arbitrary timeline or if there was an external factor that influenced that deadline. Khalid might realize his preceptor wasn't planning to review the stewardship documents until Monday morning anyway, which would allow Khalid to use the weekend to finalize. If the project timeline is not flexible, Khalid's preceptor might conclude that she will need to complete the drug shortage response or delegate the task to someone else. The bottom line is that Khalid and his preceptor can only negotiate a mutually acceptable outcome if they fully understand each other's needs as well as available alternatives.

What I have found to be successful

- **Open dialogue is critical in managing through competing priorities.** By raising awareness of the situation, your supervisor will gain an appreciation of the situation and can assist you in considering alternatives. If there is no alternative but to assume those additional responsibilities, your supervisor will have a much greater appreciation of the need to look for alternatives and help you reprioritize competing projects.

  The ability to managing competing priorities is much more complex when requests originate from more than one manager or department within your organization. This creates a scenario where you must sensitize multiple individuals of the competing priorities and will often find yourself in a position where one party is feeling neglected if a different manager's request is being more highly prioritized. Again, the key is open communication and sharing enough information so all parties fully appreciate the dilemma and the rationale for your decision regarding prioritization.

- **Offer suggestions for alternatives your supervisor may not have considered.** You may be aware of several options for shifting or delegating in an effort to achieve the desired outcome. As long as your suggestions are focused on achieving the goal and not simply focused on avoiding additional responsibilities, your supervisor will recognize your efforts as being a team player.

NEW LEADER ADVICE

The ability to prioritize multiple tasks is an essential skill for any new practitioner, whether that is prioritizing day-to-day activities to best meet patient care needs or a list of projects. Recognize that research and communication of a plan to address the drug shortage prior to the weekend is critical to the patients and the department— Khalid does believe he can finish the communication plan, note templates, and data collection forms by the due date of this Friday if he does not focus his time and efforts entirely on his major project.

Khalid should sit down with his preceptor to discuss how directing his attention to the drug shortage will likely cause him to miss the Friday deadline for his major project he and his preceptor had previously set together. The discussion should focus on the urgency of each project, whether or not the previously established deadline for Khalid's project can be extended or not, and ultimately a plan to address the drug shortage, which may or may not involve Khalid.

The last thing Khalid would want to do is to take on the additional work of researching and developing a plan and communication for the drug shortage without at least a discussion with his preceptor concerning the potential impact on his ability to complete his major project work by the Friday deadline. As a new practitioner, the temptation to just take on the additional assignment to please the preceptor can be strong; however, this may lead to an unmanageable to-do list.

What I have found to be successful

- **Develop a process for tracking to-do lists and projects, including priority, due dates, and expected time requirements for completion.** As you take on additional responsibility, I have found it very helpful to track the status of various projects I am responsible for, including priority, time requirements for completion, due date, and current status. Share this list with your managers or preceptors to update them on the status of your current workload and progress so they can assist you in prioritizing tasks to ensure your focus and efforts are in the most appropriate area. In addition, keeping your managers or preceptors updated will assist them in assigning additional projects and tasks to yourself or other team members.

CASE 2.5

When is it appropriate to say no? (Is it ever appropriate?)

PRINCIPLE ■ Negotiation

Jessica is an outgoing new practitioner who quickly has become a well-known and respected face since she joined the community of Scranton, Pennsylvania as a pharmacist at Woodhill Drug Pharmacy 3 years ago. In collaboration with the medical clinic in town, she helped set up an influenza vaccination campaign within the first few months of her beginning at Woodhill Drug Pharmacy, which led to a 75% increase in vaccinations in the community versus the prior year. She helped develop a "Medication Safety Tips" booth at the county fair, which both Woodhill Drug Pharmacy and the local medical clinic sponsored the last 2 years. She has also been working with the medical clinic providers to develop references on medications available generically to help improve affordability, accessibility, and compliance with medication therapy regimens for clinic patients.

Jessica feels strongly that all pharmacists have an obligation to train and mentor the next generation of pharmacists and has worked with her boss and the other pharmacist who works at Woodhill Drug Pharmacy to begin taking PharmD IV students for ambulatory advanced practice experiences. The first year Woodhill Drug Pharmacy had three students sign up for their rural, ambulatory care experience, and the feedback from those students was so positive they filled every rotation block this year!

Jessica's outgoing and "can-do" nature extends beyond the pharmacy profession, and she is actively involved in community activities as well. She is a den mother for the local Girl Scouts troop, is a member of the school board at the elementary school her daughter attends, and volunteers at the local food shelf twice a month.

Jessica continues to maintain close contacts with one of her pharmacotherapy professors, Richard, and last week they met up for coffee prior to a state pharmacy organization's fall meeting. Richard mentioned to Jessica during their conversation that there were many people at the college of pharmacy impressed with how much she has accomplished only 3 years out of school. He also mentioned that feedback from pharmacy students has been overwhelmingly positive and that the college board would like to extend an offer to her to sit on the college's experiential education planning committee. Jessica was speechless and honored by the offer, and Richard told her he thought this was a great opportunity and fit for her. He also mentioned that the committee would begin holding meetings in less than a month, and thus she would need to accept or decline the nomination by week's end (e.g., 5 days from the notification date). Although delighted by the opportunity, Jessica is concerned that her plate is already very full. However, she doesn't want to send the wrong message to the college of pharmacy or Richard by turning down the offer.

WHAT JESSICA MAY BE THINKING...

- I can't take on another responsibility without compromising something I am already doing.
- I don't want to offend Richard or the university by saying no.
- If I say no now, will the school of pharmacy and/or Richard ever ask me again to be part of a university committee?

ON THE OTHER HAND, JESSICA MIGHT REASON...

- What current duties at work or other volunteer activities could be transferred to someone else who would be interested in the task?
- Is there anything I could simply stop spending time toward without any consequences?
- Perhaps if I can participate in the meetings by phone, I could fit participation on experiential education planning committee into my day.

MENTOR ADVICE

When Jessica accepts a new responsibility, it is important that she clearly quantifies and articulates any suspected consequences associated with assuming the additional responsibility. This will allow her to calibrate expectations if the new responsibility will compete with other priorities. She is realizing this will likely have a negative impact on her family life unless there are hospital-related responsibilities she can either delegate or discontinue. She should consider opening this discussion with the pharmacy management team to determine what could potentially be shifted.

In entering into that discussion, it would be important for Jessica to illustrate the value she would bring back to the department based on her involvement on this committee (e.g., influence over externship rotation design, insight into high-performing students who could work at the hospital as technicians or even as new graduates, etc.). Not knowing the value placed on this type of activity, she might find that the management team is very willing to free her from other obligations in support of her involvement on the experiential education planning committee. Alternatively, she has the option of declining the offer to sit on the committee.

Jessica should note that if this was instead a request from her employer to represent the department of pharmacy on a multidisciplinary committee within the hospital, she would not likely have the option of saying no. If she is a logical option and the responsibility is essential for the organization's performance, it is certainly reasonable for her employer to ask her to assume the additional responsibility. In this case, her best bet would be to acknowledge the rationale and suggest a future date when the responsibility could be re-evaluated and potentially reassigned. This could be framed in conversation along the lines of "I understand there is no other manager who can represent our department in the short term. Perhaps we can re-evaluate this once the infectious disease pharmacist is hired and oriented later this year."

What I have found to be successful

- **Assess your capacity before taking on new commitments.** If a great opportunity arises that simply cannot fit within your current priorities, carefully assess what could be delegated or even discontinued that could increase your capacity. Unless you routinely conduct this "inventory" of responsibilities, you might not be aware of current tasks that are no longer necessary. A great example is the compilation of a workload report that you find is no longer viewed/utilized that could easily be discontinued or perhaps converted to an automated workload report.

- **Don't be afraid to test your limits.** Think of an athlete training for an event who gradually increases strength and endurance for optimal performance. Testing your capability and capacity for additional responsibilities is no different. Take additional responsibility in incremental steps. Once you reach a threshold you will then be challenged to further enhance your efficiency or regulate your acceptance of any incremental responsibilities. Simply think through a contingency plan if you were to experience an influx of time commitments and responsibilities during the short-term.

- -

NEW LEADER ADVICE

It is apparent that Jessica feels strongly that all pharmacists have an obligation to train and mentor the next generation of pharmacists, and thus the opportunity to sit on the college's experiential education planning committee seems to be a great fit for Jessica. That being said, her concern about already having a very full plate needs to be addressed before she can make a decision on whether or not to commit to participating on the committee.

First, Jessica needs to find out more from Richard on what her role would be as a member of the committee and the expected time commitments in this role. Next, she should look at the various activities she is currently involved in and decide if she would be able to commit the time and energy necessary as a member of the committee. If not, then she needs to decide if she is willing to give something else up in order to participate or respectfully decline the offer. As she works through her decision process on whether or not she will accept the offer to join the planning committee, she needs to balance the risk of becoming overly overwhelmed and stressed from taking on additional responsibilities with the need to stretch herself to continue to grow as a pharmacist and leader.

Transitioning time and effort from another commitment to focus your efforts on the committee may be another option she may choose to pursue. Again, she needs to decide what other responsibilities she can let go and have conversations with those involved to ensure a proper transition of duties if needed.

What I have found to be successful

- **Discuss the new opportunity and current obligations with your mentor(s).** When presented with a new opportunity, have a discussion with your mentor about the new opportunity, your current obligations, and your goals focusing on how each of your obligations aligns with your personal and/or professional goals.

- **Clearly articulate how your involvement in the new opportunity supports the organization and/or the profession.** With your manager, discuss any value your participation in the new opportunity would provide the department, hospital, or organization. You will also want to have a clear understanding of what type of time commitment the opportunity will require and whether or not that will affect your ability to meet current work obligations. In particular for opportunities/roles outside of your organization, it is important that you balance your work responsibilities with the new opportunity to ensure you are able to meet current responsibilities or hand some of these off to others in the department to free up time for you to participate in the new opportunity.

Summary

Becoming an effective leader requires a great deal of desire and discipline. Although each of us possesses leadership ability, a savvy leader has the ability to utilize a variety of leadership tactics and know which to use in order to achieve optimal performance from the individuals and teams he manages. To acquire these skills requires a commitment to observe others, reflect on your own successes and failures, and to increase awareness of team dynamics such as the level of competence and commitment to the project at hand. An emerging leader must gain familiarity and comfort with using a variety of leadership tactics to achieve optimal effectiveness. Along with these stylistic skills, a leader must also be proficient in tactical activities such as delegation, project management, negotiation, and time management in order to be successful.

Leadership Pearls

- No single leadership style or leadership tactic is universally superior for all scenarios. Instead, an effective leader must develop skills in a variety of leadership tactics and learn to apply the appropriate tactic depending on the situation at hand. Your effectiveness as a leader will require you to increase your awareness of your individual style as well as the factors associated with the situation you are navigating.

- Delegation is an essential skill to develop in order to continue growing as an effective leader, and it is a critically important skill that you will not exercise and fully develop until you assume informal or formal management responsibilities.

- Take charge by letting go. It is important to balance the need for clear direction setting without leaning too far toward micromanagement where you run the risk of stifling creativity and compromising your efficiency in leading the activity.

- Don't let a title, or lack thereof, limit you from pursuing new challenges and growth opportunities within your department (i.e., you can lead from both a formal and informal standpoint).

- Take the time to understand the interests and motivation of those around you. In the situation where priorities are at odds, gain an understanding of what value the other person is placing on the issue or item of debate in order to find a "win-win" outcome.

- Identify what additional responsibilities you are interested in pursuing within your organization and let your interests be known. This will open a discussion of what personal development is necessary for you to prepare for those responsibilities and ensure you are considered if and when an opportunity presents itself.

Leadership Exercises

- Identify your "default" leadership style and gain perspective on what alternative styles you use less frequently that you will need to develop in order to become a dynamic leader.

- Develop a process for prioritizing competing demands on both a professional and personal level and recognize when it is acceptable to say no.

- Actively seek out a mentor(s) and work to develop and cultivate a mentor–mentee relationship. Work with them to develop a personal plan for growth. Make it personal, attainable, measurable, visible, and expandable.

- Gain management experience in a volunteer organization whose goals align with your own interests and/or passions. This is a common venue for gaining early exposure to management practices among emerging leaders.

VETERAN MENTOR PROFILE

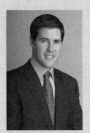

Ross W. Thompson, MS, RPh
Director of Pharmacy Services
Tufts Medical Center
Boston, Massachusetts

Why did you decide on a career in leadership? I decided to become a pharmacy leader at the same time I decided to pursue a career in pharmacy. I was motivated to leadership from the start. I had an excellent mentor, the director of pharmacy in my home town, who was instrumental in helping me determine how I could apply my various interests in business, operations, management, and medicine.

Where do you turn for advice when you are stressed? Professionally, I turn to my incredibly supportive network of colleagues and mentors. Within my personal life, my wife and family keep me grounded and add incredible perspective during difficult professional situations I've faced during my career.

What is your favorite leadership book? *The 5 Dysfunctions of a Team* by Patrick Lencioni.

From your perspective, what is the most important issue facing pharmacy leadership today? Pharmacy leadership is constantly challenged to shape not just pharmacy practice, but rather the overall patient care delivery model in the United States.

Looking back over your vast experience in pharmacy, what one or two things do you know now that you wish you would have known as a student and new practitioner? Managing fairly doesn't necessarily mean managing equally. To treat every employee exactly the same isn't going to serve you well in the long term because each employee has different needs and a different skill set to contribute. Also, we all too often assume other disciplines within health systems understand pharmacy practice. We should not take anything for granted but instead should ensure they understand our skill set and our unique contribution toward optimizing patient care.

What is your best advice for a new pharmacist today? I would encourage all new practitioners to gain experience in a variety of practice settings and responsibilities and not shy away from taking a chance and doing something out of your comfort zone.

How do you envision this publication assisting student and new practitioner leaders? This book will provide the reader with enough perspective to help them identify where they would benefit by spending more time developing their skills in management and leadership.

NEW PRACTITIONER PROFILE

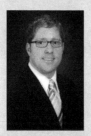

Paul R. Krogh, PharmD, MS
Pharmacy Manager
Abbott Northwestern Hospital
Minneapolis, Minnesota

Why pharmacy: I was interested in science and sports in high
school and considered physical therapy upon entering college.
After completing 100 volunteer hours necessary for application to
the physical therapy program, I realized it wasn't for me. My continued interested
in sciences, in particular chemistry and molecular biology, led me down the pharmacy path.

Advice to readers: In school I worked a lot my first couple of years and wasn't
as involved as I should have been. My advice to students is to get involved earlier in
various activities such as professional organizations because you learn what others are doing and benefit from their ideas. My biggest challenge since graduation
is applying my course work, such as underestimating the time and documentation
it takes to deal with personnel discipline issues. In starting a career, ask people you
work with to share their career experience and ask lots of questions. Consider teaching and precepting students because it will take your knowledge to another level and
provide you with practice influencing others by giving effective presentations.

Tips for work-life balance: Recognize that the balance is going to be a struggle
and organize your personal time; otherwise it is easy to lose control. Shut off all
technology (mobile phones, pagers, computers, television, etc.) and have an established "date night" every week with your significant other.

Personal career: My best career decision has been to complete an MS residency
program because of the opportunities and doors it opened in my career. It jump
started my professional network through the people I met and taught me what to
do as well as what not to do to be an effective leader. My career goal is not necessarily a title but having continual learning experiences as my responsibilities
increase. Ultimately, I would like to be a director of pharmacy in a large health
system. My career success is being excited to go to work every day because I am
passionate about what I do.

Why leadership: My interest in leadership was sparked by talking to pharmacists
and thinking about how to get where they were career-wise. In school I also had to
choose a career track, and I chose management as part of it—I had two rotations
at a procurement/distributor vendor. The preceptors saw something in me before I
did and told me I would be bored with just clinical practice so to keep my options
open. My health-system rotation preceptor discussed the various options in health-
system pharmacy. Being pushed by preceptors was instrumental in my choosing leadership. My major success so far was forming a group of pharmacists and
technicians to analyze the nonsterile dispensing system and ultimately redesign

the system to improve efficiency and turnaround time by eliminating unnecessary steps and clearly establishing roles and responsibilities to improve accountability. Having individuals who do the work on a daily basis assist in the workflow redesign and development of clear roles and responsibilities was key to gaining "buy in" and hardwiring the process changes. My favorite leadership book is Carnegie's *How To Win Friends and Influence People*.

Recommended change for pharmacy: I believe the development of standardized and required didactic and experimental training for pharmacy technicians is needed prior to being allowed to work. This would allow us to optimize the role of pharmacy technicians in the preparation/dispensing functions, provide technicians greater autonomy and job satisfaction, and allow for pharmacists to focus on clinical activities.

Using this book: I feel this book contains real world situations and applicable material that will be picked up and used for advice on practical topics, but not necessarily read cover-to-cover.

Suggested Additional Readings

Bennis W. *On Becoming A Leader.* Cambridge, MA: Perseus Books; 1989.

Blanchard K. *Leadership and the One Minute Manager: Increasing Effectiveness Through Situational Leadership.* New York, NY: William Morrow and Company; 1985.

Carnegie D. *How to Win Friends and Influence People.* New York, NY: Pocket Books; 1936.

Covey SR, Merrill AR, Merrill RR. *First Things First.* New York, NY: Simon & Schuster; 1994.

Covey SR. *Seven Habits of Highly Effective People.* New York, NY: Simon and Schuster; 1989.

Phillips DT. *Lincoln on Leadership—Executive Strategies for Tough Times.* New York, NY: Hachette Book Group USA; 1992.

Becoming A Leader: A Checklist of Key Points

- Properly executed delegation can achieve the following benefits:

  1. Enhance the engagement and confidence of employees

  2. Improve the ability of a leader to effectively coordinate multiple projects

  3. Provide team members more autonomy and creatively on how the work is organized and completed

- The most effective leaders are able to adapt their leadership style to best fit specific situations.

- When identifying a mentor:

  1. Look for someone who exemplifies the traits and skills that you want to adopt.

  2. Think about where you are in your career and where you would like to be.

  3. Outline what you want to achieve from the relationship.

- Volunteering for project involvement will lead to a broader understanding of the organizational goals and directions and make you a more attuned and valuable employee.

- Tips for prioritizing workload:

  1. Make a list.

  2. Consider time constraints.

  3. Consider people constraints.

  4. Consider the consequences.

  5. Reprioritize as necessary.

  6. Remove unimportant items.

Read "Success Skills" articles 12 and 13.

CHAPTER THREE

People, People, People!

Rafael Saenz, PharmD, MS; Sara J. White, MS, FASHP

Introduction

Within the course of an average day, pharmacists need to accomplish many tasks. In any pharmacy setting, they are relied on to ensure the successful treatment of patients, see to the business of running a pharmacy, and any other requests made by their superiors. So how do they get everything done in a single day? The answer is obvious—by working effectively with people.

The personnel working in a pharmacy are the life blood of the department. They ensure the movement of medications, the monitoring of patients' treatments, and they oversee several small tasks that one person alone could never manage due to time constraints. They are the key to success as a pharmacist, manager, or leader in pharmacy. However, harnessing their abilities for the betterment of the department is not as easy as you would hope.

People are, after all, individuals with feelings, pride, motivators and a sense of personal accomplishment. The intent of this chapter is to unravel some of the complexities you will encounter when working with people as a pharmacist. While working effectively with people has many components, for the purpose of this chapter the following principles were selected and are each illustrated by a specific case, veteran mentor, and new practitioner advice. Some of the cases you are about to read may make you feel uncomfortable, but they are realistic and they are intended to simulate the emotion and raw tension that can occur when dealing with individuals that do not see things your way. In fact, many will simply make you angry. With this being said, remember that anyone can become angry, but a pharmacist will manage those emotions to achieve a favorable outcome for all. The principles are as follows:

- **Informal leaders are necessary change agents.** Every pharmacist must be a "little L" leader or "change agent" on their shift or in their clinical practice so pharmacy services can continue to evolve and thus make the best use of the pharmacist's expertise on behalf of patients. In contrast, "big L" leaders are those that have a formal title, such as store manager, director, assistant, supervisor, coordinator, etc. Working together, "little L" and "big L" leaders will be much more effective than just the "big L" leaders alone.

  Think of this informal leadership as active and collaborative involvement with groups, team, or committees. A way for "little L" leaders to perfect their effectiveness is to observe the dynamics between the members of any group and ask themselves who seems to be able to influence others and why or how are they able to do so. Think about why certain people, even those with good ideas, are not very successful in teams. Successful leadership involves being prepared for each meeting by reviewing the agenda ahead of time for the topics to be discussed, reading any background material provided, and seeking input from colleagues and department formal leaders. Always be on time to meetings and if unable to attend arrange for a colleague to attend. During the meetings, listen carefully to the others' discussions, ask questions, and offer input (in a concise way, not just repeating what others have said). Don't be intimidated by the views of those with more experience. Ensuring different views is why various people are asked to participate. If a consensus does not develop, voting is the democratic process. Leaders vote their conscience, not just with the majority. Once a consensus or a decision has been made, whether it is the leaders' preference or not, they support it and do not lobby against it. After each meeting, leaders think about whether there are ways they could have handled things differently, and they use this learning experience to be more influential in future groups.

- **Achieving success with an angry or strong-minded person.** One of the leadership lessons is to try and understand who the influential people or informal leaders are in any workgroup. These are the people to whom others look to for guidance or approval. These people have influence because they have good people skills, such as caring about coworkers as individuals and listening to them. These people may have gained their power from years of experience and or from being liked and respected. This influence has nothing to do with whether they are pharmacists, technicians, clerks, secretaries, etc.

  Angry or strong-willed people are often just trying to be recognized for their contribution and feel valued as part of the workgroup. Remember, every job is important to getting the work accomplished. For example, without the technicians, housekeepers, etc., the pharmacist would have to do that work and thus might not have the time to fully use their clinical knowledge. An approach for a pharmacist is to frequently make a deposit in each person's "emotional bank account" that they work with. A deposit might be recognition for doing a good job, "going beyond" assisting others, having a positive attitude, bringing up possible challenges before they become problems, trading shifts, etc. Think about how you feel when someone mentions any of these things to you and thus do it for others. Never feel like "They are just doing their job and I should only mention the negative things." Like a bank account, once you have made deposits you can "withdraw." A person will often give you the benefit of the doubt if you have failed to involve them or communicate with them as a withdrawal if you acknowledge your "error." Remember to use the deposit approach not only with those you work with, but also with those "above" you.

- **Having crucial conversations when needed.** Conflicts always need to be immediately addressed as they rarely go away on their own and can fester and become worse over time. Trying to understand the issue from the other person's point of view is helpful in resolving conflict and minimizing the leader's own emotional response is critical. Crucial conversations are used to understand the other person's point of view and provide constructive feedback to people on either their behavior or performance. A leader should never assume another pharmacist understands what leadership is in relation to working with and supporting formal leaders. While there are many definitions of leadership, basically it is through influence that leaders improve patient care services and thus have an impact. Leaders should not lead to make themselves feel important, have power, or be liked by their staff but should lead to be respected for caring about others, especially patients.

- **Having influence with people who have more authority than you.** Even every pharmacist needs to be good at "practical politics" as it is how every organization functions in allocating its resources such as positions and drug dollars. Think of politics as how and by whom decisions get made. A key to being successful is "sensing" when the timing is right and making the best use of opportunities. Effective leadership involves managing yourself and controlling your emotions, so others want to work with you and thus you can influence decision makers. Think of this political leadership as working effectively with all people. A leadership key is understanding other peoples' needs so you can partner with them. Once you have assisted them in meeting their goals, you stand a much better chance of having them support your vision/passion.

- **There is no "I" in team.** A leader does not cast things as good or bad/fair or unfair but deals with them as they are. This positive attitude allows you to use your mind to find effective ways to maximize the situation versus wallowing in pity for yourself and your situation. Leadership is always a team sport because success depends on people implementing and executing no matter how carefully the planning has been done. Every pharmacist and leader must realize that they can only be successful if the people they work with succeed, "buy in," and support the plan. Effective leaders know they must first help others get what they want if people are going to follow them. Without willing followers, you are not a leader and thus are not able to be a "change agent." The team will never win if members compete with each other even if their styles are different. There is enough abundance for everyone to win without someone having to lose. The keys to sharing with others is delegation (even if just having a technician do a task), clear definitions of the desired outcome (asking the person to paraphrase back what they have heard to ensure complete communication), discussions of resources (such as time they will have available), the desired timeline, what the final product should be, how you want to be kept informed, and which decisions are entirely theirs and which you want to approve. No matter how you ask to be kept informed, it is wise to touch base and ask them how things are going, so if they need help you can provide it.

- **Don't take credit for the ideas of others.** A leader understands that their success comes from helping others feel good about themselves so always invest credit in others, even if part of the idea was the leader's idea. No matter how sharp the leader is, they need the best ideas of the all the people they work with to ensure excellent pharmacy services. People will only truly engage with and willingly support a leader they respect. To obtain respect from others, first give it to them and expect it from yourself—no matter the personal consequences.

- **Gaining respect from those with more experience than you.** Being an effective leader does not depend on being older than those you supervise or just having a title. Leadership is about developing a personal relationship with those you work with. Developing a relationship means finding out what each person thinks about their career, their personal life, what they enjoy about their current position, what they think needs to be changed, and what they would like to be doing in the future. Sharing some of your own thoughts about your career and life helps establish a mutually trusting relationship. Look for opportunities to assist each person with what they would like to be doing in the future because then they will be more willing to assist you.

If you are new, your first step should be to cover shifts and understand how the systems in your pharmacy work—remember each pharmacy functions differently. In covering your staffing requirements, be mindful of differences on evening and weekend shifts compared to weekday shifts. To work toward a "buy in" from the pharmacists for change, facilitate the staff developing its own practice vision/mission by asking them to visualize if there were no obstacles or barriers, what would be the best use of the pharmacists' efforts. Once the vision is developed, the next step is asking for input on what needs to change to move toward it. Recognize that it is not uncommon for lots of obstacles to be raised, so don't respond to them but keep the group focused on what needs to be changed as they move toward their ideal future vision.

CASE 3.1

Informal leaders as necessary change agents

PRINCIPLE ■ Being effective with different roles on a team

Kim is a clinical pharmacist at a community medical center. She has always enjoyed her work and been a team player. About 4 years ago, Kim found herself as a member of a team that was responsible for the redesign of the pharmacy practice model (how pharmacy is organized in order to provide care to patients including the role of the pharmacists and technicians, drug distribution system, etc.). She was chosen for the team because of her obvious passion for her career and her seemingly tireless work ethic. Kim had never failed to demonstrate her commitment to the department or to the profession in general during her tenure on the committee.

When the new practice model was to be implemented, Kim was assigned as a lead pharmacist who would be working side by side with other pharmacists during the course of their day. Her responsibilities were to ensure that the newly designed practice model was upheld by the other pharmacists and to provide guidance to all the pharmacists working in this practice model with regard to their interdisciplinary communication and cooperation.

Until this point in her career, Kim had been accustomed to being a team player, not a team leader. She found that the new demands made of her from her team mates were unnerving. She soon began to feel overwhelmed by the requests for assistance being made of her and insecure about the few decisions she had made so far. More importantly, she felt confused and somewhat annoyed by her new position. She had enjoyed her work so much when she was a clinical pharmacist, but her new title of lead pharmacist had stripped her of some of this passion. She wanted to be an example of a good clinical pharmacist and not be made into a "pseudomanager."

Feeling overwhelmed, insecure, confused, and most importantly embarrassed by the fact that she was unprepared for this new role, Kim seriously thought about changing jobs. She was saddened by this thought as she had helped build this new department. Why was she feeling this way? How did this situation get so bad for her?

WHAT KIM MAY BE THINKING...

- Why didn't anyone prepare me for this new role?
- Why did they come to me? Aren't there other managers who could have taken on this responsibility?
- Why wasn't I asked if I wanted this role?

- Why wasn't I made a full fledged manager/supervisor so I had the authority to direct the pharmacists?
- Maybe I should just quit. That'll teach them!

ON THE OTHER HAND, KIM MIGHT REASON...

- I should be able to do this easily. I did design the new workflow after all.
- I just need to adjust to my new role.
- I will simply find a mentor to help me with this transition.
- I need to be proactive and ask for help from my "big L" leaders.
- Who else would do a better job?

MENTOR ADVICE

Kim feels overwhelmed, insecure, confused, and embarrassed by the fact that she is unprepared for this new role; this is normal and she is already a "little L" everyday leader. She needs to view this new challenge as a way to grow and develop additional skills that will be useful for her career and in her personal life. Assisting coworkers to make changes requires informal leadership. Kim must keep in mind the ideal future/vision of the change and review how and by whom it was developed. It helps if everyone that will be affected has had input as the vision is being developed. "Change agents" should help their colleagues be successful by patiently answering questions, providing additional training, and sincerely listening to any concerns. Kim shouldn't take complaints personally even if it was her idea because it is the change, not Kim, that is making people uncomfortable. Often people don't really expect leaders to solve the concerns but just to listen and "feel their pain." If any concerns are valid, Kim should be willing to alter as appropriate and stay focused on why the changes are important and constantly talk about them. Being visible and accessible to colleagues will reinforce her true commitment to them as individuals. Kim needs to deal with issues as they arise. The leadership key is to use the feedback and experience to make the best decisions possible and keep the project moving forward. There are always ways to deal with challenges and obstacles. Informal leaders don't run away (even if they want to) from tough times but see them as a way to grow and develop their skills at being a "change agent."

What I have found to be successful

Pharmacists who find themselves feeling unprepared need to remember that leadership is an art, not a science. It is impossible—no matter the level of input and planning—to anticipate everything. The important thing is to just keep moving forward with the needed changes and work out the issues as you go.

Perseverance is a key leadership trait, which means not giving up when confronted with concerns and obstacles. There are always ways around them when you believe you can overcome them. You must believe in the vision and understand its benefits once achieved because your attitude is critical to others following you. Your attitude must be sincerely optimistic and enthusiastic so that others will assist you in making things work versus the "victim mentality" in which the belief is that nothing productive can be done.

NEW LEADER ADVICE

Although the "little L" (the leadership who is without a title but demonstrates natural leadership behavior) role is ever present with pharmacists, it is difficult to graduate to "big L" responsibilities when asked to do so. As is the case with Kim and the majority of pharmacy leaders throughout the country, most "little L" leaders are asked to assume greater responsibilities without any additional training or preparation. Following simple guidelines to leading a group of people can increase the probability of success for pharmacy leaders.

A democratic process for problem solving has always produced better results. More importantly, the end users or front-line pharmacists will feel more empowered to make decisions related to the specific problem at hand. Kim should ask her pharmacists to begin proposing their own solutions to their own problems instead of trying to solve them all by herself. Being suddenly in charge can challenge Kim's confidence. If she is successful, being in charge can test her determination and commitment as more and more people begin to depend on her. The fact that her coworkers' demands are unnerving to Kim suggests that perhaps they are a little too dependent on Kim.

What I have found to be successful

I was in a similar uncomfortable position not too long ago when I became a leader. I had to understand the sometimes overwhelming needs of staff and colleagues, especially when they are looking for guidance from someone in a leadership position. You can continue to help yourself by preparing for and systematically running group meetings. This will help your staff have confidence in you and in the work they are doing. I have found that being prepared for meetings results in a more productive and overall upbeat meeting. When there are (and there inevitably will be) disagreements, you need to learn to listen to the reasons people are disagreeing. Leaders have to be able to put their pride aside and consider all viewpoints. Most importantly, you should keep the group on task. Otherwise, the chaotic situation will produce a steady supply of upstream demands.

Lastly, when leading a large group, a leader (especially a new leader) needs to learn to manage their emotions. It is easy to become angry and exercise the "big L" authority (the authority granted to a person who has a leadership title). But great leaders will inspire others to see their vision, market their viewpoints, and be flexible with their ideas in order to produce a more desirable outcome for all.

CASE 3.2

Achieving success with an angry or strong-minded person

PRINCIPLE ■ Dealing with difficult people

Barbara is a senior pharmacy technician at a very busy and sometimes chaotic community pharmacy. Many of the technicians look to Barbara for advice, assistance, or training. She is always ready and willing to help anyone who asks her. She has, for a very long time, overseen the workflow and quality of the work that her fellow technicians perform. Barbara is also a very strong person in that her communication style, her demeanor, and her nonverbal communication often intimidate her fellow teammates.

Barbara came in to work one day to find that a change had been made to her workflow in response to a medication use error. This change would be a permanent fix to her workflow and the error was in no way Barbara's fault. Barbara, however, found the change to be annoying and of poor design. When asked about the change, she stated that it would have worked had she been included in its design and implementation. Her manager, Dick, learning of her resistance, approached her about her behavior and willingness to participate. Barbara retreated from the situation, smiled, and told her manager that she would very happily comply with the new changes and went back to work.

Over the course of the next several days, it had become apparent that Barbara was not obeying the newly designed workflow and, as a result, all the other technicians followed her lead. One night, the same error in the medication use process occurred and it was deduced that this error was a result of the technician not following the newly designed workflow. When asked why they were not performing their jobs as instructed, they simply stated that nobody was doing it because Barbara wasn't doing it.

The next day, when Barbara was again asked about the workflow, she took a very different approach to her response. Barbara quickly took a defensive stance with very aggressive communication. She stated that nothing new will work in this pharmacy unless she sanctions it. When the change was explained to her, Barbara simply stated that she did not care about the reasons and that she should have been informed of the change before it was implemented. She went on to state that she felt unappreciated and that she has been treated unfairly by leadership because of her exclusion from the design of this workflow.

WHAT DICK MAY BE THINKING...

- I should fire Barbara from her job.
- Why didn't I include her in the initial design of the workflow?
- As her leader, can't I just tell her that it needs to get done or else?
- Why is Barbara being so stubborn and throwing a tantrum?
- Why isn't she thinking about patient safety?

ON THE OTHER HAND, DICK MIGHT REASON...

- Barbara should have been informed first.
- Informal leaders have stake in their work areas, don't they?
- Why was the change made so quickly anyway?
- Shouldn't Barbara be given the opportunity to contribute to this change?

MENTOR ADVICE

A leader always needs to involve as many of the affected people as possible in planning changes, and it is critical that the informal leaders be included. Participation helps people "buy in" to the process change and helps with their willingness to make it successful. If the person is not available, it is wise to contact them before they return to work even if just by phone so they are not surprised. Dick shouldn't argue with

Barbara because it probably will "burn bridges" with her and the others. Dick should realize how valuable Barbara's insight would have been, apologize to her for leaving her out, and ask her what it would take to make amends. Dick should sincerely listen to Barbara's response and then move forward. This is a learning experience and it will help him to avoid such situations in the future.

What I have found to be successful

Getting to know people on a personal level and letting them know I care about them as unique individuals has been beneficial in my career. If someone is offended, the best approach for the leader is to apologize even if it is on behalf of the organization so the person can put it behind them and move on. No one expects a leader to be perfect, but they deserve a leader who takes responsibility for their actions and the organization. Likewise, "going to bat" for the employee with the organization if they have been wronged enhances the leader–employee relationship.

- -

NEW LEADER ADVICE

This is a classic, new leadership dilemma. Every pharmacy in the world has someone like Barbara. And with a situation like a serious medication error as fuel for action, it is easy to want to rush in and fix the problem. Dick has identified the problem and wants to be the one that potentially saves lives and keeps any more medication use errors from occurring. If he is a new leader, this fix could be his first big act that will define him and his work within the department.

Dick should view the situation from Barbara's perspective. She has probably been single-handedly preventing this problem from occurring for years by performing her job above expectations and without a single piece of recognition for having done so. Barbara's communication style and demeanor may have played a key role in the work standard being upheld until the day she was gone and the change was implemented. Suddenly, her opportunity for recognition disappeared, whether she ever realized it as an opportunity to begin with. In her mind, she may have been thinking that her character at work has made her successful and instead of being thanked, the department moved on without her.

What I have found to be successful

This case illustrates an employee who seems to be expressing raw human emotion at who they feel is responsible for their hurt. I believe that if an employee reacts this way, it was probably because Dick had not made any "deposits" into the employee's emotional bank. Therefore, he had "overdrawn" and the employee was making it known to him. It has taken me a long time to make this deposit concept discovery in my own practice. As a new leader, I have often seen many high-performing individuals give and give and give without much kudos. I have learned that the best way to keep informal leaders engaged in their work that will make them successful, and ultimately you, is to keep "depositing" into them with kudos, authority, and stake. It was a hard-learned lesson that caused me several months of frustrating communications. The employee being honest with the leader when they return regarding how they feel has helped me grow as a leader. The lessons learned from situations such as these will save time and relationships.

Having crucial conversations when needed

PRINCIPLE ■ Conflict acknowledgement, management, and resolution

Jason is a new practitioner pharmacist in the pharmacy. He has proven himself to be a very able and eager team member. Jason is a very logical person and can anticipate and solve problems before they occur. Over the last year, Jason has taken on greater responsibilities in the pharmacy. He assists his leader, Sharon, with the orientation of new employees and creates work schedules for everyone on the team.

One of Jason's stated career goals is that he would like to be a leader in the profession. He would like his journey to start by becoming a manager or assistant director at a pharmacy. Sharon agrees to help him achieve this goal by providing him with the necessary experiences and feedback that will help him grow as a leader.

In the course of leading the department of pharmacy, Jason's leader begins to encounter resistance to decisions she is making regarding the pharmacy. At a department-wide meeting, Sharon is surprised to learn that Jason is leading the charge against change in the department stating that "we are constantly bombarded with changes!" Noticing that this is behavior unbecoming of a leader, Sharon pulls Jason aside and asks him why he has been acting in such a manner. Jason simply states that he is simply reflecting the thoughts of his fellow teammates. Satisfied with that answer for the time being, she continues her development plan for Jason and confides new goals for the department.

At the next staff meeting, the same type of resistance is encountered to the plans for change and improvement that had occurred previously. This time, it is from the pharmacists Jason works with regularly. When she questions them individually about their concerns, she discovers that they know information that she has only mentioned to Jason. Once Sharon completes her description of the plans for change, the two pharmacists are excited and support the plans, but they ask that she not share their new feelings with Jason.

Then, like a lightning strike, Sharon knows her new strategy for Jason's development; however, a much needed and overdue conversation is about to occur between them.

WHAT SHARON MAY BE THINKING...

■ Why am I investing so much time in Jason when he can't be trusted?

■ Why do I care what Jason thinks? I need to confront him!

■ Why is Jason counter-detailing me with other staff?

■ Did I not share the nature of my plans for change with Jason? Why else would Jason be resisting me so much?

■ Perhaps I should also be including his team members in the planning of the changes.

ONE THE OTHER HAND, SHARON MIGHT REASON...

- Jason is smart. Is he using passive resistance to change because it is the only way I will listen?
- Should I stop trying to develop Jason?
- Do Jason and I have trust issues?
- Perhaps my new strategy for developing Jason should be to charge him with the leading of the change initiatives.

- -

MENTOR ADVICE

Sharon should have a crucial conversation with Jason. She could start by asking Jason why he is interested in a leadership position. This may reveal some dysfunctional reasons that Sharon needs to correct, especially if he expresses a need to feel important or a need to belong. Sharon could share her observations that he has leadership potential and affirm what he has done thus far. Sharon should clearly outline her view of how a leader behaves using specific examples of Jason's behavior with regard to partnering with you as his formal leader. Using "creative dissatisfaction" (thinking creatively for new ideas when you feel dissatisfied with your current circumstances) with the status quo means not complaining or resisting changes but proposing possible solutions. Sharon needs to explain to Jason the meaning of "in confidence" and why his breaking of it means she will be reluctant to share anything again and ask for his thoughts. Sharon should also explain the result of his "representing others" and the concept of not being intimidating to others, especially as it relates to his personal integrity. Sharon needs to ask for his input on what the next steps for both of them should be. She should listen carefully and paraphrase back what she hears so as to ensure that she understands his views. Sharon and Jason need to jointly develop a plan of what going forward will look like. Then Sharon should close the conversation by expressing her faith that he will improve. She must be patient with people—what they have been doing has made sense to them—as it will take them a little time to change. When Jason does make efforts to change, she needs to remember to acknowledge these efforts.

What I have found to be successful

Always give people a second chance. Investing in people is a valuable approach for a leader because most people have lots of untapped potential and passion. By investing in them, you will engage them and your workgroup will benefit from their ideas and energy. Also realize you are role modeling the appropriate attitude and behavior of a leader so always take the "high road." In my experience, more times than not, they will rise to the occasion.

- -

NEW LEADER ADVICE

Any new manager will remember the first time they had to have this important "cold, hard truth" conversation with one of their employees. A new manager may worry that it will not go as planned or sound parental. The key is a no nonsense discussion in which the proverbial gloves may need to come off.

To work effectively with others, Sharon needs to respect any confidences shared. The most important success trait Sharon has is personal integrity, which means respecting others' wishes, not being involved in gossip, and being honest and sincere in all actions.

PEOPLE, PEOPLE, PEOPLE! | 77

What I have found to be successful

As a recipient of many of these conversations, I know that I have always appreciated a leader who communicates with me in a straightforward manner and talks to me as an adult. It is in the middle of these conversations that one begins to think about all of the possible excuses you can make in order to explain your behavior and cut the conversation shorter. However, it is the truthful nature of the dialogue that has kept me engaged. The fact that I was being called out on behavior I knew was inappropriate made me think hard about my actions and about my career goals and aspirations. Most importantly, the best conversations also included a plan for improvement. Again, drawing from my own experiences, these plans have never been formal or long winded—merely honest and realistic suggestions for improvement from a person who cared about my future.

CASE 3.4

Having influence with people who have more authority than you

PRINCIPLE ■ Practical politics

Sally is the new director of pharmacy for a community hospital and has had a great working relationship with all of her colleagues and supervisors. She was appointed director after her director suddenly passed away. Sally hadn't planned on this career move quite so soon after graduation, but she has had 4 years of experience, has a great pharmacy leadership team, and feels confident she can grow into the role. Additionally Sally has a new boss, the vice president for patient care services, Beth. Beth told Sally and the other patient care services directors at a meeting that she plans on producing great savings for the organizations by reducing the overall number of resources available to each of their departments. Sally thinks "There is never a dull moment in leadership and my people and I can figure out how to assist Beth so I am successful as the pharmacy director."

WHAT SALLY MAY BE THINKING...

- Beth may not be sincere and this is just a relationship of convenience for her
- Shouldn't I feel threatened?
- Isn't Beth being a bit of a sycophant?
- If I am the director of pharmacy, I shouldn't worry about resource reductions. It is always the "little people" who go first...right?

ON THE OTHER HAND, SALLY MIGHT REASON...

- Why is pharmacy being asked to reduce since we make money for the organization through our drug charges?
- We don't have enough pharmacists now.
- I need to be proactive in my approach to resource reductions so they occurred in a planned and organized fashion.
- Do I need to get to know Beth personally and her needs so I can lead up?

MENTOR ADVICE

Sally should ask Beth for clarity of the project, such as what exactly she considers to be resources (being careful not to be inflammatory or accusative). It is important for Sally to know Beth's specific goals, such as details about the types of reductions (staff versus equipment, drug dollars, etc.) and the types of initiatives that Beth would consider worthy of further funding, so Sally can pick the most effective tactics for the pharmacy. It is important for Sally to see if Beth has a specific target for pharmacy or just an overall target for patient care services to indicate the magnitude that she is looking for.

In this type of situation, Sally should engage her leadership team and staff in where the opportunities might be so she can put together a strategy that would address all of Beth's resource cutting goals. Each of the initiatives contained in the strategy need to be designed to help Beth achieve her intended outcomes and achieve a pattern of success within the department for improving services and becoming a high performing department. At the next director's meeting, Beth could announce that she would like each of the directors to present their strategies for achieving savings and that she would expect that each department achieve a minimum amount of savings so be ready and prepared. Then, she can turn in her department's plan soon after the request and include a timeline for achieving the savings and the strategy for continued growth based on the new resource paradigm.

As time progresses, Sally needs to ensure that all the targets for savings are met as well as the timelines. She should keep Beth informed of the department's accomplishments and provide her with any necessary information she might need in order to report her successes to her superiors. Sally needs to make sure that Beth gets to know her and her department so she can come to rely on Sally for insight into more than just the pharmacy department as resources to be cut.

What I have found to be successful

A good strategy is to under promise and over deliver. When engaging your staff and leaders in where the opportunities might be, give them permission to question everything that is currently done. Questioning doesn't mean what we are doing is wrong. Rather when the decisions were made they were right, but times have changed so let's update our processes. Be sure as people brainstorm that no one "puts down" any ideas as not feasible or you will turn off peoples' creativity. Be careful how you as the leader respond as well. Ideas can be evaluated and prioritized at a later date. I have found that amazing opportunities exist when people have permission and feel safe in expressing them.

Partnering with those above me has paid off because first assisting them provides them the incentive to help me with my goals. Just because they are your boss doesn't mean they have to support you unless they want to. Knowing them on a personal level has always helped me as well.

NEW LEADER ADVICE

The politics of leadership are, without a doubt, the most difficult concept to master as a new leader. They can also be scary; however, knowing and understanding the politics of an organization is paramount to success. Politics are ever changing. Figuring out hotspots of information can make maneuvering through the politics more effortless. Failure to do so can result in project delays or a political misstep if an important political avenue is neglected.

Political influence, like money, can be "banked." If Sally always delivers and keeps her word and meets deadlines, political favors will be earned. If she is seen as a person who does none of these things, she will have a deficit of political clout that she can spend later. Sally is as good as her politics allows her to be. As a new leader, if Sally happens to be on the receiving end of bad politics, such as underperformance or a failed project, it will not always end in a complete destruction of her career. Sally, however, needs to work harder and longer to succeed. But she *can* succeed and in time political wins—such as completed projects, contributions to the goals of the organization, and different approaches to communicating—will result in a higher level of accomplishments.

Sally must understand the difference between being politically savvy and being a sycophant. Being politically savvy is an art in which you understand the needs of the organization and the people that have influence within it. They can be business needs or social needs and you address these needs from a win–win perspective. Sycophantic behavior, on the other hand, is obvious and insincere.

What I have found to be successful

My approach to interacting with my superior would be to come prepared to all meetings with the objective of clarifying their expectations of you and your department. As a new leader, I have watched as leaders above me in my department have asked specifically for the outcome desired by their superiors. This straightforward approach to identifying goals has been appreciated by people in Beth's position and made life easier for department leadership.

CASE 3.5

There is no "I" in team

PRINCIPLES ■ Competition ■ Collaboration

Don and Raul are both new managers in the pharmacy. Don is in charge of pharmacist scheduling and medication distribution. Raul is in charge of clinical services and interdisciplinary initiatives. One day, the director of their pharmacy asked that they collaborate on an important project that would revolutionize the way pharmacy is practiced at their site. Don would be responsible for the scheduling of individuals and the redesign of the medication distribution model. Raul would be in charge of the new practice design, pharmacist "buy in," and implementation of the project.

This mandate, however, has Don and Raul vying for project lead as they both have integral components of the project. Each would be required in order to succeed with project completion. The project lead will, undoubtedly, be acclaimed as the innovator of practice and the hero of the department. Don's approach is to conceptualize, plan, and implement the project within a week. Raul envisions a robust brainstorming session with input from all pertinent stakeholders, a trial period, and a systematic roll-out of the new design.

In the initial rush of the project, both Don and Raul began to work independently. Both initiated the first phase of their projects without communicating with each other. And both were eager to show the results of their work to their director. After a short time of independent work, the director of pharmacy asked (in a very public meeting) for them to give a report on their progress. After a short time, it became apparent that neither of them had any significant results worth sharing and that they had not been working together. They began to blame each other and the project seemed to be falling apart before it had begun.

WHAT DON AND RAUL MAY BE THINKING...

- Wasn't the director clear that they were to be working together?
- Why are we so eager to impress our boss?
- Why was our initial attempt such an example of independent work?
- What are we competing for? Is this a sign of our ambitions?

ON THE OTHER HAND, DON AND RAUL MIGHT REASON...

- Don is right. It needs to occur quickly and decisively.
- Raul is right. It needs to occur with stakeholder input and patience.
- The director should have been clearer when the project was delegated.
- We should have had a project start-up meeting to avoid this embarrassment.

MENTOR ADVICE

Don and Raul should treat this as a significant learning experience. They need to start over with a blank sheet of paper. While each of them has a different working style, they need to understand and accept them and decide together what the best approach should be rather than competing with each other. They must identify the key aspects (who is going to do each task) and create a timeline. Their success will come from the whole department's improvements, not just from individual performances (especially if at the expense of another person). They need to realize leaders never place blame when they experience less than desirable results. Leaders use the experience to learn from and not repeat it in the future, because blaming doesn't change the situation and wastes a lot of energy.

What I have found to be successful

As a leader when I found that my people weren't working together, I reflected on how I had delegated, coached, and maintained contact with them. My job was to set them up for success by clearly defining the desired outcome, any needed structures, and a timeline. Knowing that their work styles are very different, I either let them learn from their mistakes or asked questions to get them to think through how they can best work together. While learning from less than desirable outcomes is valuable, it wastes a lot of emotional energy that can be better used for the project. A major role of a leader is to care about each person as an individual and further enhance each person's self-confidence by acknowledging individual successes.

Don and Raul need to work collaboratively together. They should feel very lucky to be part of a large management team with a variety of skill sets and opinions. This diversity should work to augment their capacity for success rather than conceal or diminish it. They should identify the key strengths in each other and their teammates, understand their weaknesses, and determine how they can make each other stronger by complementing each others' skill set. If they obtain even a small measure of success with this strategy, they will gain political capital and professional satisfaction from the simple act of working together as a team.

If Don and Raul are in a competitive relationship, they need to "swallow their pride" and start fresh. A minor step back could help them take giant leaps forward.

What I have found to be successful

When I first became a leader, I felt alone. Not physically, as I was surrounded by people, but professionally. I felt like I was expected to lead people to success and I had to figure it out on my own. Since I was part of a large leadership team, I also felt the need to prove myself. And I can easily see how this combination of feelings leads to competition and the urge to shine above the rest.

This particular case describes a situation that I feel is very realistic and is probably observed by many of my colleagues. Several high-performing management teams in pharmacy are large and filled with very talented people. In a situation like this, I've found that creating a common vision is helpful followed by determining the steps needed to achieve that vision. I've also set ground rules upfront to establish the foundation for working together. Some suggestions may include seeking to understand an idea before judging it and respecting the opinions of others. Both Don and Raul have knowledge and expertise they could contribute to the project, and by doing so they would create a much better outcome than if either of them worked on a plan without involving the other.

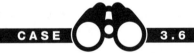

CASE 3.6

Don't take credit for the ideas of others

PRINCIPLE ■ Success comes from helping others

As a pharmacy leader, Jon relies on his staff to keep him informed of happenings in his pharmacy since he cannot be everywhere at once. One day, a staff member approaches Jon with a problem in the dispensing workflow of the pharmacy. Jon is baffled but can clearly see the problem. His staff member, a technician of only 18 months, surprises Jon with a recommended solution. After some thought, it is clear that this technician has put a lot of time and effort into solving this issue, and Jon is reluctant to implement the solution but agrees to do so on a trial basis.

It does not take long for everyone in the department to see that the technician's solution is working wonderfully. Jon himself agrees to make the change permanent and rewards the technician with a free lunch coupon to a local restaurant. Once the change is solidified into the culture of the department, fewer errors in dispensing occur and this does not go unnoticed.

Jon's supervisor summons him to his office and complements Jon on the improved results in his operations. Jon explains the new workflow but does not mention that the idea came from a technician. Jon's reasoning is that the technician got lucky and that he himself would have eventually come up with it. Besides, Jon thought, "if I hadn't sanctioned the change, it would have never occurred." Lastly, Jon thought, "I haven't had a win in such a long time. I need this for my career."

Jon received a raise and accolades at the next staff meeting from his superior. His staff, however, did not seem pleased and shot Jon a look of blatant distrust. Jon feared that he might have just done his career more harm than good.

WHAT JON MAY BE THINKING...

- What could have possessed me to lie to my boss like this?
- If I was a good leader, I would have foreseen the effect of this earlier.
- Did I think I was buying the idea with a lunch coupon?
- Wouldn't I have received credit from my boss anyway since I helped the technician develop the idea into reality?
- Am I threatened by my technicians?

ON THE OTHER HAND, JON MIGHT REASON...

- It was just an oversight on my part. What harm can that do?
- The technician might not care that I took credit for his idea.
- Since this is my direct report, I would have been given credit for this idea eventually.

MENTOR ADVICE

This is a valuable learning experience for Jon. He should immediately apologize to the technician and to his staff. Acting like he thinks his behavior is okay is worse than the short-term "loss of face." People will not expect Jon to be perfect, but they do expect him to take responsibility for his actions. He is, of course, just human and will continue to have similar learning experiences in his career, so the best approach is to do what he can to make it right and to not let it happen again.

Jon should reflect on his need to "look good" to his supervisor. He needs to examine his definition of a successful leader and be sure his measures are accomplishments and the success of others, rather than external validation. Depending on external recognition is difficult for Jon because he tends to only receive the negative comments, but he needs to be the "complaint" department if he is going to keep his people focused and productive. Jon must provide his own validation by accomplishing the leadership goals he set out for himself.

What I have found to be successful

Develop the approach that you never compete with others, only with yourself. If you compete with others, there will always be those that make you feel good and those that make you feel lousy. Competing with yourself means doing better than yesterday, last month, or last year.

Yes, occasionally you will slip, but more often than not you will be successful and thus feel good about your progress. When you feel good about yourself and keep your own score, you have no need to take credit for others' good ideas or work. Investing that credit in them will become natural as you become successful in your eyes.

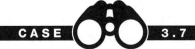

NEW LEADER ADVICE

Jon is caught in a very unique situation as a new leader. He can't be successful without his staff, so what is his worth to the organization? He may start thinking that he can be easily replaced and that any minute now, someone will figure this out. It is easy to see how some managers would then move to hoard credit for the success of others. The problem is that once Jon does this, his overall success ceases. His staff loses their trust in him and begins to see him as an unscrupulous individual.

It will be difficult for Jon, but he needs to become comfortable with the feeling of letting people take credit when and where credit is due to them. Regardless of how it makes him feel or how instrumental he is to their success, this is simultaneously one of the greatest acts of leadership and one of the greatest management challenges Jon will face.

What I have found to be successful

During leadership and management training, I was told that you can only achieve success through your people. When I became a leader, I was fortunate enough to have a mentor that warned me about this pitfall early. His advice to me was simple: "Develop your people so that they can achieve more on their own. Give credit where credit is due. At the end of the day, you will reap your rewards by having achieved a high level of success for the area for which I hold you responsible."

The instructions were simple. I was to develop and encourage those that worked for me to succeed, because I was being held responsible for my specific area. Since I could not complete my work without the people working in the area, my success rested on their shoulders. Well, I thought this would be simple to do until I saw my boss and colleagues praising my employees for the success of projects that I planned and managed by working through and with them. I did all of the textbook procedures for staff "buy in" including allowing them to provide input to projects, giving them stake in the game, etc. It has been the ultimate test of confidence.

CASE 3.7

Gaining respect from those more experienced than you

PRINCIPLE ■ Working with people who are older or have more experience than you

Sandeep has been a pharmacist for 35 years. In the course of his career, he has experienced a lot. He remembers, for example, the transition pharmacists made into the clinical arena. He remembers how he was asked to be the first clinical pharmacist in the city, and he remembers when the PharmD degree was unique and there were few that had achieved such a distinction. Mary, on the other hand was only 1 year out of her management residency. She had decided to do a residency at a prestigious hospital in the eastern United States. In this short amount of time, Mary was convinced that she had experienced enough to tackle any assignment. Her first job was leading the clinical pharmacy services at the hospital with Sandeep as the senior clinical pharmacist.

Mary's first assessment of her area of responsibility was that they had the foundation for basic clinical services, but there was more that could be done. She remembered all of the cutting edge practices at her residency site and felt very confident that she could replicate those services here, at her new job. She made a list of all of the areas that she felt could be improved and a list of the new clinical services that her pharmacists would be providing. She created a detailed plan for transition in services and she even created metrics that would ensure they were meeting their intended goals. Mary felt that her plan was sure to work and that she would create a spitting image of her residency site (which she now felt had superior clinical services).

Mary called a meeting of her staff and laid out her plan for them. At first, there were no responses. Then, as if a thunderstorm had just settled in over Mary's head, the rebuttals, skepticism, and downright refusals started pouring in on Mary. She was utterly shocked. Her plan was fool proof and they would be better off. When the room cleared, Mary sought out Sandeep and asked why he had not supported her plan. He immediately began to tell her the many different reasons why her plan would fail. She could not simply walk in one day and make changes or dictate to them how to do their work when she could not explain what they did day to day, and she forgot to include anyone in the planning of her new design. He told her that if she missed her residency site that much, she should return to it immediately.

Mary had achieved a moment that all new managers must endure. She was realizing the true nature of her new culture and how one should act if they are to be successful.

WHAT MARY MAY BE THINKING...

- I can just force the changes with my title and position power.
- I can just remove Sandeep from his position until he complies.
- I should not have mentioned my last place of work and just claimed the changes as my own.
- Maybe I should look for another job.

ON THE OTHER HAND, MARY MIGHT REASON...

- I need the support of the staff if the changes are going to be successful.
- I should have assessed the departmental culture before moving forward.
- Sandeep simply wanted to feel like his input was valued. Since he has been around for so long, people look to him for guidance and support. His approval would be key to success.

- -

MENTOR ADVICE

Mary needs to give the staff a few days to cool off and reassess her approach. She should jettison her plans, but keep her end goals in mind and realize that if she is going to be successful, she will need help from Sandeep and the other staff members. Mary could approach Sandeep and explain that she has been wrong and offer him an explanation of her desire for change and see if he becomes more receptive.

Sandeep, having been in the profession for so long, may see that you have good reasons for suggesting change. Seeking his input will help him view it as an opportunity to improve. Once he understands that Mary had no intention of altering their work just to enhance their best practices, she should demonstrate that she recognizes opportunities for his growth in contrast to his previous manager.

Mary and Sandeep should have regular meetings to discuss the process of change, and Mary should ask Sandeep to involve other clinicians as he sees fit with her approval. By successfully conveying her vision for new pharmacy services, she has made him feel valued by allowing him to contribute his experiences and wisdom to the development of change.

What I have found to be successful

Age differences will melt away if you focus on doing a good job for your workgroup and patients. Having the attitude that you don't have all the answers and never will enables you to seek out and involve others in decision making. The involvement of others not only allows you to benefit from their vast experience, but also indicates to them that you value them. Remember, as a leader you will only be successful if your workgroup is successful so always care about others and involve them.

NEW LEADER ADVICE

Mary should keep in mind that senior pharmacists want progress just like anyone else, but they have seen and experienced a lot. In fact, many will say that processes and change come in cycles. What doesn't work this year may work in 5 years, then go out of fashion only to be retried by a new manager 5 years after that. They know what works in that particular culture and organization and what can stop a successful project dead in its tracks.

Mary could coach Sandeep that he would have greater success in influencing the new changes if he would change his approach to voicing his disagreement. Being difficult just because he can is not a good example to set for younger pharmacists that will one day fill his shoes. He knows what works and what the dangers to any project are, and he needs to share this information with Mary. Sandeep, his patients, and his coworkers will all benefit from his insights and experience. If Mary chooses not to accept his advice, which is a possibility, then he can at least have the comfort of knowing that he tried and made a contribution. The ball is in his court.

As a new leader, it can be hard to admit that Mary needs help. But respecting the experience of others and allowing some guidance will gain Mary a very valuable ally. In this case, Sandeep seems like an ally with strong informal power and an inside track to your success.

What I have found to be successful

When I was a technician, I remember a senior pharmacist tell me that he hated his younger "know-it-all" boss. I have been paranoid that this is a feeling shared by some of my staff about me. I have since become more comfortable with the fact that this conversation has probably been had. My goal, however, is to respect all of my pharmacists for the individuals that they are.

An important lesson I learned is that sometimes our older pharmacists are not only great sources of information but also great sources of informal power. My advice is to seek them out as mentors—perhaps not as mentors for your job but as mentors for the pharmacy organization or culture.

Summary

This chapter was meant to give you a cross-sectional view of the complexities a pharmacist encounters when working with people. The new practitioner shared personal experiences with you regarding success and failure in dealing with people. The seasoned mentor shared some practical advice regarding the handling of specific situations and recommendations for your behavior. It goes without saying that people are as diverse as there are stars in the sky. Each situation will be different. Undoubtedly one day when dealing with a people issue you will say to yourself, "I never learned this in school" or "I never read this in any textbook, but I remember a case about it." And you will have a foundation for growth and you won't be as surprised.

It is important for new pharmacist leaders to see their new role as a challenge and an opportunity to expand their skill set. Learning how to lead will be difficult, but with the right frame of mind that includes being politically savvy, collaborative in nature, respectful, and full of integrity, you will be successful. Good luck to you—new and future leaders of pharmacy.

Leadership Pearls

- Every pharmacist needs to be an informal, "little L" everyday leader to act as a "change agent."

- Personally get to know all of the people you work with so you can assist them to be successful, which is where your success comes from. Give them credit for a job well done versus taking the credit yourself.

- Always seek input from and involve people in the decisions and changes that affect their work, thus getting their "buy in."

- If people aren't performing well, first ask yourself if your training and supervision is clear so they understand the expectations. Never put off having a candid conversation about their performance or behavior.

- Age, experience, and authority have nothing to do with being a successful leader.

Leadership Exercises

- When at work, observe the people around you and get to know them. Identify the informal leaders.

- Ask the "big L" formal leaders if you can shadow them for a day to better understand what formal leadership is all about.

- Next time you are part of a meeting, try to identify or describe how you imagine the leader prepared for that meeting. If you have questions, make it a point to ask the leader after the meeting.

- Identify someone at your practice site that most people label as "difficult." Next time you have an opportunity to speak with this person, listen to what they are saying. Determine if their behavior is in reaction to the way they are treated. If you are leading a group project, try to include this person and allow them to lead a segment of the project.

- Identify an up and coming leader in your department. Sit with them and ask them why they want to be a leader.

- Next time your preceptor or superior gives you a project, ask them to clarify the goals of the project and make sure you ask for a deadline. During the time you work on the project, make a list of the milestones you need to achieve. Provide your preceptor or superior with a report on a regular basis.

- Identify the people in your organization or department who are "in the know" about politics. Establish or improve your relationship with them and ask them how you can become more influential.

VETERAN MENTOR PROFILE

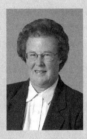

Sara J. White, MS, FASHP
(Ret.) Director of Pharmacy
Stanford Hospital and Clinics
Mountain View, California

See Chapter 1, page 32, for Sara White's profile.

NEW PRACTITIONER PROFILE

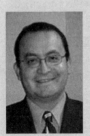

Rafael Saenz, PharmD, MS
Director, Acute Care Pharmacy Services
University of Virginia Health System
Charlottesville, Virginia

Why pharmacy: I liked chemistry in high school and knew pharmacists compounded medications, which sounded interesting. During high school I had a job at an oncology clinic and saw what pharmacists actually did and was intrigued.

Advice to readers: Don't be passive in school so you get the most out of it by looking for opportunities beyond just the class work. As a student, ask your preceptors to discuss career opportunities as it was a rotation preceptor who introduced me to MS-Residency programs. Since graduation, I have learned that the right answer to every practice problem isn't contained in books and you have to use your knowledge to develop the specific answer. Consider doing a residency because it will provide you with the foundation skills in problem solving and show you where to find information you will need in practice. In picking a job, select it for the most mentoring you can receive from those you work with, which is critical early in your career.

Tips for work-life balance: Realize that you need to give priority to having a personal life and take care of yourself. Turn off technology when you go home. Validate your expectations of having to work so hard and put in long hours because they may just be only your expectations and not your superior's.

Personal career: Professional organizations have opened doors for me that I wouldn't have considered otherwise. Through organizations I am meeting people, developing friendships, and building a professional network that I will use throughout my career. The people I meet provide me with ideas of the right way to do things and benchmarks for my practice. In my job, I am redesigning our practice model and developing and implementing an accredited MS-Residency program. I am the director for our international operation, which means I frequently spend time overseas assisting health-system pharmacies. My career goal is to be a director of pharmacy and establish a solid practice that is meaningful to the profession. Career success is making a sustained contribution and conducting educational programs that will benefit the profession.

Why leadership: My best career decision has been to get involved in professional organizations as a student because I was exposed to several types of residencies that focused on leadership and management, which sparked my interest. My favorite leadership books are Ken Blanchard's *The Secret: What Great Leaders Know and Do* and Robert Greenleaf's *Servant Leadership: A Journey into the Nature of Legitimate Power and Greatness.*

Recommended change for pharmacy: I would hope that all pharmacists would act like healthcare professionals and do what it takes to take care of patients and not just be motivated by money.

Using this book: I think this book will be a good introduction for young people so they aren't surprised by what they encounter.

Suggested Additional Readings

Abrashoff DM. *It's Your Ship.* New York, NY: Warner Business Books; 2002.

Andersen E. *Growing Great Employees.* New York; NY: Penguin; 2006.

Covey SR. *The 7 Habits of Highly Effective People.* New York, NY: Free Press; 2004.

Goffee R, Jones G. *Why Should Anyone Be Led by You? What It Takes to Be an Authentic Leader.* Boston, MA: Harvard Business School Press; 2006.

Gostick A, Elton C. *The Carrot Principle.* New York, NY: Free Press; 2007.

Patterson K, Grenny J, McMillan R, et al. *Crucial Conversations: Tools for Talking When Stakes are High.* New York, NY: McGraw-Hill; 2002.

White SJ. Success skills for pharmacists: managing yourself so others want to work with you. *Am J Health-Syst Pharm.* 2008;65:922-924.

White SJ. Success skills for pharmacists: working effectively with people. *Am J Health-Syst Pharm.* 2007;64:2221-2225.

Additional Materials

Am I Working Well With People

Checklist (check all that apply)

_____ I know the names of the spouses and children of the people I work with.

_____ I know the priorities of my superior and frequently suggest solutions to improve our services challenges.

_____ I see myself as a "little L" leader and know that to be successful I need to get along with others.

_____ On a frequent basis I recognize someone I work with for doing a good job and thus make a "deposit" in their "emotional bank account."

_____ I never take credit for what others have done and always invest it in them.

_____ I immediately address performance or behavior issues.

_____ I don't let a conflict fester but try to resolve it with the other person when it arises.

_____ If I precept or work with students or residents, I spend time individualizing their experiences to assist them in growing and developing.

_____ When I find myself about to react emotionally, I pause and ask myself, "What is my best response in this situation?"

_____ I don't let those with more experience or authority intimidate me, rather I try to understand their viewpoint.

Discuss your results with a mentor or trusted colleague and identify areas to work on.

Read "Success Skills" article 5.

CHAPTER FOUR

Motivating the Eyores

Roberta M. Barber, PharmD, MPH; Staci A. Hermann, MS, PharmD

Introduction

What is an Eeyore? Some of you may recognize the reference to the story Winnie-the-Pooh. Eeyore is a donkey and a stubborn one at that. He is generally characterized as a pessimistic, melancholic, depressed, and miserable donkey—always seeing the gloomy side of things. Well, some of you, in your professional career as a student, pharmacist, or leader may recognize the "Eeyores" in your school, workplace, and community.

This chapter discusses how to motivate these people to accomplish goals and contribute to the success of whatever project, program, or organization you have been charged to lead. Motivation is an abstract concept, but it is essential to getting a task, job, or project completed. Per *Webster's New College Dictionary, Third Edition*, motivation is "the act or an instance of motivating or the state or condition of being motivated or something that motivates; inducement; incentive."[1] Every day, decisions are made that impact one's ability to maintain or digress from one's own internal motivation—decisions such as working on a project for class so that tomorrow's group meeting is more productive; volunteering to take the lead in a committee to help advance the practice of pharmacy; or finding the information that a physician colleague requested so he doesn't have to remind you that you were charged with looking up the information.

At various points in a professional career, motivating oneself and others can prove to be a challenge. Some actions a motivated professional may take include completing projects by the appointed deadline, working well in teams, having a high impact on patient care, and providing leadership on every shift. It is not uncommon for students and new practitioners to fall into the unmotivated category in order to spend time on activities that are perceived to be more fun. A motivated individual, however, can recognize when they are doing this and can correct their behavior to meet the requirements of their responsibilities. Chronic or perceived lack of motivation can have detrimental effects on students and new practitioners as well as others around them.

Correcting one's behavior is relatively easier than influencing the behavior of others. This does not mean, however, one cannot influence the behavior of others. Some of the ways one can influence others are through the following:

1. Leading by example

2. Sharing your passion with others

3. Inspiring others to achieve a common vision

4. Developing relationships

5. Holding people accountable for their performance

6. Recognizing the importance of the "fit" of an individual to the department/organization

7. Emphasizing the importance of individual contributions to the team

Throughout this chapter, these seven basic leadership skills will be examined by way of case presentation and analysis. This introduction is intended as an overview of these leadership basics, which can be referred to while reading the following cases.

- **Leading by example.** Recognizing that you have more influence over your own behavior is particularly important because leading by example is one of the easiest yet hardest things to do when trying to motivate others. Leading by example applies to any situation where you are expected to perform in a professional way under a certain set of guidelines or rules. It requires a leader to be constantly vigilant about their own actions and ethics, as it is difficult to expect others to follow rules when the leadership is lax about them. It does not mean that a leader is supposed to be perfect, however, as that is not possible. It just means that others are watching to see how you, as the leader, handle these difficult situations. The reason that modeling is so important is that simple deeds can make a difference. One does not need to be a formal leader (i.e., a leader with a title) to demonstrate this type of activity. Another important concept to remember is that in all organizations, informal leaders can exert influence over decisions and support the vision and goals (or sometimes not). If you find yourself in one of these formal or informal roles in the future, think about your own behavior and how it influences your coworkers, the department, and the department's quality of service. All of these situations put us in leadership roles—how we handle these situations dictates whether they are a success or not.

- **Sharing your passions with others.** Another way to motivate others is by sharing your passion with them. Most people are more empathetic and willing to listen to someone who is excited and enthusiastic about a project, idea, etc. Success breeds success, and by sharing the reasons you want to lead with others, you may cause a spark, an idea, or a whole movement for those you lead. Sharing with people encourages others to get involved by propagating a feel-good message and can inspire others to want to cooperate and contribute. People in general want to do good for others. In fact, that is why many of us became pharmacists. Sharing how you contribute to your community or profession, and why, can lead others to do the same.

- **Inspiring others to achieve a common vision.** Many of us have heard the expression, "many hands make work light." This saying is also applicable in motivating oneself and others. If a new leader is able to harness the input and energy of those around them, they can achieve many great things. It is critical for leaders to not always have their own way, but to listen to the team and be flexible. Help guide the team to a win-win situation where there is some compromise, but not so much as to deter success or create patient safety issues. A key element to this concept is that "buy in" to the vision is essential—because without it nothing will get accomplished. Creating a common vision is crucial to success as it is the guidepost that moves a team or organization in a synergistic direction toward a common goal.

  Many times, the vision starts with an idea from the new leader; however, the leader must assess whether or not the goal is achievable now or if it is something that needs to wait a bit until the culture of the organization is ready for it. Ideally, the vision should be shaped by those who need to adhere to it, thus making it more likely that the followers will endear themselves to making the vision succeed.

- **Developing relationships.** Relationship building is crucial to understanding team members and what motivates them to perform at a high level. It is important to establish effective means for these relationships to develop. Multiple modes of frequent communication are best. Frequent (weekly or biweekly), one-on-one meetings between leader and student/staff member are very effective. Team meetings and social events are also good ways to establish a better understanding of "motivational triggers" and to help build rapport. However, it's important to understand the fine line drawn between socializing while holding a leadership role. Relationships can be counterproductive if not handled as collegial and professional, and leaders can get their perspective distorted if they get drawn into cliques or become too familiar with social and personal issues.

Healthy, productive, and professional relationships should not be underestimated as it can smooth over a lot of "rough edges" during times of stress or confusion. In other words, healthy relationships are very important because they can help teams achieve their goals. Effective communication is one method of building and maintaining strong working relationships. Leaders should consider not only what message is being delivered but how it is being delivered. In this age of high-tech communication, attention should be paid to the times that a more personal mode of communication is needed. For example, e-mail or written correspondence assures messages are sent but not that they are received and accurately perceived. In short, e-mail is not the best communication method for relationship building and should be reserved for minor communication or documentation purposes. Personal and direct means of communication—asking questions that will bring out answers in a nonthreatening or intimidating way—are very effective in relationship building.

As with any form of communication, keep in mind that individuals are working from their own paradigms, which can impact the tone of communication and the relationship. It is the role of the leader to be open-minded, perceptive, and to try to "read between the lines" and approach individuals with consideration as to their personal perspectives. Dealing with individuals who are deeply entrenched in their ways can be very challenging, and it requires a lot of skill and practice in relationship building.

■ **Holding people accountable for their performance.** Performance management is an essential leadership tool, which is crucial to motivation. Making the expectations clear, routinely following up, and redirecting when necessary are key elements to assuring that performance standards are met. The most important part of holding people accountable is that if expectations are not met—and met consistently throughout the team, department, or organization—then it will start to erode the motivation of others, even highly, self-motivated people.

Performance management is generally a programatic approach to personnel management, which includes activities that ensure organizational goals are consistently being met in an effective and efficient manner. Performance management may focus on the performance of individuals, a team, a department, an organization, or in some cases processes to build a product or service. The following are some characteristics of a typical performance management program:

- Expectations are set around work that is planned.

- Work performance is monitored.

- Individuals are trained and the ability to perform is developed and enhanced.

- Performance is measured and the ratings are summarized and reported.

- Top performance is rewarded.

Such programs include an organizational mission/vision and goals as well as a mechanism that motivates individuals and teams to follow guidelines for meeting goals. A corrective action component is usually included to get individuals and teams back on track or to weed these people out of organizations when they are not productive. Additionally, hiring practices should be reviewed as well as the impact that the hiring processes have on teams or an organization—both positively /negatively and culturally/financially.

- **Recognizing the importance of the "fit" of an individual to the department/organization.** Getting the right people for a job from the beginning ensures that motivation for doing a good job is inherent. The hiring process is the time to really vet a candidate for potential performance issues and to weed out any possible behavioral, philosophical, or competency issues that might get in the way of training. The hiring process should be both thoughtful and substantive. The orientation period is also a time to assess the "fit" of a prospective employee within the existing culture and whether or not that person has the capacity to do the job.

However, sometimes this process is not followed and a new leader finds that their team is lacking the right motivation, either through lack of rigor in the hiring and orientation process or even with the right people. Sometimes motivation can wane for other reasons such as erosion of team morale due to cultural, financial, and management issues. Selection of the best people will ensure that the right amount of motivation is cultivated when needed and that there is a reduction in staff turnover.

- **Emphasizing the importance of individual contributions to the team.** When trying to influence the behavior of others, it is important to recognize that there isn't one way to handle each problem but rather guiding principles that can be learned and applied to each situation. Also, not all solutions may be applicable to the new leader's situation when dealing with different personalities, etc. Similar to how each patient needs to have a customized medication regimen to meet their needs, each situation will need its own unique solution to its problems.

Throughout the chapters there is a theme of dealing with people to motivate and achieve results. One element of leadership that is not specifically addressed in any of the chapters—but is touched on in all of them—is having the sense of how to deal with people. Sometimes this is called emotional intelligence (EI). EI addresses the capacity to assess and manage the emotions of oneself and others (often teams and organizations). Sometimes it is referred to as the skill of understanding and managing other people. Much like an intelligence quotient, there have been many models proposed as to how to measure this, but all in all it is regarded as a real concept and is referred to frequently in basic leadership literature; thus, it is worth mentioning here (for further reading, references are included at the end of this chapter).

Leading by example

PRINCIPLE ■ Modeling leadership traits

Jessica is a P1 at her local school of pharmacy (SOP). She had previously been very involved in numerous activities while in high school and really enjoyed being a part of something bigger. Since being accepted into the SOP, she is struggling to find ways to become involved. She is also concerned because all of the people at school who are leaders appear to be running around like chickens with their heads cut off! She's not sure if she can handle all of the time commitments associated with school or the numerous SOP organizations.

Jessica has started hearing about the leadership crisis in pharmacy since being accepted into the SOP. She is passionate about the profession of pharmacy and does not want to see the profession suffer because of the lack of leadership. She has also noticed that the same people in leadership positions within the SOP seem to just rotate titles among all of the organizations (i.e., the president of one organization is the treasurer of another). Jessica has also noticed that even though she brought up some ideas about changing things within one of the organizations, her suggestions were not addressed and she had been told by older classmates that nothing ever changes from year to year (e.g., the organizations hold the same events, do the same fundraisers, etc.).

Office elections are being held in 2 weeks for the student chapter of American Society of Health-System Pharmacists (ASHP) at Jessica's SOP. Jessica is considering running for vice president of the organization; however, she is concerned because she has only been a member of this organization for less than a year, and she would be running against a veteran member of the organization and people might consider this to be too ambitious for a young professional. Given the lack of response about her previous suggestions, Jessica also isn't sure she wants to be part of an organization in which she has personally seen very few benefits. Lastly, Jessica is thinking that her best option is to bid her time patiently and wait for the right time to apply for a leadership position when all of the seasoned leaders have stepped aside.

WHAT JESSICA MAY BE THINKING...

- I'm scared about committing to something that I can't handle.
- How does anyone learn to balance school with extracurricular activities?
- What if people don't follow me?
- Will my grades suffer? (This is more to the point and what the writer, reader, and Jessica are really thinking!)
- I'm scared I won't get elected. How will I face my peers if this happens?

ON THE OTHER HAND, JESSICA MIGHT REASON...

- The only way to get anything done is to do it yourself.

- Employers don't really care about grades as long as you graduate from pharmacy school.
- The leadership crisis can't be that bad. There's always someone who is willing to volunteer for things.

MENTOR ADVICE

It is wonderful that Jessica has an interest in a leadership role. Not everyone has this interest, and she should consider this as a sign that she has some innate leadership ability. Jessica needs to build her skillset and confidence as well as learn to overcome any fears. Leading by example may seem like an easy enough skill, but it is not. There has been some question and controversy as to whether leadership is an innate ability or whether it is something that can be learned. There is a body of literature that addresses this subject, but in a nutshell if Jessica is thinking about leadership, she is already demonstrating a propensity toward having leadership qualities. The thought of becoming a leader can be frightening, but if she begins to build early and slowly, her skillset will become broad and strong before she knows it.

Jessica's apprehension to run for vice president of the student chapter of ASHP may be due more to her environment than from internal cues. When she observed the leaders in the school "running around like chickens with their heads cut off," this is probably due to lack of leadership skills on their part and perhaps lack of a strategy. There is never a perfect time to step forward. If Jessica waits for one, the moment may never come. She needs to assess her ability at this stage in her student career as to the amount of time she has to dedicate to being a vice president. Are her grades good enough to allow her to spend a few hours a week? If so, it would be a great opportunity for her to explore her leadership style and abilities, build her skills, learn new concepts, and make new friends. Even though she will be running against a veteran of the organization, with some fresh ideas and strong campaigning she can be successful. The best part is that she is signaling to others about her interest to get involved. If she wins she will be thrown headfirst into a leadership role with many responsibilities, and if she doesn't win there will be other opportunities to run for in the future.

Or perhaps this is not the right time to run for vice president if her grades are low or her personal life will not allow it. If so, she needs to find other ways to get involved, contribute, and continue her growth and development in the leadership arena. She could start by being observant and talking to others. She can find out what other student organizations are active and what types of activities are happening on campus. She should start slowly because it is not necessary to jump in full speed especially while still in school and trying to maintain her grades, but she can find outlets for her creative side and her internal drive to be a leader. Jessica could offer to organize a student event, get involved in the yearbook committee, or participate in other student professional organizations (statewide or national).

Jessica should also consider looking for leadership opportunities on a daily basis, such as handling difficult problems that others may shy away from or by resolving immediate operational or clinical issues. She can let her preceptor or the pharmacist-in-charge know that she is interested in helping out in any way. By doing this, she will be leading by example; other students will see this and might not be so afraid to step up to the plate in the future.

It is true that the profession of pharmacy has been lacking good, strong leaders over the past several years. There have been articles written about this in professional journals, which discuss the reasons for this as well as propose suggestions. One possible resolution is for existing leaders to encourage and mentor young, budding leaders who show an inclination toward leading. There are so many ways Jessica can hone her leadership skills while providing service to the school of pharmacy community. The more she gets involved, the more that faculty and other students will identify her as a leader.

What I have found to be successful

The most important lesson to remember is that as a leader, you are a role model. Through your years as a pharmacist leader, you will realize how important your actions are to those around you. If you are fearful of leadership, I suggest that you find a mentor or another form of support system in your workplace. It is not always easy being a leader. In my career, I remember being extremely scared when I found myself in a leadership role as the only pharmacist on the weekend shift (in a small hospital). I was right out of college and didn't feel I knew anything. The technician I worked with was truly a veteran and supported me through those early times. I could have quit that job and went somewhere else where I didn't need to be in a leadership role, but having her support was invaluable and it helped me develop my confidence* and leadership skills.

Another suggestion is that if you have a fear of getting into a leadership role, take baby steps. I got as much involved as my lifestyle allowed at the time. My message here is to get involved to the extent that you feel comfortable, but push yourself to do more as I have found that has been the key to my success.

*On that note, confidence comes with time and success. Continuing to demonstrate the behaviors that you want to see in your team, department, or organization, and doing what you know is right is something you can do on a daily basis to practice the skill of leading by example.

- -

NEW LEADER ADVICE

Jessica should take a risk and run for the vice president role. Leaders are not just individuals with titles, and this is an important concept to remember especially if Jessica does not get elected into office. Just by running for office, Jessica is proving that she is willing to take a risk to improve the organization. People do not tend to follow leaders who are sitting on the sideline. Instead, they are looking for individuals who have good ideas and are willing to work alongside them to accomplish their goals.

Jessica needs to find the best way to make changes in a professional organization or committee and volunteer to head the project herself. By doing this, she is demonstrating that the project is very important and the project will not get lost amongst all of the other activities in the organization or committee. Leading such a project can be overwhelming; however, leading does not mean that Jessica should be doing all the work herself. She should obtain the support of others. By getting other people involved in the project, Jessica will be able to stay focused on her academic as well as professional commitments.

What I have found to be successful

Developing your own mission statement is something I was encouraged to do as a student and resident. I have found this advice to be invaluable to me as I transitioned to being a new practitioner. It provides me with the framework to guide me in most of the decisions I need to make and goals that I set for myself. It also provides me with the optimal outcome that I am working toward as a pharmacist and as an individual. My personal mission statement is something that I periodically review and update.

As a new practitioner, it is indeed frightening to "put yourself out there" especially when you are new or have limited experience. Many times, I have wanted someone to tap me on the shoulder and say "You have arrived." It is important to realize that no one will do this for you and that you must have the initiative and the drive to seek out opportunities for yourself. Leading others by example is one of the most difficult aspects of leadership as it is "walking the talk" and it encompasses many different aspects of leadership such as team building, gaining support for new ideas, and being effective at getting things done.

Putting myself "out there" is the best way to get others motivated. If people see me making recommendations and then actively working on implementing those changes or volunteering to be on committees, then they see that I am dedicated to the profession as well as interested in changing things for the better. Also, passion and excitement about something new will make others more likely to assist me when I ask for help because they can see that I truly care about what I am doing.

I know that if I don't try or apply for something, I will never get to where I want to be or where I envision the profession being. Minor setbacks, such as not winning the election, should not deter me from trying to get involved. I may have to identify other ways to demonstrate leadership such as getting involved at a smaller level (e.g., leading department committees, leading a charge for the SOP or my company, or volunteering for activities at a state or chapter level). By getting involved in these smaller issues, others will notice my commitment and want my participation in larger initiatives, especially if I am successful at accomplishing the smaller tasks.

CASE 4.2

Sharing your passion with others

PRINCIPLE ■ Inspiring others

Jim is relatively new at the Uptown Hospital Pharmacy Department. He is always upbeat and a great person to work with. Many of his coworkers are always commenting on how nice it is when Jim works with them. Because of his great personality, Jim's manager has asked him to take the lead on a fundraising event for heart disease, which is important to his company.

In order for Jim to fulfill his requirements as the lead on this project, Jim needs to obtain $5,000 in fundraising (the means are up to him) as well as recruit fellow coworkers to participate in the 5k walk associated with the fundraising event. The event will be held 8 weeks from the day Jim's manager asked him to head up this event for the department. Jim has been told that this event has not gone well in previous years. The department has never been able to reach the goal of $5,000, and their participation in the walk has only been mediocre at best. Jim's manager has expressed that his goal this year is to have the best turnout ever for the walk and to meet and exceed the $5,000 fundraising goal.

Jim is particularly fond of the organization that is sponsoring this event as he had a family member who suffered from heart disease and passed away a year ago. He has also had first-hand experience with the organization and knows many people who work there.

Given his new assignment, Jim sent out an e-mail to the entire department asking for their support for the fundraising event. He also set out a tip jar in the break room where people could place their leftover change or any donations. In addition, Jim made a couple of announcements at staff meetings but received a lackluster response. With only 4 weeks left, only three people have agreed to attend the walk, and the last time he looked at the "tip jar" there was only a handful of change in it. He is extremely frustrated and not sure what to do next.

WHAT JIM MAY BE THINKING...

- I'm not in a leadership position so no one wants to join me in this endeavor.
- How can anyone get this group of individuals to do anything?
- Why doesn't anyone care?
- Why doesn't anyone put forth effort in these fundraiser events?

ON THE OTHER HAND, JIM MIGHT REASON...

- I can get my manager to back me up and require people to attend the 5k walk.
- Should I donate a significant amount of money to lead by example?
- I'm sure people will donate. They are probably waiting until the last minute before doing so.

- -

MENTOR ADVICE

Jim is struggling to understand why everyone doesn't have the same attitude toward their jobs that he does. An important aspect of getting others onboard with a program or an activity is clear communication. Jim needs to effectively communicate and share his enthusiasm for his profession. This will help him achieve "buy in" to the 5k walk. Effective communication requires information flow in multiple directions. This involves not only information being sent out, but also "feedback loop." In other words, there needs to be a sort of barometer for the level of enthusiasm that the message receives. Jim's decision to send out an e-mail only—without other measures of communication that are more personal or direct—is a recipe for disaster. This is especially important if his department is less than enthusiastic about giving back to the community.

Sometimes if team morale is low, then enthusiasm wanes. People start wondering "What's in it for me?" because they are not thinking as a team but rather as individuals. Jim should talk to team members about his personal experiences and discuss how much the organization can benefit from the greater good at some point in their lives. Individuals may not see an immediate or direct correlation to themselves, but sharing stories or igniting feelings about the common bond of community can make people soften their stance sometimes. Jim could share his passion for the organization by discussing some of his personal experiences one-on-one with his coworkers when the opportunity arises. It can be very powerful for coworkers to hear a real-life, personal story, and these stories get shared among team members without ever having to make a group presentation or sending out a communiqué. As we all know, the "grapevine" is usually is associated with gossip and negativity; however, it is a very powerful form of communication that, if used in a positive way, can be a very effective tool.

Jim needs to talk to his coworkers and ask for their input on how best to engage the team. Asking for their ideas and their support while letting them know that he cannot do it alone will be a very effective way to get "buy in." It is a very effective tool to motivate the procrastinators ("Eeyores"). In general people really do want to help, but some need to be asked as they may not be motivated to just volunteer. Jim should seek out others who might be willing to help. It may be risky because not everyone is willing to support or help, so he should be prepared to accept some opposition to his requests. There is almost always at least one naysayer in every department . Naysayers sometimes pride themselves on their informal influence over the department's thinking, culture, and progress. It is some people's nature to be negative, but when it happens to a team or a department it can be devastating. It is a leader's role to turn this around, and this is not an easy task.

Jim should arrange a kick-off event for the fundraiser, such as a benefit dinner party. It doesn't have to be elaborate, just as long as there is a broad spectrum of participation and everyone feels they have been included. Most importantly, he should remember to celebrate any successes—no matter how small or incremental—even if it is done so as to set a goal for the next event or fundraising activity. Inspiring others to follow or contribute to his passion is part art and part science. It always requires skillful and open communication, creative ideas, persistence, teamwork, and a supportive, positive culture.

What I have found to be successful

I always facilitate communication when I need to inspire passion in people. Listening is a very important component to effective communication. Finding common ground with team members is a first step, and critical listening is imperative. Talking with people to understand their viewpoints and motivations is helpful in building excitement and "buy in" to any project or program.

Personal, one-on-one communication is most effective. Providing examples of what the work means in terms of patient outcomes or staff morale can make people feel more connected to the work they are doing. At times, I have found it necessary to prompt better communication among team members by having an off-site retreat. This may seem a lot of preparation and work, but it brings a multitude of benefits. Some benefits are seen immediately and some changes take time to work themselves through to prove beneficial.

Celebrating success is important for teambuilding and morale boosting. Remember morale is something that can't be seen, but it can be felt. Don't underestimate morale or the culture of a department or organization as it can make or break success. Also, building your leadership "tool kit" can offset negativity within a team. A negative culture can kill passion and enthusiam. The old expression "We eat our young" applies here. I have seen departments go through tremendous and difficult transitions. This was always due to a negative culture. One person alone cannot resolve this. Leaders need to recognize a negative culture, decide to do something about it, and then gain support within and outside the department to change it.

Developing a positive culture takes everyone's effort. Negativity—backstabbing, complaining, and lack of teamwork—contributes to poor quality service. So recruit good people and then train them thoroughly.

- -

NEW LEADER ADVICE

Jim shouldn't get down about the current state of affairs. Instead, he should focus his energy on 1) finding people who may have had similar experiences as himself and 2) continuing to communicate with the department. Many times people tend to forget information once they hear it because of how busy they are in their personal and professional lives. Jim needs to counteract this problem by having others engage people in this activity too. If he can find people with similar experiences as himself, he will most likely find that they are more willing to contribute because they have an emotional connection to the cause.

Jim should continue to communicate to the staff. Sending one e-mail and making one announcement at a staff meeting will not engage the staff. It may take individuals a week before they can get to their e-mail, and if they were not able to make the staff meeting then they may miss that communication as well. It might behoove Jim to start having one-on-one conversations with people during the course of the day. By doing this and having further e-mail and staff communications, Jim will be able to reach more people.

What I have found to be successful

It is important to tell your story because if you do not, others will develop their own story and this could lead to frustration on both ends. Hearing your story can have a major impact on changing people's minds and perceptions. I know I am always more empathetic to a cause when it relates to someone I know, and it makes me more willing to contribute what I can to helping this individual.

Communication is the key to obtaining support for activities such as this. In general, it takes communication in three different formats (e.g., e-mail, in person, flyers) at least seven times before people really receive the message. Therefore, it is very important to recognize the importance of communication and the various types of communication that are needed when wanting to influence people's perceptions.

It is a great idea to find one to two individuals who are of like mind. One mistake many new practitioners make is in forgetting to engage others when trying to bring other people along with a decision. For example, Jim could have spoken with a few of his coworkers to see what ideas they may have had in the fundraising initiative or in getting others to participate in the 5k. By engaging these people in the decision-making process, Jim might have seen that he won their support and then been able to use their support to influence other people.

Inspiring others to achieve a common vision

PRINCIPLE ■ Encourage your team to "buy in"

Leigh is a new operations manager at LMN Hospital Pharmacy. She has just completed her residency in pharmacy administration and is very excited about her job. During Leigh's residency, she took classes in human resource management, change management, and a variety of others. She believes she has a good grasp on how she can effectively run the operational side of the department given her experiences.

During Leigh's first month of orientation, she noticed that the way the department ran in IV room was drastically different than where she did her residency. There appeared to be complete disregard for the USP 797 guidelines (no one was even wearing hair covers), the pharmacists in the IV room only checked the batched items and chemos coming out of the IV room while the triage pharmacist out front was responsible for checking first doses, and everyone kept complaining about how busy they were and that there wasn't enough staff to get people trained properly.

Leigh asked a lot of questions while she was training with the people who worked in the IV room. She wanted to know why the triage person did all the first-dose checking as well as why the IV room pharmacists only did the batch and chemo checking. The overwhelming response Leigh got was "because that's the way it's always been done." Leigh also asked what would be some of the things people would change about the IV room, and she found out that the number one item that needed to be addressed was technician training in the IV room. In fact, Leigh got so many complaints about the lack of adherence to aseptic technique during her month of training that she immediately formed an IV room task force to start addressing operational issues within the IV room.

The task force was off to a great start and was starting to make many changes in the IV room, but Leigh still thought it was odd that there was not a dedicated pharmacist to oversee the IV room. Leigh was not responsible for the pharmacists who worked in the IV room, and when she brought the idea up to the veteran manager who oversaw those people, the manager did not seem to think the idea of moving the IV room pharmacists around was of critical value as there were other "more pressing" issues she was dealing with.

WHAT LEIGH MAY BE THINKING...

- Why does the other manager just dismiss my ideas?
- Are people really satisfied with just the status quo?
- If the volumes of the IV room are going up, why am I the only one who cares about how the department is able to meet their standard turnaround times?

ON THE OTHER HAND, LEIGH MIGHT REASON...

- I haven't been here long enough to know the "big picture."
- Am I moving too fast? Should I be making changes this quickly since I just got here?

- Am I making a mountain out of a mole hill (i.e., overreacting) just because things aren't the same as what I am familiar with?

MENTOR ADVICE

Inspiring others to accomplish common goals is one of the most intriguing leadership concepts. Leigh might wonder, "How can I get others to do what I want them to do"? or "How can I convince others to do what is right for the patient? Involving others to see things the same way is basically what a common vision is all about. Some leaders have an innate, charismatic way that people naturally follow. Others, like Leigh need to work on a different approach. She needs to connect with people on a human interest level, appeal to their sense of what is good, and help them see what their work or organizational setting could be like if they join together and try to improve things. Leigh should encourage the team and continue to ask, "How you can help support the common vision?"

Leigh should start developing relationships with other managers to begin laying the foundation of a collaborative relationship. She could ask to have lunch together and then talk about common interests rather than pharmacy issues or work. Also, at some point, she might want to think about establishing a 1:1 routine meeting with the manager, who could help develop strong bonds and break down any potential barriers that might prevent communication and collaboration. Working collaboratively with her peers is critical, as working in a vacuum will create "territory wars" between managers and department staff or even between departments.

Leigh should think about the "bgger picture" and how her efforts will affect the whole. Even if her ideas are correct and well intended, it can have the opposite effect if not handled properly. She needs to include all the people who should be involved in a project and describe what she sees in the future and why. Leigh needs to cite examples of best practices, regulatory requirments, and safe-patient standards of care and then tell them how much more efficient operations can be and how this would improve their work lives. By describing in detail, Leigh will inspire others to join her and lead others in the cause.

Leigh may not gain success from simply asking for their advice or for them to sit on a committee. In fact, this is just the beginning. The departmental vision will most likely include quality and safety measures. The IV room task force needs to keep this vision in mind when determining what types of projects the group will work on. Leigh should include the task force members in decisions about where the group is heading. This way, she is more likely to motivate them into seeing things her way. Getting a team excited at this point is not hard— most people know what they would like. The frustration sets in when the reality of the hard work and the limitations arrive. This is why it is crucial to get "buy in" or consensus to the vision upfront. Leigh must remind the task force that consensus is the amount of support needed to move an initiative or program forward and that compromises are needed in order to make the program work. One of the most important aspects of leadership is persistence. Leigh should look for support from her peers, her mentors/coaches, and, most importantly, from her team.

What I have found to be successful

Widening your circle of influence can help on many levels. It helps build support for your vision from people you lead and from those you are accountable to. I myself have widened my circle of influence by talking to my manager about resolving quality/service issues with other managers. Remember to try to include as many different people and different levels of support to influence and support your vision or cause. Naysayers ("Eeyores") will generally try to influence around the "fringes" of a group, department, or organization, but having strong relationships within and outside the group will help nullify this activity. Focus your energy on people who are positive and who can share the vision and help spread enthusiam about it. Do this by talking with them, by encouraging them, and by involving them in key decisions.

Many management books speak to a shared vision, but how we get to that is the difficult part. Sometimes it is not clear that everyone does not share the same vision until the implications of such start to crop up in practice—the inattention to detail, the disregard for safety guidelines, and the noncompliance of policies and procedures with no apparent accountability or consequences. Shared goals are established by the team, generally through a goal-sharing session or visioning session. The best way to initiate a shared vision is to examine common problems, goals, and plans (not arbitrary goals set by administrators). However, the role of the leader is to guide these goals in a positive direction, providing guidance and feedback where needed. The leader should know best practices and share experiences to allow the team to make educated decisions. The leader should be willing to make hard decisions when the vision gets off course and be able to get the team back on track.

The skilled leader knows how to gain consensus to a positive outcome. Something that I learned in my practice is that the team does not always have to agree 100%. But before moving forward with any key project, I ask, "Can the entire team give some consensus to supporting the success of this program if we move forward"? This will provide you with some indication as to where the weak links or the naysayers may be, and you will hear the naysayers point of view. Try to be openminded and realize that if you don't listen, you may be in for some trouble with your project. Many times naysayers are very influential people on the team, sometimes referred to as "informal leaders." These people can either help or hinder. If approached the right way, they can be very helpful in supporting and accomplishing goals. If not approached the right way, they may be successful in railroading or halting a project that doesn't suit their vision or needs. Sometimes their motivation is that they may like the attention and prestige that comes from successfully putting up roadblocks for leaders. Not all informal leaders are naysayers, but it is important to listen and continue to work on the positive aspects of how solving this problem together will benefit all. You may need to have some separate conversations with the naysayers and informal leaders to determine motivations and engage them in a positive way. Circumventing this important step can be disasterous to your project.

There are voluminous bodies of literature on how to create a common vision, but in essence the leader needs to be clear about the message. The mission needs to be accomplished and the "how we get there" is the matter at hand. Once the vision is clear, then the leader's role is to measure the level of support. That can be by 1:1 conversations or by a pledge of support at a group meeting. It is important to hear people's concerns, especially if there is an issue of potential patient or staff safety. However, at some point the leader needs to take charge, move the decision forward, and remind everyone that the vision was created together and it is expected now that we all support it.

As we all know, organizational and departmental culture can be very strong. The old cry "Because that's the way we've always done things here" is a common cry of a culture that

Is resistant to change. Change can be fear provoking. It means learning new processes, being flexible, moving out of familiar territory, and perhaps developing some new skillsets. In pharmacy practice, it is crucial to always keep the patient's welfare at the forefront of one's perspective. Easier said than done as politics, egos, and personalities often get in the way of focusing on evidence-based, best practices. And sometimes excuses are made that "Administration will not let us do it" or "We didn't get the money budgeted that was needed for the program." If policies are disregarded and staff are directionless, then something is wrong with the leadership. Attention to the vision, mission, and goals of the organization and department is critical. Without this regard, quality will probably falter. Remember, your mission is your purpose and staying focused on this will help the vision become clearer.

Now that this project is about to be launched (unless there are significant patient safety concerns), there needs to be consensus with at least enough support by every team member to not have the project fail. Be careful with 1:1 conversations though because in my experience people may tell you what they think you will want to hear and then later you hear otherwise, especially in group settings when the informal leaders exert psychological pressure on the others so that they may not feel comfortable voicing their concerns or opinions. It may help to have 1:1 conversations with an informal leader, and if possible make that person a point person on the project.

Change theory is another concept with scientific foundation. Basically it speaks to the process that a team goes through in the midst of organizational changes. In general the leader, who helps shape the vision, is at the forefront of the change curve. Understanding this is critical for the leader to provide adequate time for the team to adjust and mold some of the changes to their comfort zone. Sometimes though, if enough resistance is created, there are backward trends. It is the leader's role to recognize this and finesse the teams way back to the point of progress. Issues may need to be ironed out at this point, but it should always be clear that the vision is the "guiding light" and without it, there will be no direction and progress will be halted. Given this, it is critical for the leader to not always have their own way, but to listen to the team and be willing to be flexible. Help guide the team to a "win-win" situation where there is some compromise, but not so much as to deter success or create patient safety issues.

- -

NEW LEADER ADVICE

Leigh should make sure the administrative team is all on the same page. There is nothing worse than trying to roll out a new project and not having the administrators on the same page, as this can lead to staff upset if they disagree with the project. Also, there may be a very good reason that Leigh's co-manager does not want to change the staffing at this point in time, and if Leigh does not understand this it could make things more difficult for her in what she is trying to accomplish.

Leigh has a long way to go in getting others to "see her vision" and should take baby steps. Making smaller changes will go farther in making a larger change more successful because Leigh will have demonstrated her ability and others will gain confidence in her ability. Another way Leigh can obtain support for her vision is by creating a shared vision with her staff by asking for their input. People tend to put up barriers to changes when they are not involved in the decision. By involving them in the changes, it will make things easier for Leigh when it is time to implement the changes.

What I have found to be successful

Creating consensus from a few key members of the staff and management team will greatly enhance your ability to achieve your vision. Include both the formal and informal leaders on your side as you start making changes, as they can help influence the naysayers and down play their negativity to your ideas. It is also important to have the leaders of change on the same page from the get-go so that the staff do not sense discord and use this to sabotage any type of consensus building.

It is also important to understand the culture of the organization in order to determine how change will be received by the members. If the organization is resistant to change, it will be very difficult to bring in new ideas to promote the growth of pharmacy practice. The idea that 1:1 meetings can be used to help influence others is very important as well as knowing the organization's vision and 5-year plan. This knowledge can be used as the basis for promoting new growth and development of pharmacy practice in your areas.

Even though you may communicate with staff, they may not see or understand why you are trying to accomplish something. This has led to frustration when I have tried to implement new changes. One thing I have learned and try to incorporate into all of my communications (e.g., e-mail, staff meetings, etc.) is the five Ws (who, what, when, where, and why). This helps to keep me focused on what I need to tell staff yet provides them with all of the back-ground information so that they can understand where we are going.

CASE 4.4

The importance of developing relationships

PRINCIPLE ■ Communication and team building

Jack is a new manager at the TCB Pharmacy and has been in his role for 5 months. He has two technician supervisors who assist him in overseeing the 40+ technician staff. One of the supervisors has been with the company for 15 years and in the technician supervisor role for 10 years. The other had been with the company for 10 years but had only recently been promoted (within the past 2 years) to a technician supervisor position. Jack spends the orientation part of his job really trying to understand the department and the organization. He participates in meetings with the technician supervisors, but really defers to them when deci-sions need to be made since they have more of a history with the decisions being made. As Jack spends time in various meetings, he starts to notice little things about his supervisors. One always completes her tasks and is able to get them done on time whereas the other one does not. One is always coming up with new ideas on how to improve the technician work-flows and the other is late for meetings, is not taking things seriously, and is not responsive to Jack's requests.

Because of the vast differences in the performance of both supervisors, Jack decides to hold weekly status meetings with each of them individually. Jack thinks this is the best course of action since it will allow him to confront the individual who is not performing as well as to maintain the relationship with the other supervisor who is performing. Two weeks after Jack implements the individual weekly meetings, things are still not improving with the inefficient technician supervisor. Jack has already confronted her about the fact she takes more smoke breaks than most of her staff; she is routinely late for meetings and does not have a good reason for being late; she is not producing any results in terms of projects Jack has assigned her; she expects her day to be exactly 8 hours long and not a minute more (yet she is a salaried employee); and she does not have accountability on her part with respect to her job. The heart-to-heart talks with this supervisor seem to be going nowhere, and Jack is at a loss as to what he should do next.

WHAT JACK MAY BE THINKING...

- I should continue to coach this person in her job as she just doesn't understand what I want her to do.
- She is a great technician, and I know she has the capabilities to perform at this level.
- I know people do not deliberately set out not to do their job, so I need to understand why she is not doing hers.

ON THE OTHER HAND, JACK MIGHT REASON...

- I don't understand why she doesn't get it and won't perform.
- I should demote her back to a technician-level position and hire someone who can perform.
- I will start following the organization's disciplinary action steps so that she will see that she is not performing and this is unacceptable.

MENTOR ADVICE

It is always frustrating dealing with others who do not have the same level of enthusiasm or care about the job the way Jack does. A key element to motivating people is developing relationships. Jack needs to understand the motivation behind people's attitudes toward their jobs. Not everyone comes to work every day to help people. The reality is that some people come to work because they need to make money, and that is all the job is to them. Sometimes these are the people that are so difficult to motivate toward a better performance level. On the opposite pole, sometimes people's motivation is tied into their ego or level of prestige associated with the job they are doing. In this case, it can also be sometimes difficult to manage highly trained, skilled workers who take a great deal of pride in the work they do. But this ego can be used to attain results. Jack should not underestimate this because many narcissistic types love to take on projects to plump up a resume.

Jack can use techniques to improve productivity through teambuilding. He should consider alternate means of dealing with performance, such as coaching, before entering into discipline. Coaching is a way of encouraging people and guiding in the right direction. It demonstrates an interest for the person as an individual rather than just someone who has to follow directions. (Disciplinary action can be effective, but it can also leave good people feeling hurt and offended and ultimately have the opposite than intended effect; however, sometimes in the performance-management process when all other leadership skills have failed, it may be necessary.) Jack will receive better results through understanding his team as individuals—understanding "what makes them tick" is a very helpful method to connecting with the team on a personal and professional level. This is not to mean that Jack should be forming friendships outside of work, but it does mean that he should see his staff and teammates as human beings with individual needs.

One benefit coaching provides is the opportunity to get to know people in a nonthreatening way and to learn their motivations, strengths, concerns, and fears. This is an opportunity to build trust and respect between employee and manager as well as opportunity to provide positive feedback and constructive direction where needed. Jack should reserve discipline as a last-line approach to a management problem because once you invoke discipline, it brings the issue to a whole new level.

It is important for Jack to not set up preferential type relationships, especially if it is perceived that he might favor one staff member over another and may have clouded judgment when dealing with performance issues. He must be fair with all he oversees—being considerate and pleasant but firm and fair.

What I have found to be successful

Get support outside of the department for personnel issues, especially when dealing with entrenched staff members that are unwilling to change. It is wise to let human resources (HR) know when problems begin to arise so as to build support for your management style and future actions. They can provide perspective and invaluable guidance as well.

The concept of coaching versus disciplining is often raised. Is coaching always preferred over disciplining? The short answer is yes but disciplining is sometimes necessary, and it is important for the leader to know when to use each. For example, I have found coaching to be more successful to improve performance when technicians know that you have their interest at heart. This requires relationship building, which the process of coaching will provide. In cases where technicians are not receptive to coaching or multiple attempts at coaching have failed, then disciplinary action must be used. Communicate in different ways through different forums with as many levels of people you come into contact with. This will help you build relationships that can assist you with tough decisions and projects later on. On the opposite spectrum, relationships can be a detriment if not dealt with appropriately and in a positive and fair manner.

- -

NEW LEADER ADVICE

Jack is on the right track by having heart-to-heart talks with the technician supervisors. He should not only focus on the expectations (or the fact that they are not being met), but should also focus on the person. What is driving this supervisor to act in such a manner? Are there home issues? Training issues? Lack of understanding Jack's expectations?

Jack needs to speak with the technician's former supervisor if possible. Her previous supervisor may be able to enlighten Jack with some ways that work best in dealing with this individual. If Jack can figure out what situations the technician excels in, he should focus on directing her into more of those situations so that she can continue to be successful.

If all else fails, Jack should involve his HR department. By working with HR, he may be able to get through to the supervisor that things are not working. Sometimes it takes this type of situation for individuals to take a hard look at what is going on at work and decide if they are in the correct job. It is also important for Jack to be resetting expectations when he HR department is around so that he, HR, and the supervisor are all on the same page.

What I have found to be successful

Everyone has a story. The only way you can learn a person's story is by getting to know the person. The story can impact the person's day-to-day work (e.g., sick kids, troubled marriage). In the book, *Crucial Conversations: Tools for Talking When Stakes are High*, the authors explain that people do not set out to fail or underperform; there is usually an underlying cause for them not completing tasks or meeting expectations. The authors state that the only way to know what is really going on is to have a conversation with people and focus on understanding where they are coming from. Getting to know someone is not an overnight accomplishment. As in any relationship, it is something both individuals must work on; however, by understanding where the other person is coming from, you will have the most complete view of what is truly happening with them.

Just as it is important to understand the other person's story, it is also important to understand the motivational triggers. There is a saying about having the right person on the right bus in the right seat—meaning that people tend to perform their best when they are doing activities that they are good at and enjoy. Managers cannot make this determination without understanding or building relationships with their staff. Having periodic conversations with the staff (e.g., "How are things going?" and "What would you like to be doing?") will allow managers to have a better understanding of their staff and allow them to move their staff into desired positions. Furthermore, in the book, *12: The Elements of Great Managing*, the authors discuss the concept of having someone at work care about me. The authors explain that when people feel that someone at work cares about them, productivity improves as well as getting "buy in" from those individuals into various types of projects.

It seems reasonable that people should know what is expected of them no matter what position they are in (e.g., officer in an organization, staff member of a department); however, that is not always the case. I find this can lead to frustration on the part of both individuals. In order to minimize frustration, I review my expectations at staff meetings. If individuals are still not meeting my expectations, I conduct one-on-one conversations with them to see 1) if they understand my expectations and 2) what may be causing them to not meet my expectations. I also find that having them tell me what my expectations are in their own words tends to help because I can assess their ability to understand what my expectations are. Lastly, I have developed a tool that assists me in following up with individuals. This tool keeps track of all my to-do lists and all of my follow-ups. By staying on top of issues early on, I can help redirect my staff back on track and meet my expectations on what they should be doing.

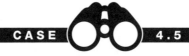

CASE 4.5

Holding people accountable for their performance

PRINCIPLE ■ Performance management

Sally is a pharmacist at ZXY Pharmacy and has been with the company for 2 years. She is very passionate about patient care and does whatever she can to assist her patients. For example, last week she spent 30 minutes counseling a patient on a new medication because she was concerned about the side effect profile of the medication. Sally's outstanding performance over the past few years has allowed her to become the lead pharmacist for the pharmacy. This means she is now participating in the hiring process for new technicians and pharmacists. She is not responsible for hiring them, but she does participate in the interview process.

Two weeks ago, Sally and her manager decided to hire a very personable technician named Barry. He was very outgoing and Sally and her manager thought he would be a great addition to the pharmacy; however, he had no prior pharmacy experience. Sally did not think this would be a big deal since many of the technician staff do not have a strong background in pharmacy and usually adapt quite quickly to the environment. Barry was doing a fantastic job during his orientation. He would perform any task any one asked him to do and was quick to learn many of the different jobs in the pharmacy. Once Barry's orientation period was over, however, Sally started hearing complaints from the other technicians. They would often come to her and inform her that Barry was taking a long time to complete basic tasks and sometimes would not even get them all done; therefore, they were doing his work plus their work. When Sally asked Barry about some of the incidents that were brought up to her, Barry told her it was just an oversight and that he had not meant to "mess up" and would do better. Weeks went by and things did not get better. Sally asked Barry why he was still late in getting his work done, but Barry again stated he would do better and that he loved his job and didn't want to lose it.

WHAT SALLY MAY BE THINKING...

- Why is it so hard for Barry to complete all of his tasks?
- All the other techs can handle the workload, so why can't he?
- I am starting to get complaints from customers because their prescriptions aren't ready when they need them. Can I have Barry fired?

ON THE OTHER HAND, SALLY MIGHT REASON...

- I know Barry is new to pharmacy and once he gets into the groove, things will get better.
- Maybe Barry just needs more training. Once he has that, things will get better.
- I know people do not deliberately set out not to do their job, so I need to understand why he is not doing his.

MENTOR ADVICE

Selecting and training new people is one of those leadership challenges. Although it is tempting to bring people onboard quickly especially in times of staffing shortages, in the long run it can be a detriment if a thorough hiring process is not followed. Many organizations utilize behavioral style interviewing by utilizing questions such as "Describe a time when you had to deal with conflict during rounds. What did you do?" This type of questioning is designed to weed out any potential characteristics or behavioral patterns that may be a poor fit for the organization. Behavioral interviewing is a style of interviewing developed by psychologists with the idea that a good predictor of future performance is found by examining past performance in similar situations. This interviewing style has become very common in today's recruitment process. Questions are developed, generally by the team of interviewers, that address specific situations and applicants are asked to give examples of how they have handled themselves in similar situations. Perhaps in this example, Sally should have included in her behavioral interview some questions to address how Barry would respond if asked how he has dealt with large volume of work, task completion, hands-off communication, and workload to other team members. Sally should review her organization's hiring process and help revise as necessary so as to prevent future hiring issues.

Sally should also review the organization's orientation program. Is it competency based and thorough? Does it require documentation (an orientation check sheet) before new technicians can move on to higher level tasks? An orientation check sheet should be reviewed with new employees to explain the expected timeline and levels of performance required to move through the entire orientation period. It should be clear what the expectations are and if they are not met what the consequences might be. To help her assess and revise the orientation program, Sally should refer to technician training guidebooks, such as those written by ASHP.

In this case, Barry successfully completed the pharmacy's current orientation training and performed well early on—but now he is not performing well. Barry has expressed a desire to remain employed, which is a positive sign. Sally needs to discuss the importance of teamwork with Barry and make it clear to him that he is part of a bigger picture and that his performance affects his coworkers (e.g., when his work is left undone, then others must pick up after him). She should also mention that his lack of attention to detail and followup is also impacting patient care; if he doesn't get his work done on time, then patients will not get their medications in a timely manner. This should be motivating enough to Barry if he really cares about his job and what he is doing.

In most cases, such one-on-one discussions will work. But it requires consistency, monitoring, and followup. Once employees realize that no one is overseeing them, their performance can slack. In fact, the strongest motivational approach in managing technicians to a higher performance level is to appeal to their sense of teamwork and the overall impact on patient care. It is important for Sally to repeatedly show her staff that she values and appreciates them for the important work they do. However, it is also important to maintain balance. She must be careful to not overpraise as this can lead to complacency too.

Finally, Sally must stress the importance of respect (respecting your job and respecting each other) to Barry and the other staff. By not doing his job, Barry is demonstrating disrespect for it and to his coworkers. Showing up late to work and slacking are other forms of disrespect. Sally's team will be strong and productive once the staff has ongoing, consistent respect for their jobs and each other.

What I have found to be successful

At the beginning of the orientation process, managers and orientees should sit down together and review the orientation check sheet and discuss performance expectations. If performance does not progress as intended or wanes after the orientation period, managers need to set the expected timeline for improvement and ask the employees if they have any concerns. Coaching methodology should be employed but good documentation at this stage is a must. If things do not improve during the orientation period, then an action plan may be needed. A major part of holding people accountable is letting them know the expectations; setting clear expectations upfront will help allay a lot of issues in the long term. Also, letting people know the consequences if these expectations are not met is another important part of holding people accountable for their performance.

Routine communication with all staff is very important, especially in the orientation process (e.g., weekly meetings with managers). A motivational factor in getting technicians to perform at a higher level might be to associate incremental skillset development with promotions and pay raises. This both recognizes and rewards improvements in performance. The type of program that I advocate and describe here is called a "Career Ladder," where several levels (usually three to four) are established for level of competency and goal attainment. Names can be associated with each level, such as generalist for entry-level training and specialist for higher-level training. Splitting generalist and specialist into more discreet levels, such as generalist 1/2/3, allows for more incentives in attaining higher levels of performance.

Generally, people who are personable and smart enough to "wow" you in an interview are capable enough to do the job. It is usually a matter of attitude and the ability to get along with others that needs to be addressed. If this behavior is not displayed until after the orientation period, managers should involve HR to determine if the probationary period can be extended and make it clear to the new employees that they must meet performance expectations within a given time period to retain employment.

NEW LEADER ADVICE

It is important for Sally to make sure that the complaints she has heard are factual. Then she needs to gather documentation of what has been done to help Barry get settled into his new environment and review his orientation program. Does he need to go back and redo some areas of training? She should talk with some of Barry's coworkers to see if they specifically know what may be slowing Barry down. After gathering information and reviewing his orientation program, Sally should schedule a meeting with Barry and reaffirm his job expectations (e.g., completing work in a timely manner).

What I have found to be successful

A technique called behavior interviewing can be extremely helpful in the hiring process. This employment screening technique allows potential employees to provide examples of how they may have handled different situations in their past, which helps to predict the types of behavior they will display in future situations. This technique is not fail safe, but it does allow interviewers to have a better understanding of the people they may be hiring. In addition to behavior interviewing, administering a basic math test and behavioral assessment allows departments to make sure they are getting the most qualified candidates, which is particularly important with the technician staff as there is no standard licensure for them.

One of the things I have heard my staff say repeatedly is that we need a better training program. During the first year in my job, I spent a lot of time working on that. It is still not perfect, but I have worked with my tech supervisors to standardize the way they do new employee orientation and training. We had found that many of our new tech hires had no pharmacy or hospital experience so we elected to have them spend their first week just shadowing in the pharmacy department. We have found that this allows the new hires to have a better picture of how the department is integrated and how their job impacts others who are working in various positions. Because the training is standardized, new hires also have set competencies that they need to complete before moving on to another area of training. Most of the training is hands-on training, but the new hires and their trainers have a set document that they follow to make sure the new hires are able to do the routine activities in the area that they are training in.

Most people are competent while they are in training and pass all of their required competencies. It is typically after the initial training period that you start to see where they may cut corners in their work or test the system. In dealing with these types of individuals and my HR department, I have been routinely recommended to counsel these employees and reset expectations. I have also found that while doing this, it is beneficial to the employee and myself to have a written action plan detailing the necessary steps the employee must accomplish to meet expectations (e.g., job requirements) as well as deadlines by which the employee must complete these items. Having a written plan allows employees to take it with them after they leave the meeting, and it is a good reference tool for managers to keep in case further issues arise.

CASE 4.6

Recognizing the fit of an individual to the department or organization

PRINCIPLE ■ When to "try and try again" versus "cutting bait"

Adam is a new manager in a hospital pharmacy. He has been on the job for 3 months and his manager just informed him that two new technician positions have been approved and are available for recruiting and hiring. Adam and his technician supervisors identify and hire two technicians. They are very excited as both of these individuals had prior pharmacy experience and seem genuinely happy to be working in the department, which has thorough orientation training for new hires. The new employees, Jim and Kate, spend their first week shadowing each of the various positions in the department so as to have a better understanding of the department as a whole. After that, they start training in one of the five different areas in the department. As Jim and Kate become competent in one area, they move on to training in other areas of the department. The cross-training allows for more flexibility from a scheduling standpoint, but it also allows them to move up the career ladder, which is associated with a pay increase.

Jim and Kate are fitting in nicely into the department. Each has passed their first area of training and is now staffing these areas by themselves. After 2 weeks of staffing, Adam starts to hear grumblings from other technicians about the poor performance of Jim. The complaints range from Jim not completing his assigned tasks by the end of the shift to Jim disappearing for periods of time with no explanation. Adam himself catches Jim clocking in one day and then sees him spend the next 15–20 minutes moving soda into his locker. Adam is also aware that the technician supervisors spent some time talking with Jim about his performance, apparently to no avail.

Adam decides to consult with the hospital's HR department to see what they recommend. Jane, an HR representative, suggests that Jim be placed on an action plan with very specific goals related to his job and strict timelines for accomplishing the goals. Adam takes Jane's advice and places Jim on an action plan, which had four goals and a month to accomplish those goals. However, 6 weeks later Adam is still hearing intermittent complaints about Jim's performance. He is unsure how to proceed.

WHAT ADAM MAY BE THINKING...

- How did I not pick up on such a poor performer during the interview?
- Why does Jim not want to complete his work?
- How could I have hired someone like this?
- Since Jim is still in his provisional period, can I just say things aren't working out?

ON THE OTHER HAND, ADAM MIGHT REASON...

- Maybe Jim doesn't like working in that one particular area. I'm sure he will improve once he starts training in a new area.
- Jim is such a personable person and everyone enjoys talking with him. Maybe this role isn't a good fit for him.
- I'm sure Jim doesn't realize how things work in this particular pharmacy. I will have to reset expectations with him.

MENTOR ADVICE

Adam will encounter many situations like this, which formal management and leadership training may not address. As the manager, Adam should develop an action plan that establishes clear and attainable goals, and there should be mutual agreement upfront. A key component of an action plan is followup. It is important to have frequent meetings during this time period, generally weekly, to assess Jim's progress. During this period, Jim's performance may improve with focused coaching.

Adam needs to delegate at least 80% of the orientation process to the technician supervisors. It is important that the supervisors be involved in the hiring process, the orientation period, and throughout the weekly followup meetings for the action plan. The technician supervisor role is an important relationship and should not be usurped or circumvented.

During the action plan period, Adam must assess whether or not Jim wants to stay in his job. Jim may feel that the job is not the right fit and may provide some indication of where this situation will end up in a very short period of time. Or Jim may not have the capability to perform the tasks required or possess the work ethic required. In this case, no amount of remedial support will salvage his employment as a pharmacy technician. The key here is for Adam to know when it is time to keep Jim and continue to train him or when it is time to terminate his employment.

What I have found to be successful

In my experience, it becomes apparent after an action plan is implemented whether or not to "continue trying or cut bait." Generally, within 1–2 weeks there will be marked improvement. If there is even moderate improvement it is probably worth trying, but if during the orientation period there are signs of deterioration of performance or no improvement at all within a week or two then it probably will not work out. A thorough assessment using an action plan may take 6 weeks to 3 months, but after that if there is no improvement then it is time to "cut bait" and consider termination. Knowing when to continue trying and mentoring or when to call it quits is not always a clear-cut process. One bit of advice is that as you develop as a manager, you begin to get a sense of what will work and what will not work.

The better the hiring process, the less the latter scenario needs to be played out. Determine the success factors for a job at the time that the job is created and prior to posting and recruitment. Develop a structured set of questions as well as key indicators of candidates' potential to perform the job successfully (i.e., their work ethic and organizational fit). Employing a process called "behavioral interviewing" is helpful in assessing and determining the applicants' chances of success by getting them to describe how they behave in certain circumstances. These interview tools enhance the hiring process, and for the most part they are very effective in selecting employees with the desired characteristics and traits; nevertheless, mistakes do happen. The key is to minimize these mistakes as there is nothing worse than a bad hire. It wastes time and is costly in many ways for the department and the organization.

Again, the best time to assess "organizational fit" is during the interview process. But sometimes this is not enough, and the orientation period is the second chance to assess, motivate, and determine if a long-term relationship can continue between employee and employer. A good fit is best for both parties—it produces a more satisfied employee and a far better quality of service.

NEW LEADER ADVICE

Adam must focus on resetting expectations first because Jim needs to understand how his performance impacts the rest of the department. Adam should also work closely with his HR department. Jim may be one of those employees who takes awhile in understanding what it is he needs to do; therefore, he may be on a couple of action plans before he gets it so Adam shouldn't get discouraged because the action plan does not work immediately. It can take 30+ days before a habit becomes a habit. If Jim was not practicing his action plan on a daily basis, it would make things more difficult for him to develop the habits the department is wanting. Adam should give Jim the benefit of the doubt because Jim is still relatively new to the department and may still be finding his way around. However, if Jim continues to remain on an action plan and there is no improvement, then it may be time for Adam to consider letting him go.

What I have found to be successful

I have found that many times people do not intentionally set out to perform poorly. If you have data that compares the work of the individual in question to others in the department, it is eye opening for them to see how they compare to their peers. By having objective data, it can take the conversation away from a negative, punishment type of conversation to one of positivity and assistance. For example, you could start the conversation out with "It appears to me that you are struggling to meet x, y, and z. Let's talk about why it is important to meet those goals and how I can help you meet them." Typically, after such a type of conversation, you will see the employee make attempts at correcting his or her behavior.

If you are in a situation where you repeat conversations with an individual about their performance, don't jump to conclusions. In my experience I have found that sometimes individuals are responsible for the problem, and sometimes they are not. It is very important for you to refrain from jumping to conclusions before you know the whole story. Obtaining all sides of the story is really important because you may be the point person to receive all of the complaints from other staff members. Wanting to assist those people should not take precedence over getting all of the information possible especially from the person in question before moving forward. Individuals who made the mistake often reason they were not able to meet expectations because the system was not designed to allow them to do so. In quite a few instances, those individuals were correct. So, instead of working with them to correct their behavior, I focus on correcting the system.

There is a fine line between coaching someone to meet expectations and deciding to let someone go. If you have had multiple conversations with someone about their performance and possibly put them on an action plan (see Case 4.5), you may need to think about letting them go. Letting someone go is never easy; however, I have found that I typically spend more time and energy following up and making sure this individual is doing their work correctly than I do focusing on the other important items that are required for my job. In struggling to find this balance, some of my mentors have told me that I should not spend more time and energy in making someone successful at their job than they are willing to spend. After reflecting on this and having excused people based on their performance, it amazes me what a difference moving this person out of the department has made. You can see an almost immediate impact on the morale of the other staff because the negativity, frustrations, and complaints associated with the individual are no longer present.

CASE 4.7

Working with individuals who do not take initiative and rely on you for productivity

PRINCIPLE ■ Emphasizing the importance of individual contributions to the team

Seth has been an operations manager at the Uppers Pharmacy for a year and a half. He completed pharmacy school and PGY-1 and PGY-2 residencies before taking this job. Having come from a different organization than the one he is currently at, Seth has been full of new ideas on ways to improve operational efficiency and has slowly been making the changes within the department. On numerous occasions, Seth has had to work with his coworker, Jen, to implement the changes (Jen oversees personnel who are impacted by the changes). Seth's latest idea for operational efficiency will impact Jen's direct reports; therefore, he set up a meeting to discuss the changes that need to be made with her. Jen agrees that the changes are necessary and in fact states that she is thinking about making changes to her areas and that this would fit right in with the changes she wants to make.

Seth was pleasantly surprised to get such quick collaboration from Jen because in the past, he was always having issues with her. Jen would routinely overstep her bounds and make decisions that would impact Seth's areas without discussing the issue with Seth first. Seth would often have to counteract the decisions that were being made because the staffing was not adequate to handle the decision or the decision was not based on complete information. After dealing with a couple of these incidents, Seth decided to have a "crucial conversation" with Jen about her behavior. When this conversation took place, Jen seemed to down play her role in the decisions and didn't seem to think this was a big deal at all. Frustrated, Seth brought this behavior up with his manager as he was unsure of what to do next.

At the next administrative meeting the following week, Seth was surprised to hear Jen talking about changes "she" was going to make to her areas. What surprised Seth the most was the fact Jen was bringing up ideas that Seth had come up with as if they were her own and was not acknowledging Seth's contribution at all. Given all the recent history with Jen, Seth was at a complete loss for words at seeing this behavior played out in front of the entire administrative staff.

WHAT SETH MAY BE THINKING...

- The entire department works in a team-like fashion, why won't Jen acknowledge my role in the upcoming change?
- How can I bring up my contribution to this project without seeming like I am whining about not being included?
- I don't understand why Jen is always using my areas/ideas as a means to make herself look better.

ON THE OTHER HAND, SETH MIGHT REASON...

- Clearly, my communication style is not working with Jen. How can I change it so that we can operate in a more team-like fashion?
- Maybe I should run things by my boss before I deal with Jen? Although this seems like it will slow everyone's productivity down.
- Maybe Jen didn't realize what she has done. I wonder if I should have another conversation with her letting her know how I feel?

MENTOR ADVICE

It is always difficult dealing with people that are not forthright and honest. Although Seth's department seems to demonstrate some teamwork, there is obviously something lacking within the team, which is a significant sign of a dysfunctional team. What is lacking is trust. Unfortunately, this is all too common among teams, and there are some measures Seth can take to try to improve things.

Seth has been communicating with his colleague on a professional level, so he is frustrated to find out that he has been undermined in such a fashion. He should take this in stride and try to remain professional in his dealings with Jen in the future. Jen may not be the traditional slacker, but she is taking credit for his ideas. It is important to healthy teamwork that Seth's individual contributions be recognized, as diversity of thought and respect for each others' differences are an important element to high performing teams. Seth needs to talk directly with Jen about this, but he may need to go back to his manager again who could suggest some motivational tools. Taking credit for someone else's idea is a type of plagiarism. The sad part about this scenario is that it happens all too often. The people who try to take credit for other people's work do not realize the damage they do to their own integrity and how much it affects their reputation and their workplace because it builds an environment based on lack of trust. All Jen had to do was acknowledge Seth as the brainstormer. This would have created strong working bonds as people feel good when they are publicly praised or credited with some good deed or work. Without trust, teams cannot be functional.

As the operations manager, Seth needs to step in and redirect this behavior. Seth could suggest some teambuilding exercises and hold some frank discussions with the team about what teamwork means (generally, the cooperative effort by the members of a group to achieve a common goal). Teambuilding takes time. It doesn't happen overnight or by chance; it takes the desire to want to be a team; and it takes hard work. Sometimes it even requires a change of team members.

Seth should develop employee goals that must be achieved within a set timeframe. An acronym that can help with this is SMART:

- **S**pecific
- **M**easurable
- **A**ttainable
- **R**ealistic
- **T**imely

Seth needs to be sure that the goals he sets up are mutual. In some cases there is no room for negotiation (e.g., competency standards, regulatory requirements), but in other cases accommodations can be made to help employees perform at a higher level. Seth should make sure that he doesn't set up any unfair standards, as the rest of the staff will notice and may take advantage of this or begin to feel resentful.

Moving Jen, a poor performing employee, to a satisfactory level of performance is a desired goal. In order to do this, Seth must have some metrics in place. Expected levels of competency must be established; adequate and thorough training must be incorporated into the orientation process; and performance must be routinely assessed with a feedback loop to the employee. Motivational factors are required at this stage to encourage the employee to want to move to the next level. Seth should not make this a threatening experience, but rather a coaching process. This is where reward and recognition are effective tools in moving the individual's quality of work to a higher level.

Rewards come in many forms. They can be immediate, simple, or they can be more planned and complex (e.g., organizationally sanctioned or departmentally created). Seth could pass out "hero cards" or "wow cards, which are used as a form of peer recognition. Anyone in the organization can recognize anyone else if they see a positive behavior that the organization wants emulated and propagated. This form of positive reinforcement is very effective. Seth uses the cards to recognize a team member that went above and beyond for their teammates—helping out in a staffing crunch or going out of their way to make sure a patient receives their medication. The downside of this type of reward program is that it can be overused. Seth needs to be careful not to dilute the meaning by giving cards out without significant reason or meaning behind them; if this happens, the staff may begin to feel that the cards are worthless and have no significant value attached to them. To prevent this from happening, Seth could turn the card into the cafeteria for a nominal monetary value for a beverage or treat.

Another type of reward is the "spot award"—Seth awards an employee on the spot for a good deed or stellar performance. Spot awards can be $5 to $25 gift cards for coffee stores, restaurants, bookstores, etc. Seth should include a personal note with the gift card as people will really appreciate the note and recognition. Seth could also initiate a standard monetary reward (a bonus would be paid out at the end of the year for those with high level performance standards) or a peer recognition award (acknowledged at special group meeting or event).

All these forms of recognition are useful, but Seth should use them wisely. The meaning gets lost in translation sometimes when they are passed out too frequently. The biggest problem is when they have the opposite effect than what is intended, such as when staff members get jealous of those being recognized and begin to act out by ostracizing the rewarded staff member or putting negative peer pressure on them.

Finally, Seth needs to examine his own communication style to assure that he is clearly communicating with coworkers. He needs to talk with Jen first before going to his manager for help (reserve this for a secondary solution if the first one is not effective). Talking with the manager may help him get some guidance, but at some point he needs to address this directly with Jen. If Jen has any integrity at all, she will see that stealing his ideas is unethical and ultimately affects the team and her future career.

What I have found to be successful

Consider generational differences when approaching a leadership issue. Sometimes people you are interacting with may just have differences in communication styles or in views based on their training. Or they may have biases in how they view issues based on their years of experience or the era they were brought up in. Consider ethnic differences. Sometimes it is hard to know what will be viewed as acceptable and what might be offensive. It is often necessary to just observe and try to communicate in order to better understand each other. Try to be clear and direct in your communication with the "Eeyores." If needed, backup your verbal communications with a written document or e-mail. Remember motivational tools and performance management processes when encouraging others to contribute to the team.

Provide recognition and staff rewards to reinforce positive behaviors (e.g., peer recognition, public praise).

- -

NEW LEADER ADVICE

Seth should pull Jen aside one more time immediately following the meeting where Jen took credit for Seth's idea. It is very important to address the issues as they arise instead of waiting until later. It is important for Seth to point out 1) how he feels when Jen does this type of activity and 2) the impact it is having on his ability to work as a teammate with Jen.

Seth should understand that confronting a peer is one of the most difficult things to do. However, it is important for Seth to make Jen aware of her behavior so that she can work on correcting it. It is also important that Seth find the balance between standing up for oneself and letting the "little things" slide. Seth should not be "criticizing" or "complaining" so much about Jen that people tend to ignore him when he speaks about her similar to the story of the little boy who cried wolf. Projects that are team-based where both parties are active participants in the completion of the project are an example of when Seth should stand up for himself. When this is the case, both parties should recognize the other on a job well done and their contributions to the project.

Lastly, Seth should keep in mind that regardless of his differences with Jen, their ultimate goal is taking care of patients. He should not let their differences get in the way of taking care of patients. It is important for both parties to keep this in the forefront when dealing with these types of issues.

What I have found to be successful

I have found that honest communication in these situations always works best. Similar to what Seth did during his first issue with Jen, I have found openly talking about this issue makes me feel better and assists the other person in seeing my point of view. Sometimes the issue is a simple miscommunication and can be instantly resolved. Other times, I have found this is not the case. If the situation continues, I would definitely open the lines of communication with your superior and the other individual's superior. It is especially important for your manager to know what struggles you are having because just as you are trying to find ways to motivate others, your boss is also trying to make sure you stay motivated in your job.

You need to understand the difference between work complaining and bringing up true concerns. You can walk into any lunchroom and hear such complaints as "I can't believe they're making us do this" or "That new process won't work." In providing honest feedback, you are bringing up true concerns and not just complaining; however, if you are always bringing up the work complaints, others will find it difficult to believe in you when you do have a true concern (e.g., the little boy who cried wolf).

In situations like this, I have found that it is vital to understand the other person's motivational triggers before tackling the problem head on. If you do not understand the other person's motivational triggers, you will never be able to understand why you are seeing a particular type of behavior. For some people, their motivational trigger may be networking with others, being involved in lots of projects, and enjoying working on new things. If these triggers conflict with a project you and the other person may be working on, you may experience some problems. The best way to understand another person's motivational triggers is through developing relationships. It is the best way to really know someone you work with. Seeing that we spend the majority of our time at work, it behooves anyone in a leadership position to cultivate as many relationships as possible.

One of the areas that many new leaders struggle is in communication. It is such an easy concept, yet it is probably one of the ones that is most difficult to excel at even if you are a veteran. Most problems that arise are usually the result of miscommunication. One of the reasons for this is because both individuals may not understand the other's communication style. Any leader should feel comfortable enough to approach others and say "I work best when others communicate to me in this fashion," and to ask the other person how they prefer to be communicated to. It is not easy, but it can help to dispel further communication issues.

Summary

As a new leader, you will need to build a toolkit filled with motivational techniques. This chapter discusses the numerous ways that employees may be motivated toward high performance as well as the benefits, potential risks, and pitfalls. Seven leadership case studies are examined in detail with key concepts compared and contrasted. The importance of effective communication in motivating individuals and teams cannot be overemphasized.

The benefits of teamwork and the difficulties of teambuilding are discussed in the context of motivating teams to higher performance levels. External influences and relationship building are explored with reference to achieving positive outcomes. Development of the leadership skillset to motivate both individuals and teams toward high performance and quality is viewed from both the perspective of the new leader and from a veteran mentor.

Leadership Pearls

- Look for opportunities to take the initiative on a project, in an organization, etc.—no matter how small or large the project/situation is even if it means you have to volunteer.

- Relationship building is critical in all leadership positions especially when you need those relationships to move others in the right direction.

- You will be more successful in getting others to "buy in" to your vision if you include them in designing the vision to begin with.

- It is important to set clear expectations with those you lead and to reset those expectations periodically if the situation warrants it.

- Remember the importance of reward and recognition in motivating those you lead.

Leadership Exercises

- Brainstorm ways in which you can lead by example in your school, workplace, or professional organizations.

- Describe a situation where you can show your leadership in a formal or informal role.

- Think of a time when you were asked to lead a project when others on the team were not interested in contributing. Describe two ways to get them involved.

- Imagine a situation where people around you are negative. Describe two ways that might foster a more positive environment.

- Identify three ways you can work collaboratively with teammates toward your department or organization's vision.

- Describe three ways to work "collaboratively" to get programs implemented.

- Describe a situation where coaching would be a better approach to disciplinary action.

- Define three ways a poor performer can affect teambuilding.

- At this time address any potential pitfalls in your orientation and training modules for your school/department/organization.

- Describe the benefits and potential pitfalls of a rewards and recognition program.

VETERAN MENTOR PROFILE

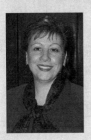

Roberta M. Barber, PharmD, MPH
Assistant Vice President of Pharmacy Services
Virtua Health System
Marlton, New Jersey
Adjunct Associate Professor of Clinical
   Pharmacy
Philadelphia College of Pharmacy
University of the Sciences in Philadelphia
Philadelphia, Pennsylvania

Why did you decide on a career in leadership? I serendipitously landed a management role at a small, New York hospital. I had some very difficult learning experiences and it look me years to learn to be a good leader and I'm still learning every day. I've always taken the opportunity to lead whether or not it was in a formal leadership position or as an informal leader in my area of strength. I have always enjoyed the challenges associated with leadership. Successfully guiding others who are passionate about pharmacy, advancing their careers, and helping the team work toward common goals doesn't happen overnight.

Where do you turn for advice when you are stressed? When I'm stressed I turn to trusted, more experienced and senior colleagues. I have leaned on my mentors during difficult times. You really need to be careful who you turn to for advice. I've found that it always helps to approach things in a trusted and positive way versus complaining. It's also been good to have a formal coach within the organization you work who can provide honest advice. Finding a trusted mentor is like finding gold. It doesn't happen very often so try not to abuse the relationship. I also turn to the literature for expert opinions. There are some great articles that stand out as gold standards when you are having issues.

What is your favorite leadership book? *The Leadership Challenge, 3rd Edition,* by James M. Kouzes and Barry Z. Posner; *The Art of Possibility: Transforming Professional and Personal Life* by Rosamund Stone Zander and Benjamin Zander.

From your perspective, what is the most important issue facing pharmacy leadership today? The biggest issue today is the leadership void. Pharmacists in the C-Suite are necessary to advance the profession. Also, from the health-system perspective, a priority area is how pharmacy is viewed by the rest of the hospital. Solid relationships with nursing and physicians are essential.

Looking back over your vast experience in pharmacy, what one to two things do you know now that you wish you would have known as a student and new practitioner? I wish I had obtained an advanced degree earlier on in my career. Also, politics can get in the way of good service, but it's a necessary evil; thus, I wish I knew how to influence an organization's capacity to function and peoples' capacity to lead.

What is your best advice for a new pharmacist today? Learn as much as you can. Take things slow and steady. Stay the course and don't try to get ahead of yourself.

How do you envision this publication assisting student and new practitioner leaders? This book will be an excellent guide to handle difficult situations. It is really a wealth of knowledge on practical issues from experienced, seasoned practitioners. It will also help to know that you are not alone in your experiences and that your colleagues are facing the same struggles every day.

NEW PRACTITIONER PROFILE

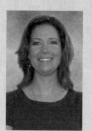

Staci A. Hermann, MS, PharmD
Pharmacy Manager, Informatics and
   Automation
The University of Kansas Hospital
Kansas City, Kansas

Why pharmacy: In high school, I had the opportunity to shadow a pharmacist and was impressed by her knowledge and passion for patient care. In addition, I saw her interact with other healthcare professionals to achieve the best outcome for her patients. Seeing those examples, I felt I also wanted to be a part of having such a positive impact on patients' lives.

Advice to readers: I would encourage students to get more exposure to leadership opportunities, informatics, and system process topics while in school. Understanding these topics is crucial for any practitioner to be successful. I would also encourage students to increase their involvement with professional organizations at the student level so you can meet people and be exposed to new ideas/hot topics. Once in practice participate in local, state, and national organizations because there is a minimal time commitment, and it provides tremendous payoffs such as learning what types of systems are available in various health systems and what the hot professional topics are so you are in the forefront of what's happening. Select your first job where people will help you grow and mature. And remember, "Rome wasn't built in a day" or in other words things will not necessarily change so you need to have patience.

Tips for work-life balance: I would encourage everyone to employ the "roles" concept from Stephen R. Covey's *First Things First* book to organize your time. In addition, try and work for people who also apply this concept, and try to have a good work-life balance.

Personal career: My best career decision so far has been my first leadership job because the people I work with are very supportive and are assisting me to grow as a professional and as a leader. Looking back, the major value of my residencies has been the connections I have made, the skillsets in learning how to process information to make the best decision possible for staff and for patients, exposure to what is possible, and understanding that not knowing everything is "okay." My major successes so far have been being active in ASHP and UHC (University Health System Consortium), seeing my staff grow over time and having others appreciate dealing with the "dead wood." My career goal is optimizing systems and integrating informatics with operations and safety while utilizing other disciplines such as human factors. Career success for me is to be challenged daily, looking at innovative processes, and taking things to the next level.

Why leadership: My interest in leadership was sparked by my dean, who saw leadership qualities in me and encouraged me to explore residencies. My favorite leadership books are *Crucial Conversations: Tools for Talking When Stakes are High* by Kerry Patterson, Joseph Grenny, Ron McMillan, et al., and *First Things First* by Steven R. Covey, A. Roger Merrill, and Rebecca R. Merrill.

Recommended change for pharmacy: I would like to see one national pharmacy voice like the the American Medical Association (AMA) that speaks for all of us.

Using this book: I feel this book's variety of different scenarios makes it applicable for many different individuals because of the principles and key points discussed.

Reference

1. *Webster's New College Dictionary, Third Edition.* Orlando, FL: Houghton Mifflin Harcourt; April 2008.

Suggested Additional Readings

Goldman D, McKee A, Boyatzis RE. *Primal Leadership: Realizing the Power of Emotional Intelligence.* Boston, MA: Harvard Business Press; 2002.

Patterson K, Grenny J, McMillan R, et al. *Crucial Conversations: Tools for Talking When Stakes are High.* New York, NY: McGraw Hill; 2002.

Wagner R, Harter JK. *12: The Elements of Great Managing.* Washington, DC: Gallup Press; 2006.

Additional Materials

Some Keys To Motivating Others

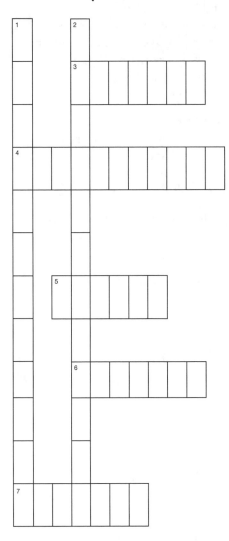

ACROSS

3. Stubborn coworker

4. Hold people _____

5. Have others contribute to the _____

6. Lead by _____

7. Share with your coworkers

DOWN

1. Personally getting to know people builds _____

2. Individual contributions should be _____

Read "Success Skills" article 5.

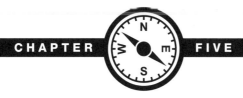

CHAPTER FIVE

Communication

Lindsey R. Kelley, PharmD, MS; Karol Wollenburg, MS, RPh

Introduction

Regardless of the practice setting or the position that pharmacists hold within an organization, good communication skills are crucial to their success as pharmacy practitioners and their effectiveness as leaders. Whether medications are being discussed with patients, plans of care with patient care teams, or new projects with members of senior management, the ability to communicate effectively is a major determinant in their ability to reduce fear, develop trust, and engage others. Compelling words and actions are required to achieve the very essence of leadership—building the commitment of others to apply their talents and skills toward a common vision.

There are many facets of communication that are important to pharmacists as they grow in leadership roles—some obvious and others more subtle. This chapter will focus on components of communication that may not be intuitive to the new practitioner. Skills required for these components of communication are often more challenging and require planning, practice, self-control, and reflection. The principles inherent in the case discussions are described below.

- **Tailoring a message to an audience.** The ability to adapt communication about a specific topic to different audiences is an important strategic skill for pharmacists to master. Just as a discharge medication list would be communicated differently to a patient than it would be to a physician, information about projects and other issues are most effective when the needs and interests of the targeted audience are carefully factored into the communication.

  Communication is most effective when the message is clear. Developing a core message that elucidates the purpose and goals of a project or initiative is an important first step that is often overlooked. This core message would be the same for any audience and may be as simple as, "In order to improve medication safety for our patients, in July, 2010, we are going to implement a bedside bar-coding system." When appropriate, it is helpful to include messaging on how the project or initiative relates to the mission, vision, or goals of the organization or group. Once the core message is clear, one can begin planning how the message could be developed for communication to different audiences, individuals, or settings. To plan a focused communication, there are numerous issues to consider.

  Whether the communication is a meeting, presentation, or written document, the purpose, goals, and desired outcomes of the communication should be clarified before work begins. Is the purpose of the communication to create awareness or provide details? Is the communication intended to push information out or to illicit feedback?

  Gaining information about the targeted audience is also important in order to adapt the message to meet the expectations and needs of the audience. Their baseline knowledge about the subject, including the knowledge range that might be expected within that group, is an important factor to consider. The timing of the presentation can also play a role in how information will be perceived. What might the emotional climate of the audience be when the presentation will be made? What might the attention span of this audience on this topic be? Characteristics such as age, gender, reading ability, health literacy, and language barriers should all be considered, especially when a presentation is made to individuals who are not part of the healthcare team.

Once purpose and audience as well as baseline informational understanding are known, one can begin consideration of how the style, format, and content of the communication might best be tailored to a particular group. What information does this specific audience need to know in order for the purpose of your presentation to be met? What materials and presentation style will best meet the goals of the communication? What combination of verbal, written, and visual materials will be most helpful for this audience? What balance of information will be needed, based on their knowledge base, to stay within the limitations of their attention span? How much time should be allowed for questions? Finance people are going to want to understand the numbers. Vice presidents (VPs) are usually interested in financial issues as well as ensuring that the benefits (such as enhancing patient care) will outweigh the risks. A condensed version of the project is usually best received by VPs. Project partners, such as nursing, will want confirmation that their needs will be met and that no new issues will arise for them. Pharmacy staff will want to know if the anticipated changes will really improve care and what the project means to them in terms of their ability to perform their job. They may also be concerned about job security or other issues that could affect them personally. Pharmacy staff is likely to want details. To best get the attention and support of any of these groups, communication must be concise and formulated to address their specific concerns in a way that they can easily comprehend.

An effective way to communicate with staff and team members is to include them in the planning process of projects so that their voice is included in decisions. This gives them a better understanding of the project, greater ownership, and provides more time for them to adjust to change. Including them in the detail stages may seem difficult at first, but in the end, it is usually a very effective strategy.

When individuals are involved, skilled communicators will also contemplate the preferences and needs of a particular individual. Some bosses prefer concepts on paper. Others prefer discussing the same issues at a meeting and will never look at paper. Some staff members need to have the big picture explained verbally so that they can intuitively understand the steps. Other staff may need the steps spelled out in a written document with flowcharts or bulleted lists before they can support the idea or process. Timing can also be important. Trying to get "buy in" from others, at a time when they may be in a bad mood or distracted by other issues, may not be prudent.

The value of focused and strategic communication is that it provides the information needed or desired by the listener in a format that is helpful to or preferred by them. An added benefit is that the effort expended to include others and to adapt the message to their needs helps to build important partnerships. These partnerships will likely be helpful when the next interaction occurs (on the same or a different topic).

- **The value of listening.** Listening is an essential component of communication that is often overlooked or undervalued. Listening provides an opportunity to understand and consider the facts and feelings expressed by others as one's own opinions, feelings, and plans are formed. It also enables the listener to consider information learned and adapt ensuing communication to be more appropriate for that person or audience. Perhaps most importantly, when sincere, listening can convey that the feelings and thoughts of the individual or audience are valued. This helps to build long-term relationships, which are valuable when the support of these individuals or groups is needed.

Listening is not a skill that comes easily to everyone. *It requires self control.* But it is a leadership skill that can be learned. All it takes is a belief in the value of listening, an understanding of some basic principles about when and how to listen, and practice. There are many subtleties to listening, including taking note of more than the spoken word. The tone, inflection, and volume of the words spoken provide obvious clues to the feelings of the speaker. The speaker's body language is another important cue to the emotional content of the communication. Leaning into the table may convey passion. Lack of eye contact may mean that the speaker is uncomfortable with talking to the listener. Things that are not said often add an important dimension for the listener to observe and consider. The ability to interpret these unspoken components of communication is a subtle, yet critical, component of effective listening.

When listening, awareness of one's own body language is crucial. Arms crossed may convey anger or a closed attitude. Looking out the window may convey lack of engagement. Leaning forward may convey intent listening. Response to what is being said is also important—not just a nod or "uh-huh," but actual engagement in the conversation. Showing interest or sympathy expresses concern for the individual. Staying calm during a heated communication conveys a willingness to listen, but also that the listener is not willing to engage in verbal warfare. Listening does not need to imply agreement with another individual. Instead, it can communicate respect for others by being willing to hear another person's feelings or point of view.

Asking questions can help to clarify issues, encourage the individual to express what has not been said, or communicate an issue one feels the individual should consider. "Did I hear you say…", "What do you think about…", or "Have you thought about…" are questions that might be asked to better understand what the individual is trying to communicate and to demonstrate an understand of their ideas and feelings.

Sensing when to listen is another important listening skill. Seeking input and understanding before talking conveys an interest in others' opinions and ideas. Even in instances when there may be a strong urge to talk about an issue, getting feedback from others first is often a wise strategy—testing the water is often helpful before jumping in!

Listening is an important means of taking in information from others about facts and emotions. If used effectively, it can be an invaluable way to build relationships by showing respect and value for others' ideas and feelings. That context is likely to be remembered and applied when these individuals listen to what is communicated in the future. It becomes a long-term investment in overall effective communication and relationships!

- **Giving, hearing, and responding to feedback.** Everyone wants their time at work to be pleasant, fulfilling, and even fun. Hard work and challenging situations can be endured and people can still feel uplifted if their work has purpose and if they feel good about their team members. On the contrary, when an individual feels that one of the members of their team is detracting from the success of their group, they may feel discouraged and unmotivated. For their well-being, the well-being of the team, and sometimes for the safety of patients, it is important to address conflict honestly and within a reasonable time frame so that the team can be steered back to a healthy state. Too often, conflict is not addressed or is handled inappropriately, resulting in heightened dysfunction within the workplace. Learning to address these issues in a productive manner is a great leadership skill that differentiates leaders from others.

When addressing concerns about the behavior of others, the outcome is often directly related to how diplomatically these issues are conveyed and discussed. Discussing the facts and not the character of the individual, careful timing, and listening are all important strategies to apply when constructively confronting another member of the team. In addition to addressing problematic issues, providing general feedback to individuals is crucial to their job satisfaction and success. Feedback provides an opportunity for team members to get a perspective on how others perceive their performance and allows them to make adjustments, grow, and improve. Positive feedback is uplifting and when offered sincerely and frequently, helps the individual to respond productively to suggestions about how they might do things better (constructive criticism). In the ideal world, feedback should be shared as close as possible to the time that the event or behavior occurred. This, however, is not always possible when the moment does not allow for a discussion or the setting is not appropriate. Periodic discussions provide an opportunity to speak to those missed opportunities and to summarize how the individual is doing and how they fit in. It is important to schedule feedback sessions at a place and time when both parties will have the time to engage in a meaningful dialogue.

The character of the feedback—such as whether it is formal or informal, spoken seriously or with humor, exchanged in private or public—will often depend on the personalities of the individuals involved. If feedback is being given, it is helpful to assess what type of delivery the other individual will respond most favorably to. An interactive dialogue regarding the feedback helps to ensure that both parties understand the perspective of the other. If communicated appropriately, feedback can be very helpful for the health and well being of the individuals involved and the organization.

Similarly, seeking and listening to feedback from others can provide insightful information about one's own performance. It can be helpful to get other's perspectives on what is working well with a team and what and how things might be improved. Listening and allowing others to express their point of view enables an honest dialogue and provides an opportunity for growth and improvement. Even when one may not agree with the feedback they receive, it is better to hear about and understand another's point of view than to try to address unrest that is not understood. As noted earlier, listening does not need to convey agreement, instead, it should convey an openness to listen and respect the other person's point of view. Thanking others for their feedback helps to keep lines of communication open.

While the diversity of human thought helps to drive progress and make our world an interesting and stimulating place to live, it can also result in different opinions and ideas that become the root of conflict. Often new ideas are appreciated. Even more often, people don't care about differences of opinions. When individuals or groups do care, they need to decide if a difference in opinion is one worth acting on. Is this issue one that is not too complicated and has the potential to be easily discussed? Is this issue worth risking partnerships and stability in order to have the differing opinion heard?

The art of successfully navigating conversations where there is not agreement with another party, especially when that individual has higher assigned authority, is often dependant on several strategic, yet sincere, practices. An individual, who has earned respect from others by being open to other's ideas and has allowed others to "win" in the past, is often seen as reasonable and willing to consider other people's ideas and opinions. In turn, others are often more willing to listen to and accept the point of view of this individual whom they have come to believe is fair. The ability to craft a discussion around common goals and remain objective during that discussion is another important skill.

Carefully thinking through the other person's point of view and preparing to respectfully address their concerns before the discussion ensues is a prudent exercise. Finally, staying open to the possibility that others might be right enables a more productive discussion and graceful conclusion, especially if you change your opinion during the discussion.

From the first greetings in the morning to the last partings in the evening, leaders use communication skills to make connections, build bridges, and develop ideas and people. By being thoughtful about the important role that effective communication plays in interactions and using it strategically and sincerely, ideas and projects can be moved forward and partnerships strengthened. Teams are motivated and inspired, and visions become a reality.

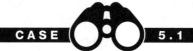

CASE 5.1

Adapting a message to a target audience

PRINCIPLE ■ Customizing a message for an audience

Becky is an accomplished pharmacist, researcher, and welcomed addition to the bariatric team. She just completed a pharmacy fellowship in internal medicine where she worked closely with surgeons evaluating absorption of medications after bariatric surgery. She has been in this current position a little under a year. The head of the bariatric surgery team, a physician, has asked her to step in and conduct the patient class next week.

All he had said in their brief initial conversation was that neither he nor his fellows were able to present the information and that he has been meaning to ask her to help change this presentation so that there is a greater focus on medication management in these classes. He felt comfortable with Becky's knowledge of the various procedures and was confident in her abilities to present the information. Additionally, he was excited to see how the patients felt about additional information on medication use both pre- and postprocedure. He did caution her, however, to make sure she kept it at the patient level; they had received poor evaluations in the past when guest presenters had not made the information both interesting as well as easy to understand. Since this was a referral business, and word of mouth was important, evaluations and patient perceptions were crucial.

Becky isn't new to giving presentations. She has given several. In fact, she was a professor at the medical school briefly in her previous job. But this was different. This wasn't her research—this was anatomy, physiology, pharmacology and this was for patients. Becky is meeting with him this afternoon one last time before he leaves the country.

WHAT BECKY MAY BE THINKING...

- How did I get myself into this?
- I'm not prepared and what if I fail?
- I can't believe I'm intimidated to talk to patients.
- Is this really a role for a pharmacist?
- How do I know how basic is too basic and when I've gone over their heads?

ON THE OTHER HAND, BECKY MIGHT REASON...

- This is a great opportunity to prove my communication and presentation skills.
- This physician really trusts my judgment.
- It is a pharmacist's role to breakdown ideas and treatments for patients.

- -

MENTOR ADVICE

Becky is prudent to set up a meeting with the surgeon familiar with the patient teaching programs in order to clarify the purpose of the classes she will be teaching as well as the characteristics of the people who will be attending the class. Are these patients who are considering surgery, patients who have decided to go forward with the surgery and need more detailed information about the surgery, or patients who have had surgery and are preparing for discharge? Is the material to be covered new to them or a refresher? If they are post-op, how many days post-op and what emotional states can she expect at this point in their recovery? Have they found it helpful in the past to use written materials to reinforce the critical content for patients after the presentation? Could she get a copy of the presentation that was used in the past and some idea of what he felt was helpful and what should be changed? Any information that Becky can obtain about this group of patients and what has worked best with similar audiences in the past will help her to adapt her content and style to produce a more successful presentation.

Changing her format and style of presentation may initially require a little effort on Becky's part, but it may also be fun to shift from her mode of a scientific presentation to one that is related to discussing bariatric surgery from the patient perspective. During her presentation, Becky should look for cues from the audience. If they look puzzled, she may be speaking above their level of understanding. If they look disinterested, they may either be lost or are already familiar with the material. Asking questions of the audience during the presentation related to their understanding and expectations could help her adapt the remainder of her presentation to their needs. The ability to adapt communication content and style to a specific audience is an important communication skill and one that can be developed with intentional and thoughtful questioning and practice. It is also a great opportunity for Becky to expand her scope of competencies and strengthen her role with the bariatric team.

What I have found to be successful

Whenever possible, organize your thoughts and materials in advance. I am amazed at the improvements I am able to make after I have let a presentation rest for a day or two. I also find it easier to find errors when I proofread a printed copy versus an online copy. It is often helpful to get feedback from appropriate individuals before and after preparation of your materials, especially if written or visual materials are used. Getting feedback on how your communication is perceived by others can be enlightening and provide an opportunity for you to improve it. Finally, practice your presentation aloud and make sure that you can complete it within the allotted time. Almost all audiences get restless when presentations go overtime. Practicing also helps to build confidence.

- -

NEW LEADER ADVICE

Being intimidated by a new audience and a new situation is normal. It is important that Becky not be too hard on herself for being intimidated by a patient audience. Even though patients are our primary concern as pharmacists, the idea of presenting to a large group of them can be overwhelming. There is great responsibility in making sure the patient understands the information so that they can be successful in their own use of medications. This is compounded, in this situation, by additional pressure from the physician group and a lack of information about the audience.

In a new or uncomfortable situation such as this, gathering more information about the patients, their needs, and their situations will immediately remove some of the pressure and fear. Practicing the presentation in front of a friend or peer can also help alleviate some of the intimidation and allow for feedback about unclear areas before the actual presentation. It will also build confidence to be comfortable with the information. Becky may want to anticipate questions from the audience and prepare answers ahead of time. Some topics may come up but may not have a place in the presentation. Preparing the topics ahead of time can allow Becky to gain additional comfort with related material, but it also decreases the chances of awkward moments during question and answer periods.

What I have found to be successful

Oftentimes, experienced presenters will begin to "wing it" or become comfortable with content and style, which results in few notes necessary and minimal preparation needed. Whenever adapting a routine message to a new audience, it can be helpful to gather input from multiple sources. Examples of ways to do this include preparing a handwritten outline with a list of anticipated questions or additional thoughts, making more notes than usual, reviewing the topic verbally with someone outside the healthcare field, or sending your slides to a colleague who can be trusted to give a fair and objective evaluation.

It can also be incredibly helpful to observe a colleague who presents to a similar audience. By observing what the audience is accustomed to seeing will allow you to prepare in a way that meets their presuppositions of how the material will be presented. This allows the audience to focus on the content and not the construct. It is also important to gather feedback from the audience after the presentation is over to evaluate any future areas for improvement.

Tailoring a message to accommodate individual needs and preferences

PRINCIPLE ■ Customizing a message for an individual

Luke is a new manager at a medium-sized community hospital. He has taken on a leadership role in the implementation of new automated distribution cabinets in the ambulatory surgery center (ASC). He is excited about the opportunity to utilize technology to provide better customer service to the ASC. Because of the expense, selling this project to senior management has been an ongoing struggle. Getting their approval for automation in the ASC was a big win, although most pharmacy staff is unaware of the work required to accomplish this.

This morning Luke met with the staff to review new operational changes and discuss upcoming plans. His head is reeling. There are so many details he shared with the staff, and he feels he did not go over everything. The new automated distribution cabinet process is scheduled to be implemented in 2 weeks. There will be changes to shift times, responsibilities, and working areas. It will also require many aspects of daily responsibilities to move and shift for both pharmacists and technicians. This will certainly be a big change for the staff, but if it works the way they anticipate they will see decreased patient wait times for their medications, not to mention the strides it will make with nursing relationships. As Luke left the staff meeting, he was stopped by a staff pharmacist who had been at the staff meeting and was very concerned about the new implementation and the accompanying changes. Luke agreed to meet with her when he returned from his next meeting.

As Luke stepped onto the elevator, he began to feel overwhelmed. There are so many things to do and he feels the success of the project is on his shoulders. He has to get the pharmacy staff to understand and get on board, and he has to start working through the details. He was in the middle of reviewing the details in his head when he was joined by the vice president responsible for pharmacy (a key champion in the move to get new cabinets and a definite big-picture thinker). Luke was caught off guard when the VP asked "So, how are the new cabinets in ASC looking?"

WHAT LUKE MAY BE THINKING...

■ I'm too distracted to do this right now.

■ What should I really tell the VP? How optimistic can I be?

■ There are so many moving pieces to this project.

■ What am I going to do with the concerned staff pharmacist?

ON THE OTHER HAND, LUKE MIGHT REASON...

■ This is a great opportunity to let the VP know we are grateful for the help.

■ I want to present a positive image for the project and my department.

■ This is a great time for me to explain all of the hard work that is going into these cabinets.

MENTOR ADVICE

With Luke's head spinning from the interactive staff meeting, he might easily slide into the details of the issues discussed at the staff meeting when he is asked about the project by the VP. The most effective way to respond, however, might be in terms of the issues that the VP has shown interest in or expressed concerns about in the past. Is the project on schedule? Is there any news, positive or negative, that the VP might want to know about? If so, Luke might give a brief summary based on issues he knows will be of interest to the VP. He might also ask the VP if he would like for the pharmacy team to meet with him for a briefing on the project or ask if he would like regular written updates.

The followup with the concerned staff member is *equally important*. Luke's suggestion that the two of them meet is a great strategy. He can then listen to and better understand this staff person's issues and address them to the best of his ability. Their discussion may help Luke decide if these concerns are specific to this individual or representative of the feelings of the larger group. He can then use this information to shape future communication. Luke should expect that several meetings will be required before staff members are comfortable with the proposed changes.

From a more general perspective, it appears that staff may not have been included in the planning process for this project and are now just learning about changes that will have a major impact on their work and their lives. In future projects, Luke should consider keeping all groups informed about projects and asking for staff input as a project is planned. This ensures that the valuable "front line" perspective of staff is factored into the decisions that are made. This also gives them more time to plan for and adjust to changes. Staff members are more likely to support a change that includes their input than one without their input. Luke is learning that in order to move projects forward, there can be numerous groups involved that have very different concerns. Astute leaders learn to adapt communication to all of these groups and to address their specific needs.

What I have found to be successful

Include staff members in the planning process whenever possible. This enables them to provide valuable input into decisions related to a project, develop a sense of ownership for the project, adjust to the idea of change over a longer period of time, and reduce anxiety when rollouts are implemented. When speaking to senior leadership, you must be brief and concise to be heard. Often, the less time you have to communicate your message, the more time it takes to prepare your communication.

NEW LEADER ADVICE

Even though Luke would love to consult a mentor before engaging in this conversation, he may not have time. Primary risk points for Luke are that he will either say too much or too little. It is important to communicate to the VP how everything is going, but as mentioned, giving too much detail is likely more information than the VP is really looking for. Transitioning from detail-oriented checklists and processes to the big picture gains for the project can be difficult. Letting go of a particular problem being processed (in this case the concerned pharmacist) can be hard as well. Sometimes getting out of our own heads can be the biggest barrier to successful conversation.

In this situation, Luke should focus on the big picture as much as possible—making a point to discuss deliverables (e.g., decreased nursing and ultimately patient wait times for medications). When he meets with the staff pharmacist, he should be very detail oriented (e.g., discuss workflow changes, how they will be managed, and what that will mean to the pharmacist's day-to-day work). It may be helpful to prepare documents ahead of time so that the pharmacist can visualize the changes while Luke is discussing them. It is important for Luke to engage the pharmacist on his own level and ask information-gathering questions. This will allow Luke to be sure he is addressing the right concerns.

What I have found to be successful

When working with projects where multiple parties have an investment, it is common that each party is interested in their own piece of the pie. To make tailoring messages easier, when working through project details, subconsciously assign each project component or detail to a bucket assigned to an individual party. For example, as a piece of interest to senior management is reviewed think to yourself, "this goes in the management bucket" and review the remainder of the details in that bucket. In doing this it allows quick transition from topic to topic when approached with a situation as described above. Additional components can then be added as they are discovered. Thus when approached by a stakeholder, begin with a simple statement about the progress of the project, and then discuss the appropriate bucket and tie it back to the stakeholder's priorities.

When confronted with a tense or unexpected conversation, focus on factual information. If a quick conversation with a mentor is not possible or you haven't had the chance to touch base to confirm direction, let the other person talk. This works especially well with peers and staff. Rather than answering with information that may be questionable, delve further into the concerns that are voiced. The additional information provided can then be used to identify means to alleviate mentioned concerns.

CASE 5.3

The importance of listening

PRINCIPLE ■ Listening skills

Diane is a new pharmacist working a central pharmacy shift. Even though she is new, she has taken initiative and been involved in a workgroup on building a new service. Diane currently works on the pharmacist piece and Levi leads the technician piece. Levi approaches Diane and asks if they could talk when she has a minute.

Diane and Levi have had their share of struggles implementing the new service. Technicians who weren't involved have been stirring the pot and grumbling. Every time technicians involved in the new service enter the central pharmacy, they are met with rolling eyes, questions about where they have been, and general disapproval (and it isn't just from other technicians). It is frustrating being undermined by people in their own department (not even considering the challenges with paradigm shifts in outside departments). Diane certainly sees why Levi might want to talk. Diane thinks to herself how perfect this is. Levi has really been getting under her skin lately, and this is the perfect opportunity to chat with him. Diane has issues she wants to discuss too—issues she feels are contributing to the struggles the service is facing. There have been reports of complaining and frustration about how the team is being led, and Levi is part of this grumbling group. The unrest and irritation have been heard by many—both on the floors and in central pharmacy. And Levi has been heard questioning Diane's vision multiple times, which upsets her.

Diane doesn't understand what is going wrong. She wants to question Levi's commitment to the project and tell him she is disappointed in his recent lack of professionalism. Additionally, she wants to say how she feels betrayed that her own teammate would sell her out to the rest of the staff, especially during this crucial time when they need the rest of the staff to support their cause. But should she?

Levi is an incredibly high-performing technician. He has already completed one degree and is working on his second, and he is usually very enthusiastic and is always looking for ways to improve any situation. Diane is really relying on him to help build the new service and wants his collaboration.

WHAT DIANE MAY BE THINKING...

- I can't wait to give him a piece of my mind.
- What is his problem?
- I can't believe he is undermining our project!
- He is not a team player.
- What has Levi done to enhance the project?

ON THE OTHER HAND, DIANE MIGHT REASON...

- How is this ever going to be successful?
- What am I doing wrong?
- Maybe I'm too new to be involved in such a big project.
- What clues did I miss?

- -

MENTOR ADVICE

Many of us can empathize with Diane's feelings of frustration and her strong urge to "set him straight." But Diane needs Levi as a partner in this project and setting him straight is not likely to produce effective results. Diane does not need Levi to just follow direction. She needs his support and "buy in." She needs to gain his respect and trust. Listening is an opportunity to help build her relationship with Levi. A more productive approach to this situation might be for Diane to test the waters and listen first to what Levi has to say. Perhaps the things she has heard are not true. Perhaps there are issues that Diane has not fully recognized or appreciated. Levi might even have helpful suggestions that Diane had not previously considered.

It may not be easy for Diane to listen when she has strong feelings herself. She will need to watch her body language and ensure that her facial expressions and body posture communicate that she respects and is interested in what Levi has to say. Repeating back what she thinks she has heard will help to ensure that she fully understands all the information she is processing. Asking questions can help Levi think through the issues and take greater responsibility for his ideas and opinions. On the other hand, jumping in too quickly with her issues may cause Levi to shut down, preventing her from hearing his concerns and losing an opportunity to build the trust and respect that she needs. After listening to Levi's concerns, Diane may then express her own thoughts and concerns. Another option is to set up another time when they can talk. This option reinforces that she really listened to and wants to give some thought to what Levi has to say. It also gives her the opportunity to think more carefully about how she can respectfully respond to his concerns and tailor her communication to him without being aggressive or defensive.

Diane has the opportunity to feel good about her self-control, her willingness to understand the issues, and her investment in her relationship with Levi. It is likely that Diane and Levi will need to work together in the future. People who trust and respect one another have more fun and are more likely to be successful than those who have not been heard, only do what they are told, and do not have passion for the greater vision.

What I have found to be successful

When I feel it is important to speak to someone with whom there might be disagreement, there are several strategies I have found to be helpful:

- Try to allow others to speak first. Once your opinion is expressed, you may never have the opportunity to hear what the other person was thinking or feeling.
- For situations where there may be conflict or emotionally charged issues, find a private place for the discussion. Choose a location that is not threatening to the individual. Privacy is usually important, but a setting outside of your office (which may be associated with authority) should also be considered.
- If there is considerable animosity toward you, you may want to consider asking a third person to sit in on the conversation.
- Whenever possible, select a time for the conversation that will allow adequate time to listen to the issue(s). Cutting a conversation short may convey that you are not interested in listening.
- When another person requests to speak to you about their concerns, try to schedule time for the conversation as soon as possible. Issues can fester if left unchecked and it is often helpful to get them out in the open as soon as possible so that misunderstandings can be addressed and solutions can be implemented. Conversely, if the speaker is so worked up that they cannot speak with some degree of civility, scheduling a meeting for a later time may allow the speaker the opportunity to enter into the conversation more calmly and rationally.

NEW LEADER ADVICE

Taking risk and investing in a project leaves anyone open to the chance for failure. This risk creates a dynamic where Diane is open for disappointment if the project doesn't go well. In this situation, frustration and concern can be expected. It is normal to want to communicate that frustration to her partner in the project, but Diane should be careful how she approaches the situation. Letting her emotion drive the interaction is likely to prevent Diane from concentrating on the facts and details and puts her at risk for directing the conversation toward Levi and not focusing on his behavior.

The other side of the coin is self-doubt. Self-doubt is common for all practitioners, but as a new practitioner Diane may feel a need to be the best and prove her knowledge. In this emotionally charged situation, the best thing she can do is take a minute. This can be done by finding a quiet place, such as a cafeteria or even the bathroom, and evaluating thoughtfully what the real issues are. This is also a great opportunity to seek out a mentor for advice.

Diane should find somewhere private and quiet where she and Levi can talk. It is important for Diane to let Levi know that this conversation is important to her and that she is not willing to be interrupted. The second crucial step is letting Levi tell his story first. This gives him the opportunity to answer some of the questions she may have had about his behavior without forcing a question. It also gives him some time to vent and Diane additional time to process and think about her response. The worst thing Diane can do is immediately launch into a tirade about all the ways Levi has let her down and put him in a defensive position.

What I have found to be successful

As stated above, it is very important to address conflicts quickly, respectfully, and as objectively as possible. When someone needs to talk, it is crucial to let them know that they are important. This can be done by prioritizing them in your day. If possible, rearrange meetings or tasks to take time to listen. It is also advantageous to leave busy times of the day open to allow for times when people want to "pop in." If meeting immediately isn't possible, then reschedule quickly. Remember, if you are emotionally charged, it is a good reason to reschedule. When engaged in a situation where there is potential for discord, such as a team member or peer wanting to talk, I suggest asking a simple question upfront that will save time and anxiety: "Before we begin, is this a problem you want me to solve or would you just like me to listen?" People sometimes just need to vent and many project leaders have an instinct to immediately begin the problem-solving process. By asking what is expected, it can save you from working on a problem you really just needed to listen to or wasting energy. The next question that makes a big difference is "have you already thought about how you would solve this or want this solved?" Many times those that desire a solution have already thought about it and will gladly tell you their ideas. It makes for easy partnership in solutions and a feeling that both of you are on the same page. When the conversation has come to a close, say "These are my next steps. Is this what you had in mind?"

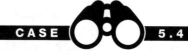

CASE 5.4

General approaches to feedback

PRINCIPLE ■ Feedback

Josh is excited to meet with the director of the department. He has just about completed his orientation and is meeting with his supervisor to go over all the required documentation and mandatory paperwork that had been completed during the last 3 months. The director has indicated that this would be a good time for the two of them to discuss feedback. In his short time with the department, Josh has seen the director regularly. He likes the way he communicates with staff and feels the staff appreciates it as well. There is a clear emphasis on communication and feedback from the staff.

Josh has been giving this meeting a great deal of thought. He has noticed many things during his short time with the company, and he is looking forward to getting a chance to ask questions and talk. There are many processes he thinks could be improved and several staff members he feels are way behind the times—something needs to be done about these things. Additionally, Josh can't remember anyone asking him about feedback, and he isn't sure what type of information he should prepare for the meeting. Would he even have a chance to talk about his observations?

WHAT JOSH MAY BE THINKING...

- There sure is a lot of opportunity for improvement.
- The staff here could benefit from my expertise.
- My boss needs to know how dangerous some of these processes/people are.
- This is a great time for me to learn my weaknesses and strengths.

ON THE OTHER HAND, JOSH MIGHT REASON...

- Who am I to tell someone else what to do?
- The director has so much experience and expertise. Why would he want my input?
- How do I even know what type of feedback I like?
- What if the director doesn't like to give feedback in the way I prefer? What if he thinks I am "high maintenance"?

MENTOR ADVICE

While it may be expected that a boss should regularly meet with a new employee to give and receive feedback, this standard is not always held to. Josh is fortunate to have a boss who has scheduled time to meet with him to discuss how things are going. He is even more fortunate that his boss is seeking input on how Josh would like to continue this dialogue as he grows with the organization. Assuming that his boss means two-way feedback, Josh should let his boss provide feedback first and wait until his boss opens the door for Josh to offer his opinions. Josh should ask clarifying questions to ensure he understands the feedback he is given.

When the door is open for Josh to share his insight, his comments should be clear and respectful. I would encourage him to start with the positive things he sees. When discussing the issues that he feels need improvement, he should try to steer the conversation to processes and systems. If he is having difficulty with individuals, he should refrain from bashing specific people. Instead, he should describe the behaviors that are troubling to him, using specific examples, and explain the impact he feels their actions have on him or the organization. He should avoid generalizing these negative interactions and defaming the character of the individual in question.

Confirming the best mechanisms for ongoing feedback, as suggested by his boss, is an excellent way to conclude the meeting. Regularly scheduled meetings, e-mail, and dropping by his boss's office are all options that could work for them. Frank and ongoing feedback is a great way to build strong relationships and to develop an organization that thrives on continual improvement.

What I have found to be successful

When feedback has been delivered constructively, be sure to thank the person for sharing his or her views with you. It is not easy for all people in leadership positions to deliver feedback, and letting them know that you appreciate it will encourage them to let you know how you are doing on an ongoing basis.

Prepare notes on what you want to say. A concise message is much easier to hear than a rambling one. In addition, it may help you remember all the points you want to get across. Be cautious with your use of e-mail. Assume that any e-mail you send could wind up in anyone's mailbox, including the box of someone who may not agree with your views. Also, an e-mail can be misconstrued and taken the wrong way. Without the ability to see the other person's response to your e-mail, you are not afforded the opportunity to immediately clarify your message. Meeting face-to-face is a better forum for feedback and communication.

NEW LEADER ADVICE

As a new pharmacist in this situation, Josh is excited to have this time set aside with his new boss. He is concerned that he is doing a good job and is in line with the department vision and goals, and he wants to get feedback about his performance. This meeting with the director provides an additional opportunity for him to let his new boss know how he likes to receive feedback. This might be a bit overwhelming since many people do not know what their individual feedback preferences are. In order to set expectations and be successful in interactions going forward, Josh needs to let the director know if he prefers a lot of feedback or a little, and whether he prefers feedback to be formal or informal, written, or verbal. Taking some time to self-reflect will also help Josh identify the answers to these questions about preference. It may be helpful to think back over previous work experience and performance during his academic career or residency.

Even though Josh is excited to discuss all the opportunities for improvements in the department, he needs to be careful. If he begins the conversation with improvements he may run the risk of alienating his new boss. The feedback may be interpreted as disapproval or rejection of their services—services the department has likely worked hard to provide in the past. There is a good chance that these services have been implemented under the current director's leadership. Josh should also be wary to not compare the new department to previous experiences. It is unfair to limit himself to what he is accustomed to—doing so runs the risk of never embracing a new way of doing things and missing learning opportunities. It is also smart to take time to fully evaluate each process so that he can be clear in his feedback when he is ready to give it. As suggested, providing clear feedback about a process will help make the process better and can prevent Josh from making any inappropriate personal attacks.

What I have found to be successful

In situations where you might be the newest member of a team, there is a risk that your suggestions can be misunderstood and that confidence can be seen as arrogance. In either case such perceptions hinder any interest in changing practice and should be avoided. Where multiple issues exist, prioritize them so that if only one gets heard it's the right one. It may also be helpful to come with solutions in mind to avoid looking like a complainer, but wait until asked before proposing and changes in service. Especially when joining a longstanding team or service with many existing members, it is beneficial to ask about history and motivation (e.g., Is the originator of the "backwards" process still on your team?). Remember that in the past certain processes made sense, but recent advances in departmental structure, patient care, or technology may have made that process less effective. It is helpful to identify the communication style of the person you are proposing changes to and, once in the middle of discussion, pay attention to body language as a surrogate marker for reception and agreement.

CASE 5.5

Giving feedback to an individual

PRINCIPLE ■ Delivering feedback

Christie is new to her current store. She was with the company as an intern and stayed when she received her licensure. There weren't any positions available at the store where she had completed her internship, so she accepted a position at a nearby store. She picked up hours as a student and knew several of the staff members as well as the manager. Somehow, that didn't seem to make her current situation any easier. The way the scheduling was done her shift consistently follows one of the more experienced pharmacists, Dave. She notices repeatedly that "problem prescriptions" were being left until she came in. Even though the manager had clearly explained that each pharmacist was to take care of as many aspects of a problem prescription as possible (including calling patients), for the last 4 months the problems she received had not had any action taken. Frustration was setting in and it was getting to the point where she dreaded coming to work.

Dave was a nice guy and a good pharmacist. He was kind to her and never seemed to mind when she asked questions. He always volunteered to stay a few minutes when she needed to come in a bit late and she appreciated his help. She wanted to connect with Dave and discuss, but she wasn't sure how to approach him. She knew the manager would be receptive, but she wanted to speak with Dave before she went above him. She just wasn't sure how he would react, and she didn't want to ruin a good working relationship.

WHAT CHRISTIE MAY BE THINKING...

- I thought we left this behavior in grade school. This is so immature.
- I need to take care of this soon before it escalates.
- I want to be respectful.
- This should not be an issue and is inexcusable.

ON THE OTHER HAND, CHRISTIE MIGHT REASON...

- Should I let someone else handle this?
- Am I overstepping my boundaries?
- Should I go to management or to Dave first? I don't want to be a "snitch."
- What if this turns out badly? Will I be blamed?

MENTOR ADVICE

Christie has waited long enough to determine that the issues are a pattern and not just the result of a couple of bad days. Although Dave has more seniority, Christie should still convey her concerns to Dave. It is usually best to address these issues when she is not angry or upset, and it is also helpful to discuss them when there are fresh examples to cite in the discussion. It is preferable to discuss issues in private so that Dave does not feel he is being publicly chided.

Christie should focus their discussion on the things that Dave has done and the impact that his actions have on her, their patients, or the goals of their team. She should avoid characterizing him as lazy or incompetent. After she discusses her concerns with Dave, she should seek feedback from him on his perspective of the problem. Perhaps he processes twice the volume of prescriptions that she fills on her shift and does not have time to follow up on the problems. Maybe he is having trouble with the technicians that are working with him. Dave might acknowledge the issue, convey that he is not comfortable with calling patients, and offer to offset his shortcomings by agreeing to pick up the slack in other ways. Christie should make sure she understands his perspective and considers his suggestions.

Dave will likely appreciate that Christie has chosen to discuss this issue with him first, instead of going directly to the manager to complain about him. This discussion, if managed appropriately, could actually build a positive relationship between Christie and Dave.

What I have found to be successful

Try to be open to changing your opinion about other people. I can cite countless examples where I or others have changed their minds about another person when we stopped to listen to his or her point of view. Learning to approach conflict with coworkers is difficult. All of us can remember a situation that we wish we had handled differently. Mistakes are okay if we learn from them. Developing the skills for a productive confrontation takes a lot of practice. If an attempted discussion does not go well, think about what you might have done differently that might have produced a better outcome.

Unless your coworkers are doing something illegal or unethical or you have a strong reason to believe that another person will not listen to you, it is generally better to discuss your concerns with your peers before you go to your supervisor. You may be able to build partners instead of enemies!

NEW LEADER ADVICE

Confronting another staff member is never a desirable situation, but it can be even more overwhelming for new practitioners. This situation is tough because of Christie's need to be respectful of Dave, but his behavior hasn't really made her want to respect him. It is important for Christie to address the behavior and leave the emotions out of the conversation. There is a risk that Dave will not be receptive to the conversation, but hopefully discussing his actions and the results of those actions will help maintain a mature dialogue.

There may be reasons for the behavior that Christie does not see. Addressing the issue from a patient care perspective will help avoid accusatory or attacking statements, and asking questions may also add some clarity.

If Christie begins the dialogue and feels like Dave is beginning to become defensive, she should restate that she is not intending to accuse him. Restating what her goal is, seeking to understand why these issues are left unresolved, and reminding him that she is on his side will help bridge the gap. Keeping an open mind and operating under the philosophy that people don't try to do a poor job is crucial to understanding and success.

What I have found to be successful

Confronting someone is never fun, but it can be rewarding and it *must* be done. If the conversation is productive and respectful, you may even gain some additional respect from or for the other individual. When thinking about having a conversation of great weight or importance even subtle things can make big differences; always make sure you are well-rested, not hungry or irritable, and that your level of stress is not above average.

When approaching an individual about an issue that you would consider a difference in work ethic, ask yourself "Is it that they are not doing their job or is it that they are doing it differently than I would? Are the desired outcomes the same? Is it a patient safety issue?" These questions can help—first by assisting in establishing a sound reason for engagement and, second by helping outline a fair and objective argument that brings the conversation back to patient care or delays in therapy.

CASE 5.6

Hearing and responding to feedback

PRINCIPLE ■ Receiving feedback

Julie is a new pharmacist within the Ramsey Health System. She has completed both a pharmacy practice and critical care specialty residency and considers herself a strong practitioner. Additionally, Julie has been involved in professional organizations and leadership for the past several years, beginning while she was in pharmacy school. She was recently elected as president-elect of one of the regional chapters of her state organization and is excited for the opportunity to develop future leaders and further the profession.

Working with her in the health system is a leader she has admired for the past several years, John. In fact, having access to this mentorship was one of the reasons she took the job. The relationship between the two of them seems to be going well, but Julie has definitely noticed that there are issues that she and John just do not see eye-to-eye on. Julie attributes these to differences in learning styles and generations. The most recent issue they don't seem to agree on is how students should be tracking and following patients while on acute care rotations.

John asked Julie to come to his office after she was done with rounds where he insisted that students should be utilizing a paper patient profile tracking form. The students are to fill these out every day reflecting changes in the patient's medications and status. Julie respects her mentor but just doesn't agree. She is a strong proponent of utilizing all technologies available and just does not see the need to use a paper form. Their medical records are all electronic, and many of the lab values can be imported directly into spreadsheets. She agrees that part of the students experience should include learning the best way to gather and compile information from the various systems used within the hospital, but a paper form is so outdated (not to mention the trees they could be saving by using electronic methods).

WHAT JULIE MAY BE THINKING...

- I hate being micromanaged.
- They're my students. I should be able to teach in whatever manner I wish.
- Doesn't my boss trust my abilities?
- Maybe I haven't explained my point of view well enough.
- What is the benefit of the paper forms?

ON THE OTHER HAND, JULIE MIGHT REASON...

- How important is this issue to me?
- Should I just give in?
- If I give in on this, will it make me look soft?
- If I stand my ground, will I be perceived as stubborn and hard to work with?
- There must be a reason John wants the students to do it this way so I should just drop it.

MENTOR ADVICE

It sounds like John feels pretty strongly about the use of the paper form. Before going to John's office, Julie might consider how important this issue is to her. Does she want to back off on this and save her political capital for another time or try to convince John that her point of view is valid and achieves the same outcomes as his paper form?

Julie needs to put herself in John's shoes and figure out why he insists on paper charts. Is John angry because he feels that the form promotes an essential part of learning for pharmacy students or because he feels that that experience with electronic charting is not needed for the student's success? Perhaps John is angry because Julie did not require her students to follow the process that he felt was so important, thus making him feel that she was undermining his authority. Sometimes the main issue in a conflict is not around the difference in opinion or core issue, but rather it is tangled with the emotions of *how* something was done. In this type of situation it is important to tease the issues apart and strategically decide how to address each one. For instance, if Julie apologizes to John about not first checking with him about not requiring the students to use the paper form, it may help to make a conversation about the merits of each patient tracking method a little easier. If she ignores that issue, he may unconsciously dig in his heels even harder when they discuss his paper form.

When the discussion does get to the paper form, it might be helpful for Julie to first clarify with John what objectives he feels are met by using the form. Perhaps there are goals that Julie had not considered. If John struggles to provide a reasonable objective, he may back off from his position of requiring students to use the form. Even if neither one changes their position initially, coming to a common understanding of the desired outcome is critical when beginning a discussion if you want to try to keep the discussion objective. Different options can then be discussed considering each person's perception of the option and then evaluated by how likely it is that each option will deliver the desired outcome. If neither party can agree on whether an option will produce the desired outcome, a pilot might be suggested where the option can be tested. Another option might be for students to learn by rotating between both formats. Listening carefully to John's opinions will show that Julie respects his thoughts, even though she has a different point of view.

If John backs down or compromises during the discussion, Julie should express her gratitude and respect for his willingness to hear and accept her ideas. On the other hand, she may need to decide during the discussion if this is a battle that is important for her to win, or if it is easier to let it go and focus on issues that are more important to her. In that case, she might express that she still has a different point of view, but respects his and will ask her students to use the paper form. Learning to let things of lesser importance go is difficult for many of us, but an important skill for leaders to cultivate. Willingness to loose smaller battles can often contribute to a more positive outcome in the bigger picture.

What I have found to be successful

In preparing for a conversation where there may be a difference of opinion, try to anticipate the other party's concerns and think about how to best respond to and address their issues. In the conversation, use clarifying questions to help ensure that you understand their point of view. Questions can also be used to ensure that others provide justification for their positions and take responsibility for their stance, but this should be reserved for instances when you feel there may be no justification for their view. You should be particularly careful in using this strategy with people who hold positions higher than yours in the organization since it may upset them and cause downstream consequences.

Staying open to other people's point of view is a leadership trait that helps to build trust and respect. Providing latitude for others to change their mind without embarrassment is another helpful leadership tactic. We can't all be "right" all of the time. Confrontation can help to resolve issues, but it can also waste energy and time and relationships. Try to remember the big picture as you are finding your way through the weeds.

- -

NEW LEADER ADVICE

This is a tough situation, and as a new practitioner Julie may certainly feel a need to defend her position and preferences. However, as a great mentor might advise, it is important to ask "Is this battle is worth it?" Julie may also be wondering what implications this will have for her career and perception going forward if she continues to pursue it. She needs to maintain a clear and respectful line of communication, working to get to the center of what the issue is.

Before going into the conversation she should take some time to evaluate and decide just how important the issue is to her. Now might not be the time to engage John in conversation about a pilot, but a later opportunity may present itself and it will be good to be prepared with background information. Asking John to identify his desired outcomes will help her to start brainstorming the next steps to a compromise in the future. Additionally, this may be a great opportunity for her. If John is committed to his way then it may be beneficial to let go of the argument and be seen as a team player. John may also be more willing to meet her halfway on future endeavors.

What I have found to be successful

In situations where the words and ideas you put forth seemingly fall on "deaf ears," it can be incredibly frustrating. Remember that people don't start out the day aiming to frustrate a coworker. Getting to the heart of why a particular method is so important can help in brainstorming compromises. Identify what each desired outcome is and work toward a solution that satisfies both parties. Pilots or trials offer good opportunities to show another person the evidence behind your conviction, and they can be great learning opportunities when you are the one that is "wrong." Whenever possible, evaluate your environment, departmental goals, personal goals, and then choose your battles.

Summary

Communication, relationships, and trust are all intricately interrelated. Sincere and thoughtful communication builds relationships and trust. Additionally, good relationships and trust create an environment where communication is much simpler to accomplish. All of these factors affect our ability to get things done, our happiness at work and home, and even how we feel about ourselves. The key points in this chapter—tailoring communication to an audience or individual, understanding the importance of listening and nonverbal communication, and constructing communication so that it is carried out with respect—all support the development of strong relationships and trust. Emerging practitioners who set their minds to developing effective communication skills will find that strong relationships and trust from others will follow, putting them well on their way to becoming great leaders.

Leadership Pearls

- Much of communication is nonverbal. Learn to read it and use it. And remember what you do speaks louder than what you say.

- Find as many opportunities as possible to provide positive feedback. But don't be afraid to give constructive negative feedback too.

- Keep constructive criticism focused on the actions or behavior of an individual. Stay away defaming his or her character.

- Learn to pick your battles. You can't get your way all the time.

- When you do disagree, begin the discussion by establishing the desired outcome and evaluate the effects of different ideas on that outcome.

Leadership Exercises

- When working on a project, write down on a note card or memorize three to five important points to convey to senior management.

- Evaluate the top 10 people you encounter everyday for their preferred communication and learning styles.

- Practice active listening, such as noticing body language and asking informative questions, daily until it becomes automatic.

- Ask/identify among the people you work with most everyday what type of feedback they prefer and try to accommodate their preferences.

- Set up a meeting with your superior to discuss preferred feedback styles for both of you. Ask about the goals and values of the department and how you fit in.

- Develop a pattern of ongoing feedback with the people you work with everyday.

- Consciously use communication skills to build relationships.

VETERAN MENTOR PROFILE

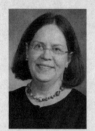

Karol Wollenburg, MS, RPh
Vice President and Apothecary-in-Chief
NewYork-Presbyterian Hospital
New York, New York

Why did you decide on a career in leadership? I did not consciously choose leadership as a career, it just evolved for me. I never set a goal of wanting to be a director of pharmacy or vice president, but I did pursue it when it became an option. Throughout my life I have often found myself in leadership positions. I think this has happened to me, in part, because when things are not the way I believe they should be, I feel compelled to try to make things better—it's just my personality. Those urgings can naturally pull you into a leadership role and you learn to work with people to get things done. I've worked in the same organization, following my residency, for my entire career. The opportunities made available to me by my bosses provided me with huge exposure and challenges, and I was able to try many different things and grow. I have had a lot of great people mentoring me and providing me with opportunities, so my career evolved.

Where do you turn for advice when you are stressed? My husband is my best friend so he is usually the first person I turn to. In addition, through professional organizations in pharmacy I have met many talented people, and when I have a problem I am struggling with, I call peers and ask for their experience and ideas in order to gain insight.

What is your favorite leadership book? There are a lot of books I have enjoyed, but *The Leadership Challenge* by James Kouzes and Barry Posner is one of my favorites because I like how it approaches leadership. I also like *Leading with Soul* by Lee Bolman and Terrence Deal because it reflects on spiritual issues related to leadership. The authors express a belief that leaders need to find what makes individuals tick. As leaders, we should help people we work with discover what provides fulfillment to them and then find a role in the organization that helps them feed their soul.

From your perspective, what is the most important issue facing pharmacy leadership today? We need to continue to demonstrate the value of pharmacy services. There are many competing priorities in healthcare today, and it's important to keep pharmacy issues at the forefront. Another important issue is that we have so many factions in the profession (clinical, informatics, educators, etc.) and the challenge is to find a way to make really good use of the diversity and use this diversity to build synergy and a strong pharmacy team.

Looking back over your vast experience in pharmacy, what one to two things do you know now that you wish you would have known as a student and new practitioner?

1. Understanding the importance of process when you are trying to complete a project. You have to think about who all the key stakeholders are and the process you must go through to be successful. For example, if you want frontline staff to do something and you feel you know how to do it, you still need to involve the staff and work through their ideas before you can get to an outcome that everyone buys into.

2. You can be a leader even when you do not have a formal position of authority. There are influential leaders with no positional authority, and people in both formal and informal leadership roles can be leaders.

What is your best advice for a new pharmacist today? Keep in perspective that you can learn as much from a negative experience as you can from a positive one. Don't look at negative experiences as failures, but look at them as a learning experience. Be open to new opportunities and experiences and look for new ways to step outside of your routines. View new challenges as a way to grow instead of feeling like you are taking on an unfair amount of work. Even if you aren't in a position of formal authority, you can develop your leadership skills without a formal title. Taking time to understand different leadership skills is important for everyone, even if you don't want to assume a formal leadership role.

How do you envision this publication assisting student and new practitioner leaders? The book provides a way for students and new practitioners to get a jump start in thinking about issues that are everyday challenges. It is structured to illustrate how leadership skills can be applied to situations that many of us have been in and ones that students and new practitioners can reflect on and learn from. The reflections and advice from the new practitioners and veteran leaders allow you to start thinking differently about leadership concepts and circumstances.

NEW PRACTITIONER PROFILE

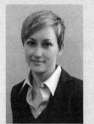

Lindsey R. Kelley, PharmD, MS
Manager, Pharmacy Operations
Department of Pharmacy and Therapeutics
UPMC Shadyside Hospital
Pittsburgh, Pennsylvania

Why pharmacy: In college I was enrolled in prenursing and I enjoyed chemistry. A fellow chemistry student discussed pharmacy as a professional option. A friend's mother was a retail pharmacist. She spoke highly of pharmacy and how good she felt helping people. Helping people in pharmacy made sense to me.

Advice to readers: In school I would encourage building bridges with other student leaders versus competing with them. Learn what makes them successful as once you are in practice everyone works together. As a student I focused more on professional organizations because of the support and network they can provide. The people I have met through organizations are still colleagues I can contact if I don't know how to do something or how to handle a sticky situation. Organizations also provide ideas from outside your practice. It is important to meet people who are professionally ahead of you and who have paved the way. Your network becomes a professional family who can be contacts for life. My biggest learning since graduation is that there is a fine line between confidence and arrogance. It's important not to have a constant need to prove yourself and know when to ask for help. In starting your career make friends and learn from colleagues who preceded you. Always build bridges with people because you won't be successful as an island.

Tips for work-life balance: Don't compromise your personal life too much for work. I set boundaries. For example, when I go home I don't take work with me or answer work e-mails. I turn off my personal digital assistant/phone when I go out biking. Our leadership team has negotiated our availabilities and work together to cover issues.

Personal career: My best career decision so far has been to do a residency because it stimulated me to leave my comfort zone and truly learn my strengths. It also provided me personal maturation and refinement through constant feedback so I could improve. This feedback was in the form of suggestions (such as "You might try this or that"), which I could adopt or not. My career goal and success is developing people and moving the profession forward versus achieving a specific leadership title. I also want to build bridges throughout the profession and someday hope to be the president of ASHP.

Why leadership: My interest in leadership was sparked by our chapter ASP president asking if I would want to run for president elect, which I had never thought about doing. Now I can't get enough of leadership. My major successes so far have involved making a difference and the personal development of others. My favorite leadership books are Peck's *Road Less Traveled*, Collin's *Good to Great*, Wooden's *Wooden on Leadership*, and Chapman's *Five Love Languages*.

Recommended change for pharmacy: I would like to see the breakdown of the divide between how retail and health-system pharmacists are perceived. I would also change the laws to increase pharmacy technicians' roles. We need to overcome ourselves as the barriers to doing things differently.

Using this book: I think this book will be viewed as a situational reference that answers many of the readers' questions. It will also be useful for those who haven't yet found the right mentor.

Suggested Additional Readings

Collins J. *Good to Great: Why Some Companies Make the Leap…and Others Don't*. New York, NY: HarperBusiness; 2001.

Covey S. *The 7 Habits of Highly Effective People*. New York, NY: Simon & Schuster; 1990.

Goleman D, Boyatzis R, McKee A. *Primal Leadership: Realizing the Power of Emotional Intelligence*. Boston, MA: Harvard Business School Press; 2002.

Kouzes JM, Posner BZ. *The Leadership Challenge*. San Francisco, CA: Wiley Johns and Sons; 2002.

Patterson K, Grenny J, McMillan R, et al. *Crucial Confrontations*. New York, NY: McGraw-Hill; 2005.

Additional Materials

Word Search

O	I	C	D	M	D	K	B	R	D	Y
Y	M	O	W	D	N	O	P	S	E	R
E	Y	M	Y	P	M	Z	V	X	J	M
Q	Z	M	G	M	C	X	D	N	M	M
P	B	U	K	C	A	B	D	E	E	F
Q	D	N	R	T	V	X	F	T	S	V
Z	M	I	O	P	D	Z	A	S	S	B
J	A	C	L	A	U	W	Z	I	A	B
S	T	A	I	D	V	Y	D	L	G	G
N	Q	T	A	A	M	C	I	X	E	A
M	E	E	T	W	N	L	J	N	S	B

Adapt

Communicate

Feedback

Listen

Message

Respond

Tailor

Read "Success Skills" article 14.

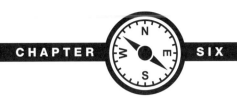

Embracing Change

Kyra Corbett, PharmD; Jeanne R. Ezell, MS, FASHP

Introduction

Pharmacy will always be challenged and blessed with change. We do not choose this great profession because we want each day to be the same as the last or because we expect the status quo. Our success correlates with our ability to cope and excel in ever changing environments. With the rapid rate of change faced by pharmacists today, we cannot sit idly by and wait to be impacted. Instead, every pharmacist should expect change to occur and strive to identify the resulting new opportunities. While there is comfort in routine, we stop growing professionally and become stagnant when we become comfortable in our daily tasks. When this occurs, it is necessary to seek out a change leader in practice who can identify the reasons for and effects of new system/process implementations in patient care. Most importantly, we must manage our psychological well-being and acknowledge that there is an emotional impact with every physical change in our daily lives. Our attitudes, beliefs, and values shape how we view transitions, and it is up to each of us to envision change in a positive and optimistic, albeit realistic, manner.

"The ability to successfully manage change has become one of the most important skills needed for personal happiness, propriety of organizations, and health of the planet."[1] The changes in the past 5–10 years are enormous in pharmacy. For instance, upon entering pharmacy school the prospect of providing immunizations may not have been apparent. Now many of our pharmacy sites thrive on their burst of sales administering flu shots each year. Change continues in the profession with ongoing new medications, new delivery methods, and new information to utilize during patient counseling. Chemotherapy agents are entering and gaining prevalence in retail and ambulatory settings as oral agents. Other changes include $4 generics programs and mail-order pharmacy. Biotech drugs, often targeted for rare diseases or with the promise of design for specific patients has been an exciting area of drug development, but most pharmacists in practice today in the United States learn very little about these medications. DNA testing to guide medication selection/dosing, such as with warfarin, is another potentially innovative service that pharmacists may be recommending to patients or offering soon. How is a pharmacist to survive or thrive with so much change happening around them? Everyone must learn to adapt to change.

The following are the change management principles discussed in the cases:

- **Change is a constant.** Even when you know change is desperately needed and will be coming, it may be difficult to embrace. When a decision for a change is made, it is important to find out everything you can about the objectives and timeline. Keeping your mind open to the positives of a change, even while being realistic about the difficulties that may be encountered during the change process, is a sign of a true workplace leader.

- **Expect methods to outmode quickly.** "I do not believe you can do today's job with yesterday's methods and be in business tomorrow."[2] Despite what may appear to be doom and gloom with the competitive nature of the retail prescription business, pharmacists should look at the public's cry for more affordable medications as an opportunity to improve medication outcomes in the United States. Changes in the marketplace drive an urgency to act to avoid being left out in the cold. Sometimes a business can delay responding to a new stimulus, but it is important to make a game plan based on possible "what ifs." Health-system pharmacists also constantly deal with changes, such as accreditation standards, core measures, and reimbursement requirements.

Networking with other pharmacists in your state will provide you with ideas and potential tools to tackle these new challenges in a positive manner. As a new practitioner, your openness to fresh ideas and your own professional dreams and goals can lead to new ways to practice and new services. While some independent pharmacies have struggled with marketplace changes in the past decade, others have thrived by more effectively meeting the needs of their customers. The $4 generic plans may be just the stimulus needed if a pharmacy is to move away from a focus on prescription profit to the roots of pharmacy services to our patients.

Even great role models, who have had wonderful successes in their professional lives, need to learn from others. Seasoned pharmacists often seek bright young practitioners when they have openings on their staff, in order to bring in "fresh blood" with new ideas.

- **To grow we must change.** "If we don't change, we don't grow. If we don't grow, we aren't really living."[3] Although some leaders seem to have been born with inherent traits for leadership, the reality is that people grow and develop into leaders by building on lifelong experiences. To be a good leader, you must be willing to expose yourself to situations in which you are not comfortable (and in fact may be afraid of). When tackling such fears head-on, time and time again, you become comfortable with the uncomfortable situations and perhaps even go on to become an expert at leading with the unexpected.

How people deal with uncomfortable situations is often a sign of leadership potential or ability. Those who are willing to face their fears and tackle the issue are usually driven by an inner desire to do the right thing for the right reasons. The more a person deals with uncomfortable situations, the more they become comfortable dealing with these situations (i.e., it does get easier to step up and take needed actions, tackle new problems, or whatever the situation may be). Most uncomfortable situations we encounter in pharmacy practice are usually due to our own lack of confidence in handling the situation (i.e., having limited drug therapy knowledge, being unsure how to handle a difficult drug-related problem, or having a conflict with a physician, nurse or fellow employee).

Many graduates from pharmacy school will become good pharmacists, but great pharmacists are those who lead the way when it's not easy.

- **All pharmacists must be "little L" leaders on their shift or in their practice.**[4] Pharmacists demonstrate leadership traits in all kinds of practice settings by taking responsibility for the pharmacy care services they provide, making decisions about everything they do, and in supervising technicians and interns with whom they work. Pharmacists can become agents of change by proactively suggesting and initiating new improved ways to perform their work.

A workplace may be ripe for change, and a pharmacist just has to speak up and voice opinions on what might be feasible. Speaking up is usually the first step, as action will need to follow the opinion. Building support for a change can be effective when accomplished through one-on-one discussions with other staff. Once the momentum builds among the staff, it starts to swing over to widespread support for a change.

More and more opportunities are coming open in the pharmacy profession for formal leadership positions, but many X and Y generation pharmacists do not want to give up their clinical, direct patient care roles to assume management or "big L" leadership roles. "Little L" pharmacists can also have a great deal of influence by becoming agents of change within their workplace, proactively engaging in changes that improve patient care and job satisfaction.

- **Change is both exciting and stressful.** Starting a new internship, residency program, or job can be exciting, but also very stressful. With all there is to learn (names of people, computer system, procedures, protocols), it can be overwhelming in the first few weeks. How you manage yourself and the stress of something new is the key to how successful you will be in your career and in your life.

People respond to change in different ways and at different rates. Adoption of Stephen Covey's *Seven Habits for Highly Successful People* can be a great methodology to help you be happy and secure with your life choices. "Begin with the End in Mind" is the first habit that emphasizes the importance of being goal-oriented. Deciding to complete a postgraduate residency program is an excellent path for new pharmacists. A residency program is founded on the principles of goals and objectives. Breaking down each rotation into its specific objectives will help each resident not to be overwhelmed by the multitude of goals to be accomplished throughout the year.

"Put First Things First" is all about practicing effective self management, while staying focused on your goals and objectives. Effective time management goes hand in hand with effective self management. New residents often struggle with competing priorities during the residency year. What has perhaps worked during pharmacy school to manage their time may no longer seem to be effective, as residents try to manage daily, weekly, monthly, quarterly, and residency year objectives. Many tools are available to help new residents with time management. One of the traits of a leader is being able to distinguish how to use your time effectively to accomplish your goals versus a good manager who may be great at using time efficiently to accomplish a multitude of tasks and responsibilities.

Another Covey important habit is to successfully manage oneself or to "Sharpen the Saw." You must make time for yourself to cultivate your own mental and physical health. Even if you get your priorities straight, you must work at nurturing them, and you can't be effective without maintaining a healthy body, mind, and soul. The psychological process you go through with a significant change in your life is sometimes the most challenging to manage. Staying focused on your priorities and making time for recreation, rest and renewal will allow you to manage yourself so that you can accomplish your goals.

Expect change to occur

PRINCIPLE ■ Envisioning change

From day 1 at this job, Rob has complained how the pharmacy's computer system is poorly designed and difficult to use. In fact, he is sure his experience with the system is partly how he landed the job at the local, small-chain pharmacy. He has worked there as a technician for 3 years before graduating and taking on a new role as a pharmacist. The company loved the fact that he needed no formal training to begin his first day as a pharmacist. He has watched new hires and rotation pharmacy students struggle for weeks before they could even tell a patient if their prescription was ready. Finally, the corporate office has approved the new Windows-based version of the same program, and it will be implemented in 2 weeks. Rob hopes the new system will improve functionality and will be more user-friendly but wonders why the company didn't look at all the other versions of software available on the market. Rob has heard great things about the computer software at different hospitals around the country as well as some of the larger chain stores and would have liked the opportunity to compare the options on behalf of his company.

After attending a quick seminar about the new system, he learns that while it is easy to learn and can enhance daily reports, there isn't anything else the system can do better than the old system, and it costs a ton of money. Another store in his chain has already made the switch and is reassuring him that it will be much smoother than he anticipates.

The staff at Rob's pharmacy is very accustomed to the computer system. Several members have used it for upwards of 20 years and are very set in their ways and resistant to change. This was clear to Rob when he worked here as a technician. He vividly remembers the uproar that happened when his manager implemented a process to staple a piece of paper to the patients' prescription bag if a product ordered was not included. This was a great idea, but the technicians complained they were too busy to attach the piece of paper. All they had to do was check a box if a medication was out of refills or needed a prior authorization or the drug was not in stock until the next day. These papers have been an enormous help to the clerks who could not communicate to the patient why something is missing from their order; nevertheless, the change was resisted and the process was implemented without the consent of the lead technician. Everyone appreciates the benefit now—even the lead technician. If that little piece of paper is such an issue, how is the staff going to handle this computer system change?

Rob has been asked to prepare the pharmacy technician staff for the switch to the new computer system. He has been informed that it is his responsibility to mentally prepare them for the switch, have everyone attend special training sessions, and complete a training DVD. He is concerned about his own competency with the new system and doesn't know how he will accomplish teaching others in such a short time frame. Now besides getting his feet wet as a pharmacist and working on the responsibilities of his position, he is now in charge of technician staffing and training.

WHAT ROB MAY BE THINKING...

- Why would they do such a drastic change without discussing it with us first?
- How am I going to find time to train all these technicians?
- Who will I ask when I have a question?
- I'll just tell my manager that I'm not dealing with teaching the system to anybody but myself.
- Maybe it's time to drop this gig and work for the big chains with better technology.

ON THE OTHER HAND, ROB MIGHT REASON...

- The end-of-day reports will be nice, especially for our billing specialist who handles deposits and sends bills to the few patients still allowed to charge their meds and have a monthly bill.
- At least in the summer time we have extra staff to make the change as smooth as possible.
- The other stores seem to think it was not so bad after all.
- Maybe the other little managerial things will ultimately help me with my job now that I am a pharmacist.

- -

MENTOR ADVICE

Rob's response to the news of the coming new system and the expectation that he will be the lead trainer is not unusual, especially when he wasn't involved in the decision process. Finding out the reasons for selecting this specific pharmacy software would be a positive start to tackling this sticky situation. As Rob's mentor, I would advise him to thank his supervisor for the opportunity to lead the other staff in training on the new system but tell his supervisor that he will need more information about the project in order to effectively prepare. Rob should concentrate on becoming more informed about the computer system by finding out details on functionality and key benefits that led to this system's selection, what the vendor offers for training and support, and what management support is available during the training and implementation.

Given the short lead time before implementation, Rob should request time away from his usual responsibilities in order to learn the new system and develop his training plan. He could point out to his superiors that a 2-week lead time may not be realistic for such a major change that involves all staff and is so vital to efficient prescription process flow. Pharmacy staff will also need support in order to get some time away from their usual responsibilities for training. Rob must be open and honest about his concerns with the change, rather than agree to take on the lead trainer role and be unsuccessful in meeting unrealistic deadlines. If he is enthusiastic about the need for change in the computer system, then his superiors will more likely listen to his suggestions for how the training and implementation could be accomplished.

Considering a job change over a new computer system is probably a waste of mental energy. All jobs have challenges with changes, but Rob needs to have control over how he perceives and reacts to the changes. Rob could engage other staff members by getting their input on the current flow of computer processes and where breakdowns and problems occur. Rob could also work with the computer vendor to flow chart the new system processes to look for tasks or processes that will need to change with the new system. Involving the other staff will build a positive team attitude, even if the new system doesn't have as many positive attributes as hoped. Learning the pros and cons of the new system could be useful to Rob later, as the management group may look to Rob to lead a team for selection of the next computer system upgrade.

Complaining to the CEO about the choice of software is not a good idea. When faced with a change that appears to make no sense to Rob, an immediate reaction might be to make the higher ups aware that they have no idea what's really needed by the rank-and-file employees. Although you may wonder what in the world were they (corporate office) thinking, there are probably some good reasons for the software choice. If Rob takes time to learn why the software was chosen and how it will work, his willingness to adapt to change will be seen by his superiors, and Rob may evolve into a change leader in the workplace.

What I have found to be successful

I have always found that it is better to be part of the solution than the problem, so a positive outlook to the potential advantages of a new system is a key way you can demonstrate value to the company. Digging into the details on the upcoming change and sharing your findings with other staff allows a person to focus on the positives of the change and avoid wasting time on the negatives. Most young practitioners may have some inner fears about their own ability to successfully fulfill a new challenge, such as training all the other staff on a new pharmacy system, but keeping your focus on the outcome of the change and breaking the change process into small steps will help make a *big* project more doable.

NEW LEADER ADVICE

Everyone knew this system was out of date and I would be surprised if Rob was not aware that someday there would be a switch to a more in-vogue system all together, not just an updated version of the same old system. There are many advantages to a new system. For example, this system could make it easier to organize file data so it can be retrieved and utilized at a later date. The customer service technicians would be the same people Rob's always worked with, and because of the similarities to the old system it should be the easiest transition possible as far as training is concerned.

Rob needs to understand the main objective for the switch over and learn more about the time frame and training options available with the new system. He should thank his manager for having the confidence in him to take on such a huge project in a short amount of time and ask him about the resources available for training the rest of the staff (perhaps the manager would be willing to let people complete the training DVD at home and pay them for their time so as to reduce staff shortage). Rob could also ask the vendors for two separate training seminars to assist the technicians in learning the basic functions before going live. Additionally, he could see if the IT department is willing to install the system on a backroom computer so the technicians can try out various tasks and become more familiar with the system. After 2 weeks of training, the system will be ready to go live.

What I have found to be successful

By working with my manager and the computer system vendors to communicate our training needs, we have developed a plan for the change and feel more comfortable with the tasks we need to accomplish in the short timeframe we have been given. When faced with a change, I have found it is often easier to determine the objective tasks and timelines I need to deal with instead of spending time worrying. By doing so, I can work constructively through the change and not spend needless time emotionally reacting to not knowing what lies ahead.

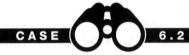

CASE 6.2

View change as a positive opportunity

PRINCIPLE ■ Envisioning change

Kim worked at a big chain pharmacy for 2 years right out of college and gave that up for the dream of working at a small-town, independent pharmacy. She is excited to work with Marla, her manager, who has been running the pharmacy for 20 years and has always been on the cutting edge of new pharmacy programs. Kim has seen articles about Marla starting the first headache clinic in the area. There are awards all over the pharmacy from her work with smoking cessation classes, precepting many pharmacy students, and even being one of the first accredited pharmacies in the area. The most recent change in pharmacy, however, has Marla very distressed and Kim has never seen her so upset. Within the last year, all the big chain pharmacies have launched $4 generic programs. Marla has looked over the program many times, and it just looks awful. She thinks the pharmacy needs to average $9 to $10 profit on every script, and the ideal profit number keeps shooting up when insurance companies decide that pharmacies should receive only $0.50 on a prescription for amoxicillin. She knows many of the drugs cost less than $4, but with the overhead of staff wages, the rent on the leased building, and other standard operating costs, there's no way to make this work.

Kim, on the other hand, had previously worked at a pharmacy that offered the $4 generics. She doesn't completely understand Marla's panic. She didn't see any immediate problems. She remembers being busy as ever when the plan first took off. Marla assured her that her big store made money because they were also selling groceries that made up for pharmacy losses. Kim didn't notice any drops in her pharmacy sales reviews with her old manager, but she wasn't about to argue this with her mentor. In fact, she's starting to feel Marla's panic spread to herself.

A whole year has passed and Marla has done nothing. Now, the local large chain pharmacy leaked the news that they will be breaking ground less than a mile away and will be up and running within 8 months. Kim knows it's time to get their $4 program running. She wants her customers to know that their little store can do everything the big chains can, including competitive pricing and customer services. She figures they'll lose the patients' business anyway if they do nothing and thinks they might as well turn to a minimal profit than no profit at all.

WHAT KIM MAY BE THINKING...

- There's nothing I can do to fix this. I'm still a new practitioner with limited experience setting up new programs, especially ones dealing with reimbursement issues.
- How can I influence Marla's decision on this? I need her onboard to make this happen.
- Will we still be able to offer the same quality service with the resources left once we bring a low price, generic plan into effect?

- We only make $1 on most of these prescriptions when we run them through insurance anyway!

ON THE OTHER HAND, KIM MIGHT REASON...

- Is there something else we can do to compete with the big chains besides this program?
- Has Marla thought about the opportunities to reach more patients? She may get a few patients back that left for the $4 generics already if she continues with the same services.
- Will we have to take a pay cut? Will we see more opportunities for medication therapy management (MTM), diabetic footwear, flu shots, and other vaccination programs?
- I could research the prices of these medications and look for less expensive options from other suppliers.

- -

MENTOR ADVICE

To continue to be successful, Marla's pharmacy must be proactive to changes in the marketplace. Kim is in an interesting position—somewhat in awe of Marla's accomplishments, but with the opportunity to put forth her own ideas for tackling the issue at hand. Kim has chosen an innovative practice with this job change to Marla's pharmacy. Marla probably would not have hired Kim, if she had not seen her potential to become a mover and shaker in the profession. But even seasoned innovators can have a dry period or have difficulty finding the silver lining in looming clouds. This is an opportunity for Kim to get creative and propose possible ways Marla's pharmacy can tackle the competition's $4 generic prescription plans. Kim has already started doing some homework on the issue, in finding out that most of the generic medications they purchase cost about $2 per prescription filled. She could network with other pharmacists across the state and do some research on how other independent pharmacies have increased their business when faced with tough economic challenges.

Since Marla is no stranger to innovation, she will probably be quite receptive to Kim's ideas for expanding patient services, such as improving medication compliance, which in turn may mean more prescription refills. Perhaps Kim can suggest ways to utilize technicians more fully, which could enhance their job satisfaction while decreasing the time demands on the pharmacists and the costs for prescription filling. Kim could consider proposing a new angle on the low-cost, generic medications such as a 90-day plan or a pharmacy-specific, frequent-user plan. With Kim's fresh ideas and Marla's proven leadership, a positive outcome is sure to result.

Kim could also request time outside of the pharmacy's regular hours for all of the staff to sit down and do some brainstorming with Marla. A true brainstorming session involves listing all kinds of ideas without initially discussing them. The purpose is to generate lots of ideas that can be further discussed, ranked for feasibility, and explored in more detail. This would be the first step in strategic planning for changes. By capitalizing on the experience and positive energy of all the pharmacy staff, Kim will likely produce an effective plan for the future. Involving all the staff empowers each individual to invest more time and energy into the success of the organization.

Changes in our profession, the marketplace, in reimbursement services, and in legal or accreditation requirements can be very challenging. It is hard being optimistic during difficult times, but Kim needs to break down the problem and find at least one new positive that can result.

What I have found to be successful

Try something new that others in the profession have found to be successful. I have found that most of the "innovative" practices we adopt in pharmacy are modifications or enhancements of a practice done somewhere else. Present the problem to the staff. Engage each person in brainstorming ideas to address the problem and give consideration to every idea proposed. Engaging everyone for input on this new challenge can build synergy for an effective solution.

NEW LEADER ADVICE

It's understandable for a pharmacy to get distressed when something threatens its livelihood, such as decreasing reimbursement nearly in half on the most popular medications. But this is the way the profession is moving and it is time to step up and accept the challenge of staying in business. Seasoned pharmacists, new practitioners, students, and technicians all represent different points of view and should collaborate in brainstorming and identifying innovative solutions to pharmacy problems.

One of the reasons Kim may have been hired as a new practitioner is because of her fresh mindset and ability to think outside of the box. Kim needs to focus on customer needs and what patient-centered services her pharmacy can provide that the big-chain competitors cannot. This is an opportunity to really help some of her favorite customers. Providing more comprehensive, patient-centered care can give her pharmacy a competitive edge.

Kim should begin by involving staff in problem-solving activities to find ways to retain and attract customers while implementing the $4 generic prescription plan. This could lead to new pharmacy services such as vaccinations, medication therapy management [MTM], 90-day prescription plans (patients receive one bottle, one label, and one trip to the store every 90 days, which decreases overhead costs of the savings plan), and "call backs" (automatic phone calls to patients letting them know their medications are ready for pick up, which will increase compliance and leading to increased revenue).

After the brainstorming is done, Kim should meet with Marla to discuss the various solutions. This meeting will help Marla shift her focus from what has happened to what the pharmacy can do next.

What I have found to be successful

One positive thing about pharmacy is that it is a "small world." I've noticed this in the interview process with new hires, through transferred prescription phone calls, and in association with colleges of pharmacy. We need to use our "small world" connections to our advantage by networking, collaborating, and learning from others' experience.

Being comfortable with being uncomfortable

PRINCIPLE ■ Incorporating change

Rudy entered pharmacy school because he wanted to work in healthcare and help patients, but he detested anything to do with blood or needles. He really thought he'd picked the perfect profession until the day he interviewed for a clinical pharmacy intern position at a large chain store. He would be an intern assisting with implementing clinical programs like diabetes day, heel bone density screenings, and diabetic shoe programs at all the retail stores within a 30-mile radius. He would be based out of one store in particular and that was the interview he had to knock out of the park.

The pharmacy manager asked if he was certified to give vaccinations. Eager to please in his new role, he quickly answered, "Yes, of course." The pharmacy manager went on to explain that the corporate offices made it mandatory to have at least one pharmacist to give flu shots at each location. Rudy wasn't listening at this point. He instead flashed back to that dreadful day in lab when he received his certification. It was all he could do to get through that day. He remembered his fear, the way he shook, how he promised himself he'd never have to give another shot again if he could just get this certification on his resume. He never dreamed he would have to use his certification again, but the job market kept pushing toward clinical pharmacy and the older retail pharmacists didn't seem to want to deal with any of that. So he knew it would give him an edge for a job if he ever needed it. He had not intended to discuss vaccinations. He was so excited for this job opportunity. He knew he would be perfect at it. There were 30 applicants for this position and it wasn't going to be easy.

Rudy's mind snapped back to the interview when the pharmacy manager informed him that the other three pharmacists were not willing to become trained in vaccinations. They instead have decided its time to add another pharmacist to the team so they are looking specifically for someone to lead the immunization program at their store besides the clinical routine of the corporate side of the job. Rudy just nodded and smiled.

The following week, Rudy got news that he had passed his boards with flying colors and he received the clinical pharmacy intern position he'd so badly wanted. Now if he could only get past his fear for giving immunizations.

WHAT RUDY MAY BE THINKING...

- Why did I ever get that certification?
- Is this requirement setting me up for failure with all eyes on me?
- What if I hurt someone?
- I suppose they'll want an intern who has more experience giving vaccinations.

ON THE OTHER HAND, RUDY MIGHT REASON...

- Maybe I'll become more comfortable if I get more practice.

- If I develop a niche with giving vaccinations, I would really boost how attractive I am as a candidate next year when I apply as a pharmacist.
- I earned good grades with the vaccination class and I remember the material well, which can only help me with this experience.
- I know I will learn from this experience and be a better pharmacist as a result of facing my fears and concerns.

MENTOR ADVICE

Rudy is in a tough spot. He could abandon his objective of interning with this organization, or he could face his fears head on. Telling the store manager and pharmacy director that he's not sure he can perform immunizations may mean losing the internship position. Not revealing his secret fears may not cause any immediate problem, but it could eventually undermine the trust the managers have in Rudy or even result in his being fired if he refuses to perform immunizations. There have been times in my career when I have avoided confronting a situation head on, hoping that the issue might go away or resolve itself. Typically the issue eventually comes to a head and becomes a bigger problem than if I had taken action when I initially became aware of the problem.

If Rudy swallows his fears and is willing to "give it a shot," he could seek professional help from a counselor who can help him overcome this obstacle to his future success with this company. By coming to terms with his fears, Rudy may find vaccinating patients a rewarding endeavor, and at the same time give a boost to his self-confidence.

What Rudy likely needs most is to practice or to gain more immunization experience in order to improve his comfort level with this valuable patient service. I would advise Rudy to sign up for influenza vaccine clinics in which his ASP chapter is participating. Peer pressure can often provide the support and motivation to overcome uncomfortable situations. Seeking assistance from faculty who coordinate the immunization course is another possible avenue Rudy might take.

Once Rudy finds he can overcome these fears, he can become a role model and lead the way for the pharmacists to take on this new challenge. He will probably earn even more respect from other pharmacy staff when he shares his personal story about overcoming his fears.

What I have found to be successful

When encountering an uncomfortable situation, I try to ask myself "What is the *right* thing to do in this situation?" or "What is the outcome we need from this situation?" I usually find within a few minutes that I'm breathing easier and the situation isn't so bad after all. Afterwards I often feel a new boost of confidence that I managed to handle the situation okay. It really does get easier with any new situation that arises. Always be open and honest with your superiors so that you never have to regret what you may have said or done.

NEW LEADER ADVICE

Part of the reason I took on my current position was to be challenged. Rudy seems aware of the benefits and risks associated with influenza vaccinations; he just lacks the confidence to administer them based on a bad experience in his past. I would suggest to Rudy that this is too small of a reason to give up on such an amazing opportunity. If he reviews the vaccination protocols and practices his technique, he may find the experience is better than he anticipated. Rudy could also ask his lab instructor to spend some time reviewing materials with him and make suggestions for how he can become more proficient with his vaccination skills. She may also have some tips for enhancing his experience, such as making sure both he and his patient are seated during the vaccination. Because he is uncomfortable with the situation, Rudy will learn from the experience and build confidence.

What I have found to be successful

I remember my apprehension as an intern when I was asked to assist in a vaccination program at a local flu clinic. The pharmacist asked me to administer his flu shot before we even started. I felt my hands shake and start sweating but didn't want to ruin this experience that had been set up for me, so I accomplished the task. I was surprised to see a flawless delivery and a smile on the pharmacist's face. I breathed a sigh of relief when it was over. He then told me I was in charge of the first five people who walked through the door. After that, we'd alternate customers. It was amazing. I felt the fear going away with each injection I performed. The people were so nice. "Wow, I didn't feel a thing. Thank you!" I kept hearing from each person, and my confidence with the skill grew.

While you may feel uncomfortable and uncertain when stretched outside of your comfort zone, it's amazingly refreshing when you say that you accomplished the task and you know that you are a stronger professional for it.

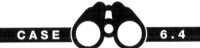

CASE 6.4

Change agent/change leader

PRINCIPLE ■ Incorporating change

After completing her hospital residency and winning over all of the staff, Mary has accepted a new position at the same hospital. Because her residency involved her working within all areas of the pharmacy, both the centralized staff pharmacists as well as the clinical specialist pharmacists were competing for her to work with them when she was done with her residency. The pharmacy director offered Mary a position working about 50% of her time in the central pharmacy and about 50% of the time on the patient units.

Mary was thrilled with the opportunity. She knew what was expected of her, she already knew most all of the staff, the pay was going to be better, but what about the schedule? Mary wasn't sure what would be expected of her for weekend hours. The central pharmacists all worked every other weekend while the clinical specialist pharmacists only worked a weekend every 5–6 weeks. She certainly didn't think it was fair to have to work every other weekend if she was only working with central pharmacy 50% of her time.

As Mary contemplated how she would make her case to the pharmacy director to consider her as a clinical pharmacist for scheduling purposes, she realized the huge inequity that was taking place. All of the pharmacists in both rotations are perfectly capable to cover the week-ond shifts. Why do the clinical specialists get more weekends off? Why doesn't everyone work the same amount of weekends?

The next day, Mary was told that she was required to work every other weekend just like all the central pharmacists. Mary quickly responded with her questions about the current schedule in place and asked why they don't allow everyone to be equal in the rotation. The director suggested she draft a schedule that makes sense and is fair for the scheduling supervisor to review.

Mary worked all night and had it all figured out by morning. She hurried into the supervisor's office to show her the draft. As she walked through the pharmacy, everyone seemed to get very quiet and stared at her. She wasn't sure if they knew what she was up to or if it was all in her head. The supervisor was impressed that Mary could draft a new schedule so quickly. Mary had developed a schedule where each pharmacist is on a 5-week rotation with only two to three extra weekend shifts per person per year. The schedule even included an extra pharmacist on the weekend to handle the workload that had steadily increased during the past year. Her supervisor didn't make any promises but said she was willing to take a look at the draft and get feedback from all of the pharmacists.

Pharmacists meetings were held to review the new schedule draft and get feedback on the changes. Mary's excitement about the new schedule faded away when she realized she was seen as a hero to the central pharmacists, but an outcast to the clinical pharmacists. That wasn't how she wanted to start her new job. But Mary felt that she had improved her hospital, helped out some of her fellow coworkers, and increased the level of care provided for their patients. She did not feel like apologizing for that.

WHAT MARY MAY BE THINKING...

- It wasn't my place to suggest such changes.
- I've ruined all of my connections with the clinical specialists.
- Maybe I should just accept every other weekend and tell my supervisor to forget the whole thing.

ON THE OTHER HAND, MARY MIGHT REASON...

- Maybe once they see the schedule, the clinical pharmacists will see that it's not as bad as they thought and it is fairer to the whole team.
- It was long overdue to change this unfair system.
- Everyone will feel more like a team unit this way.

MENTOR ADVICE

Mary may be motivated by her desire to avoid working so many weekends, but she is demonstrating leadership by suggesting a major change in the weekend work schedule. I would suggest Mary initially approach the department supervisor who prepares the work schedules and share her concerns and thoughts about possible changes. She will need to be aware that the supervisor may initially respond in a defensive manner, as she may perceive Mary to be critical of how the current schedule is done. Mary should not be surprised to perhaps get a "why don't you try to make out a schedule and see how hard it is" type remark, but hopefully the supervisor will be mature and empathetic in responding to Mary's proposal.

Sometimes I have found that pharmacists hesitate to speak up in support of a change because they don't want to make other staff "mad" at them. It seems to be human nature to avoid conflict. We want other people to "like" us and we don't want to "ruffle any feathers." Mary could just complain to some of the pharmacists about how often she has to work weekends, or as demonstrated in this case she can do something about the situation. Taking initiative shows that she cares enough to take action, and it will build respect for her among the staff, regardless of whether they agree with her suggestion or not.

What I have found to be successful

Taking the initiative to propose a change in the work schedule is a potentially risky action, as schedules are near and dear to most people's hearts. Testing the waters with one or two other staff first before sharing your idea with everyone can be effective at building support before exposing yourself to full force onslaught of feedback.

- -

NEW LEADER ADVICE

As a new practitioner, making suggestions for change and being willing to lead a change effort can sometimes be difficult. I've often wondered how I am viewed by experienced pharmacists who pass comments about the "young whippersnapper" (me) who is full of idealistic thoughts and ideas. I've often heard that I will become more realistic as I gain more experience. Mary has shown strong leadership in her willingness to propose a solution and work on a schedule to try to influence her manager to schedule more equitably. By taking the high road and presenting solutions, rather than complaining about the unfair system, she will likely be successful in achieving her desire for everyone to work the same number of weekend shifts.

In order to gain more trust and respect from her peers, Mary could share her ideas and draft schedule with them before taking it to her manager, informing them that she would appreciate constructive feedback and may incorporate their ideas as well. By actively listening to her peers and involving them in revising the schedule, she will likely appear more caring about their concerns.

What I have found to be successful

Sometimes criticism and complaints are aimed at a change leader when they are working toward an unpopular action. I have found that listening to my gut and doing the "right thing" often helps me land on high ground and influence positive changes for our department. I have also noticed that the complaints and criticism go away after awhile when the change isn't so fresh to my peers. Most importantly, I have found it incredibly gratifying to work with some of my peers when they too want to make changes and they ask for my advice.

Successfully managing yourself during change

PRINCIPLE ■ Managing change

Josh has recently graduated and accepted a residency position at State University Hospital. He's excited for his first rotation in infectious disease. He loved his hospital internal medicine rotation back at the university where he went to school. He has only a 20-minute commute from his new studio apartment, and he has already been introduced to the other residents. They all seem to know each other and he believes they all went to school here together at State University. They seem very knowledgeable about all those little local details; for instance, he heard them joking about the salad bar in the cafeteria (apparently, it recently had a run-in with a couple of big green caterpillars). He won't see much of these other residents as they all work at different sections of the hospital for this rotation. Instead, his main contact for his infectious disease rotation is a part-time, mentor pharmacist who is filling in for the regular infectious disease preceptor while she is on maternity leave, as well as the infectious disease team of doctors who range in age from med students up to fellows.

After the first week, Josh is completely overwhelmed. He thought he knew this stuff pretty well but finds himself looking like a fool over and over again. He remembered back to the second day when he forgot they were meeting 30 minutes earlier and walked into rounds late. The third day he offered to run to the patient's room to see if the patient had a fever overnight. Apparently, the vital signs and labs are available on the computer right behind him. He felt like every question they asked him required him to go look it up in a reference and get the answer back to them later that day. He wasn't even sure where he could look things up, so he waited until the doctors left for lunch to use the computer in the room where they had rounds. He thought he knew his drug antibiotic classes and coverages pretty well, but that was in a different setting. Josh had 4 years of experience in retail pharmacy while in school. He had numerous pharmacists tell him he was the best student they'd ever had. They said he was more driven and self-motivated than any of his classmates and he would be a wonderful resident.

Josh didn't feel any of those things today and he just doesn't know if this is the right setting for him to work in. He couldn't get a grip on his schedule or his role on the team. He feels as though his infectious disease background is so weak that he'll have to bone up on "bugs and drugs" every night at home. There is a meeting with the residency coordinator every 2 weeks, but he's not sure he can make it that long and he doesn't want to confess that he's failing to meet his rotational and personal goals.

WHAT JOSH MAY BE THINKING...

■ Are any of the other residents having this much trouble?

■ I can't work with a part-time mentor when the preceptor is still on maternity leave.

■ Am I supposed to have my own laptop or go home and use my computer to research information?

■ How can I possibly learn everything I need to know for this rotation in the little free time I have at home at night?

ON THE OTHER HAND, JOSH MIGHT REASON...

- Let's see what the Monday resident meeting offers for information.
- Maybe I could ask one of the other residents where I can look up research material.
- Maybe my mentor will offer some helpful advice. The infectious disease preceptor will be back in 2 weeks from maternity leave. She may offer more help.
- At least now, I know where to look up labs on the computer.
- My inadequacies may be normal and with time I may show great improvement.

MENTOR ADVICE

I would advise Josh to contact his chief resident or residency coordinator immediately and set up a time today or tomorrow to share his fears and concerns. We have all been in Josh's shoes and the chief resident or residency coordinator will gladly offer Josh advice and tips on how to become successful in this rotation and throughout the residency year. These mentors will likely reassure Josh that what he is feeling is normal, and even though he may have a slightly steeper learning curve in the hospital setting than other residents who have had more hospital rotations, he would not have matched with their program if they weren't confident he could be successful.

I believe it is wise to start the residency year with an exercise in writing out your personal goals and objectives, and in fact, this is a requirement in the residency learning system (RLS). Josh could also use Stephen Covey's "7 habits" methodology to list his priorities and designate specific activities dedicated to those priorities on his calendar. A well-managed calendar is a key to Josh's success in managing himself. Notating every meeting as well as their time and location and perhaps utilizing alarms on a personal digital device can help ensure he won't be late to rounds or meetings. Plotting residency project and presentation dates on his calendar and assigning key deadlines for drafts and finalization will break the big responsibilities down into workable units. Maintaining daily, weekly, and monthly to-do lists can empower your confidence as you see steps toward your bigger goals completed.

Josh needs to be careful that he doesn't over schedule himself and end up frustrated by failure to complete the daily to-do list. Even after many years in a management position, I still go home some days frustrated by all the things I didn't accomplish on my calendar. If I take even a few moments to go back into my calendar and fill in how my time was spent and reschedule what wasn't completed, I have a sense that the day clearly wasn't wasted, just different priorities took over. Taking time to look at my calendar a day ahead also helps me prepare for a fresh start the next morning and helps me decide what to wear the next day!

Self-renewal is the key to personal effectiveness. Josh should plan for and carry out activities that are relaxing and enjoyable, such as spending time with family, getting in some recreation, or reading a book. I believe a healthy diet and exercise are keys to good physical health and maximizing your mental capacity. Josh should put these activities to "sharpen his saw" directly on his calendar as reminders.

What I have found to be successful

Change is stressful and can lead to self-doubts about your ability to handle the change. Keeping your ultimate goals and priorities in the forefront of your everyday activities will help you deal successfully with the change. Write down your goals and priorities and review them often.

Planning for and proactively carrying out recreational, renewal, and healthy activities will lead to a healthy mental attitude and the capacity to overcome the stress of major changes and challenges in your life. Put these activities on your calendar and avoid skipping them, especially when you're tired.

- -

NEW LEADER ADVICE

Struggling to achieve success during a major career change is a common and normal feeling for students and new practitioners. Fear of failure can be overwhelming to the point where we prevent ourselves from rationally thinking through our circumstances. Josh should take the advice of his mentor and meet with his chief resident or residency advisor to relay his fears and struggles. These individuals have worked with other residents sharing Josh's current feelings, and they will likely be able to help him with lessons for success. They could also help him identify a computer he could work on and ways to become more efficient while on rotation.

What I have found to be successful

As a resident, I worked with my advisor to set residency priorities, and she helped me develop my rotational and residency goals. By establishing these goals I was able to proactively work on improving the skills I felt I needed to improve on, in addition to trying to meet the expectations of my rotation preceptor and team. By becoming more organized, I was able to develop morning routines so I could review my patients before rounds and follow up with the team at a later time when questions arose that I could not answer.

Scheduling and prioritizing time for self-renewal ("Sharpening the Saw") is very important to keep your mind focused and to prevent burnout. I used to schedule time in my residency to go golfing, bike riding, join a softball team, or take a trip to Wrigley field to watch my favorite team, the Chicago Cubs. Try to include one thing each day, or at least every few days, that is just for you. This will keep your mind clear and help you to unwind from the day in addition to helping you focus on the next day.

Summary

When installed as president of ASHP in 2008, Kevin Colgan said "Let us be the champions of change. We have the history, the stature, the credibility, and the obligation to lead the charge for better healthcare."[5] Successfully embracing change is the key to a fulfilling career as a pharmacist. Young pharmacy practitioners who can envision positive outcomes from changes that occur in our profession are our future leaders in pharmacy. Being willing to tackle uncomfortable tasks and situations helps strengthen your abilities to incorporate change in your life and lead the change process in your workplace. Young practitioners need to develop effective methods for managing their own physical and mental health so that they can successfully adapt to change.

Leadership Pearls

- You only grow professionally if you are stretched beyond the normal routine of your comfort zone by consistently exposing yourself to new experiences. This will help you grow as a practitioner and leader.

- Effective time management goes hand-in-hand with effective self-management.

- "Put first things first." Maintain daily, weekly, monthly to-do lists. This will empower your confidence as you see steps toward your bigger goals being completed.

- Take control of your future by being the change agent. It can be a huge self esteem booster to be the leader helping others to change.

- Many graduates from pharmacy school will become good pharmacists, but great pharmacists are those who lead the way when it's not easy.

Leadership Exercises

- Identify a change by thinking about something new that you have heard is coming in the pharmacy profession. Gather information from your peers and more seasoned practitioners about their concerns for this new change. List as many potential positives that could result from the change.

- List a change you would like to see for yourself, such as a new job, becoming an expert in a particular area, or learning a new sport or game. Inform yourself as much as possible about the new job, area of expertise, sport, or game. Keep your focus on the outcome of the change or new challenge, and break the change/learning process into small steps to determine how the goal can be accomplished.

- Take a situation you have heard students, residents, or coworkers complain about. Set up a brainstorming session to generate possible ideas on how the situation can be improved. Take the lead to work on at least one change action plan.

- Read the literature on the heritage of pharmacy service development to see how others have successfully managed change.

- Seek out veterans and ask about the change they have seen during their careers.

VETERAN MENTOR PROFILE

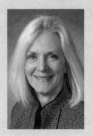

Jeanne R. Ezell, MS, FASHP
Director of Pharmacy and Residency Program
Blount Memorial Hospital
Maryville, Tennessee

Career highlights: The greatest decision I made was to complete the 2-year Health System Pharmacy Administration/MS Residency program at the University of Kansas after being in practice for 6 years. I've been at Blount Memorial Hospital as Director of Pharmacy for 20 years and one of my proudest moments was establishing our residency program. Also, I was humbled to receive the Tom Sharp Award for Contributions to Pharmacy Practice in Tennessee.

Why did you decide on a career in leadership? Leadership was appealing to me as I saw great potential in so many pharmacists and wanted to help motivate them to realize that potential. I also saw that pharmacy services could have a greater impact on overall patient care with strong leadership at the helm, and I wanted to be a part of leading that process.

Where do you turn for advice when you are stressed? I turn to my husband. His perspective and attitude are always refreshing. It's also important to keep a good routine with personal fitness.

What is your favorite leadership book? Stephen Covey's *7 Habits of Highly Effective People*.

From your perspective, what is the most important issue facing pharmacy leadership today? I think the greatest issue(s) are finding capable leaders who want to take on the work, juggle all the demands, and be responsible for the high-level decision making that comes along with being a pharmacy leader today.

Looking back over your vast experience in pharmacy, what one to two things do you know now that you wish you would have known as a student and new practitioner?

1. I wish I had had a better understanding of the whole picture of healthcare early on. It is so essential to understand how pharmacy fits broadly into healthcare and the healthcare industry.
2. It's so easy to just view oneself on one specific career path and to be too afraid to deviate. I think the importance of having a vision for the future cannot be overstated. There are so many different career paths that are out there for a pharmacist that each of us owes it to ourselves to explore the opportunities.

What is your best advice for a new pharmacist today? Complete a residency program. Take a chance on a job that could be a stretch—that you haven't thought you would do or that might be outside of your comfort zone. Depending on your circumstance, consider relocating. See how pharmacy is practiced elsewhere in the country. There is no better time than when you're young in your career to explore the possibilities.

How do you envision this publication assisting student and new practitioner leaders?

1. I see this publication used in pharmacy school classes to enhance management courses.
2. I hope it will be utilized with residents during management rotations and throughout the entire residency year.
3. I also believe it will be a great tool for all new managers or supervisors within a pharmacy department.

NEW PRACTITIONER PROFILE

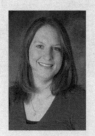

Kyra Corbett, PharmD
Community Pharmacist
Liberty Pharmacy
North Liberty, Iowa

Why pharmacy: Retail pharmacy has always been my interest. It's one part of healthcare where you can see your customers on an average of every 30 days. I love really knowing almost every customer.

Advice to readers: Communication is the key to all aspects of leadership. Learn to separate emotions from reactions. Ask the right questions to complete projects delegated to you. Know that it's more important to know where to find the correct answers than memorizing all the right answers.

Tips for work-life balance: Enjoy the juggling act. If it becomes overwhelming, it's time to limit additional projects and concentrate on what matters most to you.

Personal career: My best career decision is to work for a small chain versus a corporation because of the store's flexibility in allowing me to implement changes. My career goal as I raise my two children is to continue to deliver quality care with reduced errors.

Why leadership: Leadership skills are important to all aspects of life, not just the workplace. Pharmacists are often seen as pillars of the community. It is important to recognize this and participate in city councils, church committees, chamber of commerce, etc.

Recommended change for pharmacy: One thing in pharmacy that needs to change is the reimbursement from third parties. More third parties need to offer reimbursement for pharmacists consults resulting in therapy changes to better a patient's regimen or to save money.

Using this book: This book will be a wonderful resource to new practitioners that choose to use it. If it is read early on in a pharmacist's career, the overall lessons can be learned using these examples rather than in the real workplace.

References

1. Conner DR. *Managing at the Speed of Change.* 2nd ed. New York, NY: Random House; 2006.

2. Jackson N. Quotations book. Available at www.quotationsbook.com/quote/5275. Accessed September 15, 2009.

3. Sheehy G. Brainy quote. Available at www.brainyquote.com/quotes/topics/topic_change.html. Accessed September 15, 2009.

4. White SJ. Leadership: successful alchemy. *Am J Health-Syst Pharm.* 2006;63:1497-1503.

5. Colgan K. Inaugural address of the president-elect: pharmacy's tipping point: finding our way to the future. *Am J Health-Syst Pharm.* 2008;65:1571-1576.

6. Rate your readiness to change. Available at: http://www.goldstandardmanagement.org/OrganizeRenewal/AssessSituation/RatingOrgReadinessFortune.pdf. Accessed September 20, 2009.

Force Field Analysis

The *force field diagram* is a model built on the idea that forces—people, habits, customs, attitudes—both drive and restrain change. It can be used at any level (personal, project, organizational, network) to visualize the forces that may work in favor and against change initiatives. The diagram helps users picture the "tug-of-war" between forces around a given issue. Usually, there is a planned change issue described at the top and two columns below. Driving forces are listed in the left column and restraining forces in the right column. Arrows are drawn toward the middle. Longer arrows indicate stronger forces. The idea is to understand and make explicit all the forces acting on a given issue.

How to Conduct a Force Field Analysis?

Typically, the following steps are taken:

1. Describe the current situation.

2. Describe the desired situation.

3. Identify where the current situation will go if no action is taken.

4. List all the forces driving change toward the desired situation.

5. List all the forces resisting change toward the desired situation.

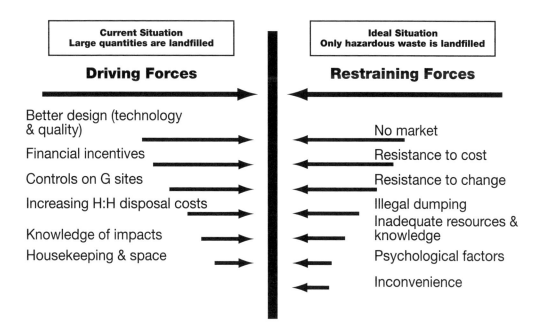

Figure 6-1. Example of a force field diagram. (Reproduced from kharahais.gov.za/files/waste/ewaste.htm.)

6. Discuss and interrogate all of the forces. Are they valid? Can they be changed? Which are the critical ones?

7. Allocate a score to each of the forces using a numerical scale (e.g., 1 = extremely weak and 10 = extremely strong).

8. Chart the forces by listing (to strength scale) the driving forces on the left and restraining forces on the right.

9. Determine whether change is viable and progress can occur.

10. Discuss how the change can be affected by decreasing the strength of the restraining forces or by increasing the strength of driving forces.

11. Keep in mind that increasing the driving forces or decreasing the restraining forces may increase or decrease other forces or even create new ones.

Tips for Change Leaders

- Keep your mind open to the positives of a change, even while being realistic about the difficulties that may be encountered during the change process.

- Networking with other pharmacists will provide you with ideas and potential tools to tackle new challenges in a positive manner.

- Include others with whom you work to brainstorm ideas to overcome a new challenge and give consideration to each of the ideas.

- Build support for a change, one person at a time.

- Pharmacists can become agents of change by proactively suggesting and initiating new improved ways to perform their work.

- Agents of change who help others solve their own problems create an independent workforce.

- Taking initiative to implement a change shows that you care enough to take action, and it will build respect for you among the staff, regardless of whether they agree with your suggestion or not.

- Routinely expose yourself to experiences out of your comfort zone. This will keep you growing as a practitioner and leader.

- Once you feel that you've overcome a new fear or challenge, help others to do the same. It's easier to learn from someone who has walked in their shoes.

- Take control of your future by being the change agent. It can be a huge self-esteem booster to be the leader helping others to change.

Rate Your Readiness To Change

Below are 17 key elements of change readiness. Rate your organization on each item. Give three points for a high ranking ("We're good at this; I'm confident of our skills here"); two for medium score ("We're spotty here; we could use improvement or more experience"); and one point for a low score ("We've had problems with this; this is new to our organization"). Be honest. Don't trust only your own perspective; ask others in the organization, at all levels, to rate the company too. It sometimes helps to have an outsider do the assessment with you. Readiness scoring: HIGH=3; MEDIUM=2; LOW=1.

CATEGORY   **SCORE**

Sponsorship   _____

The sponsor of change is not necessarily its day-to-day leader; he or she is the visionary, chief cheerleader, and bill payer—the person with the power to help the team change when it meets resistance. Give three points—change will be easier—if sponsorship comes at a senior level; for example, CEO, COO, or the head of an autonomous business unit. Weakest sponsors: midlevel executives or staff officers.

Leadership   _____

This means the day-to-day leadership—the people who call the meetings, set the goals, work till midnight. Successful change is more likely if leadership is high level, has "ownership" (that is, direct responsibility for what's to be changed) and has clear business results in mind. Low-level leadership, or leadership that is not well connected throughout the organization (across departments) or that comes from the staff, is less likely to succeed and should be scored low.

Motivation   _____

High points for a strong sense of urgency from senior management, which is shared by the rest of the company, and for a corporate culture that already emphasizes continuous improvement. Negative: tradition-bound managers and workers, many of whom have been in their jobs for more than 15 years, a conservative culture that discourages risk taking.

Direction   _____

Does senior management strongly believe that the future should look different from the present? How clear is management's picture of the future? Can management mobilize all relevant parties—employees, the board, customers, etc.—for action? High points for positive answers to those questions. If senior management thinks only minor change is needed, the likely outcome is no change at all; score yourself low.

Measurements   _____

Or in consultant-speak, "metrics." Three points if you already use performance measures of the sort encouraged by total quality management (defect rates, time to market, etc.) and if these express the economics of the business. Two points if some measures exist but compensation and reward systems do not explicitly reinforce them. If you don't have measures in place or don't know what we're talking about, one point.

Organizational Context

How does the change effort connect to other major goings-on in the organization? (For example: Does it dovetail with a continuing total quality management process? Does it fit with strategic actions such as acquisitions or new product lines?) Trouble lies ahead for a change effort that is isolated or if there are multiple change efforts whose relationships are not linked strategically.

Process/Functions

Major changes almost invariably require redesigning business processes that cut across functions such as purchasing, accounts payable, or marketing. If functional executives are rigidly turf conscious, change will be difficult. Give yourself more points the more willing they—and the organization as a whole–are to change critical processes and sacrifice perks or power for the good of the group.

Competitor Benchmarking

Whether you are a leader in your industry or a laggard, give yourself points for a continuing program that objectively compares your company's performance with that of competitors and systematically examines changes in your market. Give yourself one point if knowledge of competitors' abilities is primarily anecdotal—what salesman say at the bar.

Customer Focus

The more everyone in the company is imbued with knowledge of customers, the more likely that the organization can agree to change to serve them better. Three points if everyone in the work force knows who his or her customers are, knows their needs, and has had direct contact with them. Take away points if that knowledge is confined to pockets of the organization (sales and marketing, senior executives).

Rewards

Change is easier if managers and employees are rewarded for taking risks, being innovative, and looking for new solutions. Team-based rewards are better than rewards based solely on individual achievement. Reduce points if your company, like most, rewards continuity over change. If managers become heroes for making budget, they won't take risks even if you say you want them to. Also, if employees believe failure will be punished, reduce points.

Organizational Structure

The best situation is a flexible churn—that is, reorganization with little churn—that is, reorganizations are rare and well received. Score yourself lower if you have a rigid structure that has been unchanged for more than five years or has undergone frequent reorganization with little success; that may signal a cynical company culture that fights change by waiting it out.

Communication

A company will adapt to change most readily if it has many means of two-way communication that reach all levels of the organization and that all employees use and understand. If communications media are few, often trashed unread, and almost exclusively one-way and top-down, change will be more difficult.

Organizational Hierarchy   _____

The fewer levels of hierarchy and the fewer employee grade levels, the more likely an effort to change will succeed. Thick layers of middle management and staff not only slows decision-making but also creates large numbers of people with the power to block change.

Prior Experience with Change   _____

Score three if the organization has successfully implemented major changes in the recent past. Score one if there is no prior experience with major change or if change efforts failed or left a legacy of anger or resentment. Most companies will score two, acknowledging equivocal success in previous attempts to change.

Morale   _____

Change is easier if employees enjoy working in the organization and the level of individual responsibility is high. Signs of unreadiness to change: low team spirit, little voluntary extra effort, and mistrust. Look for two types of mistrust: between management and employees, and between or among departments.

Innovation   _____

Best situation: the company is always experimenting; new ideas are implemented with seemingly little effort; employees work across internal boundaries without much trouble. Bad signs: multiple signoffs are required before new ideas are tried; employees must go through channels and are discouraged from working with colleagues from other departments or divisions.

Decision-making   _____

Rate yourself high if decisions are made quickly, taking into account a wide variety of suggestions; it is clear where decisions are made. Give yourself a low grade if decisions come slowly and are made by a mysterious "them"; there is a lot of conflict during the process, and confusion and finger pointing after decisions are announced.

TOTAL SCORE: _____

If Your Score Is:

41–51   *Implementing change is most likely to succeed. Focus resources on lagging factors (your ones and twos) to accelerate the process.*

28–40   *Change is possible but may be difficult, especially if you have low scores in the first seven readiness dimensions. Bring those up to speed before attempting to implement large-scale change.*

17–27   *Implementing change will be virtually impossible without a precipitating catastrophe. Focus instead on (1) building change readiness in the dimensions above and (2) effecting change through skunkworks or pilot programs separate from the organization at large.*

—Taken from "Rate Your Readiness to Change," Fortune Magazine, February 7, 1994

 *Read "Success Skills" article 9.*

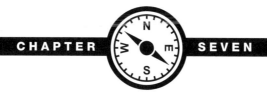

CHAPTER SEVEN

Working Efficiently

Katherine A. Miller, PharmD; Cindi Brennan, PharmD, MHA, FASHP

Introduction

Working efficiently is one of the most overlooked qualities in a leader. One of the first leadership lessons that busy health professionals learn is that they cannot do everything, even those who are incredibly productive. Time management guru Brian Tracy coined the Law of Forced Efficiency[1] that says "There will never be enough time to do everything you have to do, but there is always enough time to do the most important thing." The trick is to determine what those most important things are to your long-term success and to structure your day around them. One tool used in this process is to review your to-do list and answer three questions:

1. What are my highest value activities?

2. What can I and only I do that if done well will make a real difference?

3. What is the most valuable use of my time right now?

The ability to select the most important task and to focus on completing that one first is a distinguishing characteristic of someone who has mastered their time management skills. The key to time management includes clarifying your goals and continually prioritizing your activities to achieve those goals. When your goals align with those of the organization, you help the organization move forward and your value to the organization grows. You are seen as a leader because you can get important things done.

Although this sounds quite simple, it is very easy to get derailed by all sorts of distractions. As you read through the cases in this chapter, you will realize that different leaders get derailed by different distractions and have different downfalls in managing their time and providing results in a timely manner. You may not yet know how you can improve your time management techniques; after reading this chapter you may have a better idea. Consider all of the steps along the way to project completion. Creating the idea, breaking it into tasks, delegating tasks, prioritizing tasks, balancing tasks against other responsibilities, and completing tasks have pitfalls that may prevent you from reaching the finish line. Take time to assess how you react in each of these stages of completing a project to determine where you can improve your time management. Try one or two of the techniques we share with you, and see how much you are able to accomplish in a shorter amount of time.

Cases 7.1 and 7.2 discuss how a good leader understands the value of continuously developing his or her leadership skills to remain effective. If you have honestly evaluated your talents as well as your limitations, you can set your long-term goals for your leadership development plan. That self-assessment drives your choice of books, articles, tools, and seminars on leadership development. What resources will provide you with the best learning opportunities and will be most important to your growth? Are there resources that you can borrow or trade for? Look for every possible opportunity. Application of the lessons learned can significantly improve your efficiency by increasing your confidence in tackling that difficult project or issue. However, it is a good practice to periodically ask yourself three questions:

1. What can I be doing with what I'm learning?

2. Is this book/seminar/article telling me anything new?

3. Does the message resonate with my professional development plan?

If the answer is no, you may be overdoing it. Practice some of the new techniques you've learned about. To develop a new behavior, it takes several weeks of repeatedly using that behavior before it becomes a permanent change, so give yourself time to make these changes. As the saying goes "practice makes perfect" but only tackle one new technique at a time until it becomes ingrained into your leadership practice.

The purpose of new technology and gadgets is to support the efficiency, speed, and accuracy of finding and communicating information. Case 7.3 validates that technology can be leveraged to improve your time management skills. These tools can be used for scheduling projects, creating and sorting to-do lists, prioritizing your activities, and organizing your day. They also facilitate access to drug information, publications, and internet searches for the most current information. However, there is a reason they may be referred to as "crackberries." Many of us feel compelled to remain completely connected to friends, colleagues, and the latest information 24/7/365 at the expense of being fully engaged and participating in whatever is occurring around you. Creating a balance between being connected and being "in the moment" is a critical skill to nurture. Remember that technology is a tool and *you* are in charge of how you use your tools. It is easy to become overwhelmed with the constant flow of information that can distract you from your current task or priority.

One aspect of leadership development is taking advantage of specific opportunities to build your skills. The key is to align those opportunities with your personal/professional goals and select, if possible, those that support this alignment. Case 7.4 demonstrates that choosing whether or not to take advantage of various opportunities is not always an option, but setting or negotiating deadlines may be. When faced with multiple, competing deadlines it is critical to identify the most important or most valuable task and get going on that one first. Those tasks that have serious consequences to you or your career need to be priority number one. But the real priority is the tasks that are most crucial to the patient. Those tasks that you should do but are less consequential should only be tackled after completion of your top priority projects.

A related skill is learning how to politely say no—no to opportunities, no to your colleagues, no to your boss. There are both good and bad reasons to say no and you should evaluate those before you make your case. To help you find a good reason to say no, ask yourself the following:

- Are you already working on several important projects that don't allow extra time for this one?

- Can you delegate other projects for this one?

- Can you slide other deadlines?

- Do you have the skills for this project?

- Are you the only person who can complete this project?

Prepare a list of your projects and share that with your boss. Many times, your boss is unaware of your project list, especially if not all of the projects were assigned by her. Even if all of your assignments have come from your boss, share your list and ask for help reprioritizing.

One of the most elusive issues in today's environment is work and family balance due to the individual variability of one's needs, motivations, requirements, and economic situation. Although there is no universal solution to work-life balance, Case 7.5 identifies some solutions. Many professionals' identity is tightly linked to their work life while others derive meaning and purpose from various activities including family and friends. While many workplaces have become more "family friendly" with alternative work schedules, job sharing, and other innovations, creating the appropriate balance in your life is ultimately your issue to solve.

Making choices to balance work or school with your personal life can be emotionally challenging so it is important to be as objective and practical as possible. One approach is to write down all of the issues you are struggling to balance then review them one by one. Ask yourself "Why is this issue a challenge for me? Why is it important for me to do it? And, how much time do I need to devote to it?" As you work through your list objectively, you will probably identify some activities that are essential and others that are optional. To maintain your objectivity, you might want to share your list and thoughts about that list with your mentor.

Stephen Covey, author of *The 7 Habits of Highly Effective People*, has developed a framework for personal effectiveness.[2] Case 7.6 explores the first habit he describes, which is to *be proactive*. Proactive people use their initiative and problem-solving skills to find solutions. They are seen as positive and do not allow the situation to drag them down. On the other hand, *reactive* people complain and blame others for the situation. They are seen as negative and allow the situation to dictate how they will feel or respond. To become highly effective, proactive people focus on things they can actually influence. They generally have a positive attitude and are effective within their circle of influence, which actually expands that influence. Reactive people have a negative attitude and their complaining often reduces their circle of influence. Effective proactive leaders will determine what they can influence and focus their time and energy where they can make a difference.

A highly useful time management concept is called the *80/20 rule* or the *Pareto Principle* named for its founder Vilfredo Pareto, a 19th century economist who identified a pattern where 20% of one's activities account for 80% of one's results. Pareto aptly called these top 20% of activities the "vital few" and the other 80% the "trivial many." Case 7.7 shows you that although it is tempting to clean up the trivial issues first in order to cross things off your to-do list, you will greatly improve your efficiency by focusing on the most valuable tasks first. Since many of your tasks take the same amount of time and energy to complete, you will want to prioritize those projects that add the most value to your department and your organization. Your value lies in identifying and completing the "vital few" before you touch the rest of your projects.

We all know that some of our "vital few" are huge projects and cannot be completed at once. How do we assure that our highest priority projects receive constant attention while completing other vital tasks that pop up? This is where breaking a large project into discreet steps can really help. Once you've written out each step of a large project, you can plot them on your project timeline and make sure each one rises to your "vital few" at the appropriate time. This is the concrete application of the old saying "take it one step at a time." You will be energized by your daily progress on that huge project that initially looked so daunting.

Meeting multiple, near-term deadlines requires you to evaluate the long-term consequences of doing or not doing something. When an activity has a positive consequence for you, making that activity a priority drives how you spend your time and what you can delegate. Since no one person can do it all, effective leaders recognize that delegation skills are vital to their success. Training others so that you can effectively delegate what should be delegated will free up your time to focus on tasks where you can add the most value and it provides your colleagues an opportunity to build their skills and abilities in a new area. Case 7.8 reveals that delegation is one of those leadership skills that can be learned and must be practiced.

To delegate effectively, you need to know when to delegate, choose the right tasks to delegate, identify the right people to delegate to, and delegate in the right way. To determine if you should delegate, ask yourself if there are others with the ability to do the task, if they will build their skills by performing the task, and if you can provide the needed oversight for them. To determine the right people to delegate to, consider their previous experience with similar projects, how well they work with you, and how busy they are. To delegate most effectively, make sure you are clear about the goals, scope, timeline, and limits of the project; provide support without micromanaging the project; monitor progress routinely; and provide recognition for a job well done. Good delegation skills create highly efficient leaders and successful teams as participation in projects adds meaning to a group's work.

Now is the time to begin practicing and learning new time management techniques. This is a skill that will benefit you no matter where your career or life takes you. Improving your time management and utilization of the time you have available will have many positive impacts on your life. You may create more time for family and friends, more time for optional projects, more time to improve the work you have already completed, more time to learn from mentors or provide learning to students and new practitioners, or more time to spend increasing your clinical or leadership skills. Whatever you choose to do with your free time, be sure to use it efficiently to produce the most beneficial outcomes for you.

CASE 7.1

Tackling the most challenging task of your day

PRINCIPLE ■ Learning how to become the "master of your time" to better prioritize your tasks

Susanne has been working as an inpatient pharmacy operations manager at a local, 400-bed medical center. This is her first job after completing two residencies, a pharmacy practice, and a specialized pharmacy administration residency. While Susanne loves her job, she has been noticing lately that the work has been piling up more than usual—and more than expected after becoming involved in the state pharmacy society. On top of this, Susanne recently bought a new home with her husband and she cannot wait to start a family.

At work, Susanne is the go-to person for many technicians, pharmacists, and managers and always takes on new projects, even when she may not have the time to complete them. Susanne is often viewed by her coworkers as a role model and hard worker. However, she always feels overwhelmed by her work and though she's always busy working on projects, she never feels like she's getting anything done. Susanne has tried to prioritize her projects, but it never seems to fall in line with what others expect of her. She tends to focus on projects based on when they are due, but not always based on how much work they will entail. She makes sure that she's using every spare minute she has to check her e-mails or voice mail, but it just adds to her project list and often the e-mails sit in her inbox for days, having been read but pushed aside to address at a later time.

Not only is Susanne highly involved at work, but she also sits on the board of her state pharmacy society and is knee-deep in home improvement projects. She completes the committee and home improvement projects sooner than the other projects she has at work. They are fun and help her interact with some of the most important people in her life—her husband and other pharmacists with similar interests and goals. However, this doesn't mean that her coworkers aren't also important to her, but they are tasks assigned to her and she may not be fully vested in their outcomes.

WHAT SUSANNE MAY BE THINKING...

- Why am I unable to focus on the tasks I'm assigned to at work?
- I need to plan ahead more and prioritize based on project size.
- Can I ask my boss for fewer projects or more project time?
- Maybe I should resign from the state pharmacy society to get my job done.
- Why did we buy a house this year?

ON THE OTHER HAND, SUSANNE MIGHT REASON...

- I might as well get the more interesting and fun tasks done first. At least I'm getting something done!
- My home and family may be more important to me.
- I'm doing so much more for the pharmacy profession by helping the state pharmacy society than at my job!
- It's important to give back to the profession that has provided me with such a great career.

- -

MENTOR ADVICE

Susanne's thoughts are very common, especially for someone who prides themselves on over-achieving. If her mentor asks, she would probably admit to feeling a bit guilty for not meeting others' expectations and letting work-related projects slide while her home remodeling and state society committee work gets completed early. Her mentor could help her explore options for organizing her workday to improve productivity and her sense of accomplishment.

As her mentor, I would share my own challenges of balancing work with professional society and home life. I would ask her if she is clear about her own career goals and expectations. I would also question her motivation to take on new projects without considering their value and alignment with her goals and job expectations. It is difficult to answer the three time management questions without a clear understanding of these.

- What are my highest value activities?

- What can I and only I do that if done well will make a real difference?
- What is the most valuable use of my time right now?

I'd try to point out that the projects she enjoys most are the ones where she shares common interests and goals with the most important people in her life and see if she has had a conversation with her coworkers about these aspirations. Susanne might be surprised to learn that others at work share her perspective on the profession and would be happy to collaborate on work-related projects instead of trying to "dump" more projects on her. The result should increase productivity and create greater personal satisfaction for Susanne as she focuses on the projects that are most important to her.

What I have found to be successful

My advice is to develop an open line of communication with your manager and develop time management skills. Talk with your boss. Make sure you understand the job expectations and check that they are aligned with your career objectives. Your manager's priorities will help you set your priorities and focus on the most important activities for the department.

- Develop your time management skills.
- Explore the techniques described in leadership literature to find ones that work for you.
- Prioritize your work based on the value you bring to it and it brings to you.

NEW LEADER ADVICE

Although it is often perceived as a compliment, always being the go-to person for coworkers can become overwhelming. It is important for Susanne, a new practitioner in a management role, to learn how to prioritize the daily requests for assistance. She needs to understand which tasks are vital to the function of the pharmacy at a specific moment in time in order to begin the prioritization process. Susanne should ask some of her coworkers to talk this through with her.

Susanne could also lighten her workload by taking time to understand the ultimate goals and needs of her coworkers. They may be willing to work through their tasks by themselves and just need Susanne's help in getting the tasks started. If Susanne notices that some of her employees constantly need her assistance, it might be beneficial for her to walk them through the task so they can complete it on their own in the future. Another way to increase productivity is for Susanne to schedule specific points throughout the day for checking e-mails and voice messages. She should focus on topics that appear more time sensitive rather than the routine departmental, institutional, or organizational updates. It may also be useful to schedule time specifically to complete the largest, most challenging tasks of the day, such as projects assigned by her manager.

Finally, Susanne should begin focusing on the mundane tasks on her to-do list rather than the more exciting ones. Finding a way to get the larger projects done will prove to her that she can accomplish the big tasks, which can jump-start her energy to work on other tasks.

What I have found to be successful

The most important thing I have learned as a new leader is to think about scheduling time for the most important parts of my day. Some days this may be the project my boss just asslgned, returning an important e-mail, the massage I've been dying to have, or dinner with a friend that I haven't seen in months. Picking the one thing that is the most vital to me each day and ensuring that I've found the time to complete it provides a sense of accomplishment. It also helps me create a work-life balance by prioritizing extracurricular activities with the same or higher importance than other projects from time to time.

Another way to organize my projects is to create a to-do list with the big, overwhelming projects at the top. Categorizing projects into long-term or short-term lists (including personal tasks such as paying bills or scheduling doctor appointments as well as listing important project pieces separately) can effectively prioritize your list for you. One thing to avoid, however, is too many lists, which can be time-consuming and create more confusion.

A final suggestion for improving time management that I've come to appreciate falls directly in line with Susanne's experience in this case—being involved in professional organizations. I have found that the more activities I'm participating in, the more organized and on time with projects I am. Keeping busy prevents "downtime" where projects may get lost or forgotten about, and helps me keep on track with deadlines. While it may add to the tasks on my to-do list, it creates new experiences and opportunities to learn from while enhancing my project management skills.

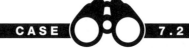

CASE 7.2

How to implement the techniques

PRINCIPLE ■ Identifying bad habits and practicing good ones

Luke has been a staff pharmacist at a local pharmacy in a retail chain for several years and was recently promoted to a new manager position. The first month on the job was a smooth transition. He was given ample time to meet his new staff, incorporate himself into the management team, and to familiarize himself with the other managers. His calendar is rarely full, which means plenty of planning time for ways to improve the pharmacy. Luke spends very little time taking his work home with him and is looking forward to putting his new plans into motion.

Luke decides to take advantage of his free time and reads several books that were recommended to him by local managers. The recommendations include books on managing people, leadership skills, time management, and how to get involved. He can't understand why some people avoid these kinds of books. After a week, Luke has already read three books and has more suggestions on how to improve every aspect of his career and personal life than he ever imagined. He has five more recommended books to read and the list of recommendations keeps growing. He only has one problem. How can he actually use all of these self-improvement techniques?

Finally, Luke has an idea! He could begin to pick specific techniques for improving his leadership, people management, and time management skills and see how well they work. If he likes one idea, after a week he will try to add a new one. Luke began testing his new techniques at work, a day at a time. The first day he worked on his empathy—taking extra time to listen to his employees, ask questions, and understand their concerns. The next day he focused on the patients he was helping. He tries to immerse himself into their view of the pharmacy and how he can improve it. During this experience, Luke notices some of his bad habits. He often forgets important things that people tell him so he begins to carry around a notebook and takes notes. He includes a to-do list in his notebook to make sure he doesn't miss any deadlines or new book suggestions. Every day before leaving work, Luke updates his to-do list of projects, short-term tasks and goals, and personal plans. Before long, Luke has a list longer than his arm of ways to improve the pharmacy. As he begins to schedule project times into his daily calendar, his employees become worried. Luke has spent so much time figuring out what is wrong with the pharmacy that he hasn't noticed how the employees feel. Furthermore, in his attempt to improve his management and leadership skills, Luke has become immersed by trying too many self-improvement techniques instead of perfecting one.

WHAT LUKE MAY BE THINKING...

- These books are crazy. No one actually does this stuff!
- Keeping a list of projects takes more time than actually doing the projects.
- Why can't I keep adding techniques to improve my worn-out techniques?
- There are too many techniques! Where do I even start?
- How do I decide which technique is the best to use with this new group of employees?

ON THE OTHER HAND, LUKE MIGHT REASON...

- Trying out new techniques is a great idea! What's next?
- The more techniques I use, the more organized I will become.
- Techniques may contradict each other, and I need to find a happy medium.
- The more techniques I practice, the more effective I will be.

- -

MENTOR ADVICE

Luke has a very positive attitude and seems committed to continuous professional development. It is common for those coming into new management positions to want to demonstrate their competence as leaders by improving the workplace. However, they may go overboard trying to integrate every new leadership technique into every interaction with their new staff. I had a similar situation early in my career. I wanted to make a good impression on new colleagues so I spent all of my time improving my management skills instead of talking with staff who had worked there for years. I was reminded by a more seasoned pharmacist that all of the self-improvement in the world did not compensate for a true understanding of the concerns of one's colleagues. Luke is eager to fix everything that is wrong in the pharmacy, but he has been so busy with self-improvement that he hasn't spent much time developing the professional relationships he needs to make these changes. He runs the risk of alienating himself from the very people he is trying to help.

There is no substitute for developing strong professional relationships when it comes to leading change. New managers need to demonstrate their understanding of and empathy for staff concerns as well as learning from the other managers' experience. Luke needs to identify the informal leaders and then share his ideas with them. He may be pleasantly surprised to find that others share his vision for some of the improvements, and thus he can leverage that informal network to achieve his goals.

What I have found to be successful

This is such a common experience for new leaders. Below is some advice:

- Take a deep breath. Although you've identified lots of personal and workplace changes that need to be made, your new staff members have not had time to keep up with you. Change can be disruptive and too many changes too quickly can have an adverse effect on staff.

- Demonstrate your empathy. Since you are new, you'll want to demonstrate your understanding of staff concerns by focusing your energy on them. You will gain their cooperation and regard as you drive changes in response to shared concerns. Encourage staff dialogue.

NEW LEADER ADVICE

Most new practitioners are not as lucky as Luke (often, the transition to a new role is not this smooth). Luke should consider trying one new technique at a time so he can discover how it is truly working. If he is completing a research study, for example, he wouldn't want any confounding variables to skew his results. He should think of the opportunities to try the new techniques as a research study by trying each one individually and then determine if it is successful or not before moving on to the next new idea.

Luke should also consider his transition to a new role. Being an outsider to a situation or process will most definitely provide insight that those currently in the process will not see. While this may be a positive discovery, the way the discovery is presented or adjusted may not be welcomed by the current users. It is important for Luke to put himself in the shoes of those he is evaluating (to attempt to fully understand why things are the way they are before he tries to change them). One of his new ideas may have been tried in the past, and without asking those involved he might spend a great deal of time implementing a process that has already failed.

Does Luke have mentors to talk through the implementation of a new technique? Discussing his action plan with his mentors can prevent negative outcomes. Then, after trying the new technique, he can evaluate the successes and failures of them with his mentors. Not only will his mentors be honest with him about the successes—and more importantly the failures—but they will also assist him to think through all of the other possibilities. And they won't hesitate to tell him when he's gone too far!

Finally, it's important for Luke to remember to go slow. He is in a new pharmacy, with new staff, new plans, and new techniques to utilize. Changing too many things at once has the potential to disrupt the good things that are occurring as well. Waiting until Luke more fully understands the systems in place before he attempts to change them can improve outcomes.

What I have found to be successful

As a new leader, I've found that I should spend more time trying to understand the current processes before I analyze what parts of the process could be improved. Asking questions of the pharmacists, technicians, and others involved in the project I'm working on is very beneficial to evaluate why things are they way they are before planning improvements. This technique may not be successful in all situations, but it is one I will need to keep in my back pocket for future use.

Sometimes it's hard to decide whether you should jump in and try your new processes or sit back and enjoy the ride for a while. A good suggestion I've received is to keep a notebook full of ideas and analyze them with my mentor before implementing them. Making a list of all of the techniques you think may work for you is a good way to start building your repertoire of leadership techniques. When I encounter a new situation that I may not know how to handle, I could review the list of techniques I've discovered and then talk with my mentor to determine which is the most likely to work. It's important to remember to discuss with my mentor why I was successful or why the technique failed in order to improve next time.

Luke's idea to keep a journal or folder to store articles, notes, and lessons learned from trying new techniques is a good one. When you're struggling with a new situation, take a moment to page through this information to search for something new. It may also help to write about experiences that you learned from and things you want to emulate or avoid as you become a better leader.

CASE 7.3

Life in the techno age

PRINCIPLE ■ Optimizing technology utilization without becoming "addicted"

John has always been somewhat technologically advanced. Before he became a pharmacy intern he had already purchased a personal digital assistant (PDA) with the most up-to-date electronic pharmacy resources. He had calculators to help him determine creatinine clearance, could run drug interaction checks, and knew exactly where to find obscure adverse events. Not only did he have dose recommendations for adult patients, but pediatric dosing, renal dose adjustments, herbal medications, and even some international medications. All he was missing was a drug identifier!

Now that John is in his last year of rotations, he has advanced to using a smartphone as his electronic reference of choice. Not only does John stay up-to-date on his drug interactions, newly approved medications, and dose adjustments, but he never misses a beat in his personal life with the constantly updated e-mails, text messages, and online networking websites.

John receives several daily pharmacy e-mail updates, and he gathers plenty of useful information from all of his classmates' experiences at different rotation sites. He also appreciates knowing where all of his friends are and where they are headed after work, not to mention the quips about patients they are each interacting with.

A few days into a new rotation, John's preceptor comments on his incessant use of his smartphone. John brushes the comment off and, although he continues to provide prompt drug information to his patients and coworkers, he occasionally appears to be paying closer attention to his friends' status updates than the FDA updates. Although John is always on top of the correct drug information to provide to patients and he never misses an assignment or project from school, he may not always be focusing 100% of his time on his patients. This was apparent during a very serious conversation with a patient about her new cardiac medications. John had set his smartphone on the counter after providing some adverse event information. At the same time, his friend sent him a picture of a few guys out having a good time on their boat. Not only was the picture offensive to John's patient, but she was no longer impressed by his pharmacy knowledge and asked to speak to a "real" pharmacist.

WHAT JOHN MAY BE THINKING...

- Is the information really any better than this book printed last year?
- Why can't other people adapt to the new age of technology? Why should I try to move back into the dark ages?
- So what if I happen to check my e-mail a couple times a day? I'm still saving time when I'm looking up the information.
- Everyone else is using their smartphone, so what's the difference?

ON THE OTHER HAND, JOHN MIGHT REASON...

- I should really shut off access to text messaging and e-mails while I'm at work.
- Is this too tempting? Should I take a step back and curtail the use of my smartphone?
- My patients need to be my main focus. How can I ensure they feel like I'm focusing my attention on them?

MENTOR ADVICE

Like many students, new practitioners, and even some seasoned practitioners, John is technologically savvy and has integrated various tools into his day-to-day life with generally positive results. Having the answers to drug information questions at one's fingertips when the questions are asked is a great contribution to the healthcare team and to the care of patients; however, John's constant attention to his smartphone has created a negative impact with his preceptor as well as with his patient. Is John truly listening to patient concerns? Is he fully engaged in the decisions being made on rounds? This could be a major barrier to patient care. The purpose of modern technology is to supplement one's knowledge, not to replace it. John needs to limit his access of personal e-mails, text messages, and networking sites during rotation time while maintaining the connection to drug information and other professional data. The bottom line is that balancing the connect/disconnect time in his day is an important leadership skill.

What I have found to be successful

I know, how can you be effective if you are not connected? Here are a couple of ideas to maintain a healthy balance:

- Turn off the technology. Of course not all day, but certainly separate work from play. With fewer distractions, you will be more engaged in the clinical discussions and learn more during your rotations. Keep personal technology separate from professional.
- Maintain a professional image. Focusing on patient care issues during the workday will greatly enhance the image you project as a healthcare professional. Leave the personal networking to nonpatient care times.

NEW LEADER ADVICE

It is important to realize that not everyone is as tied to their electronic devices as John is. Respecting patients' wishes, privacy, and time is an important concept John must consider. If he was visiting his healthcare provider, he would probably want his provider to be completely focused on him and not on pictures the provider's friends had just sent. John needs to think about his nonverbal communication with his patients, such as maintaining eye contact, because it will demonstrate that he is engaged.

John should also reflect how lucky he is to have access to such electronic resources and how other pharmacists whom he works with do not have access to electronics. Are they able to provide patient care just as well as John? Sometimes hardcopy references have their benefits— they can't freeze the page or prevent turning of pages too quickly. Understanding the pros and cons of hardcopy versus electronic references is an important first step to defending one's electronic addictions. Handheld electronic devices definitely have their upside. Having access to appointment changes, e-mails, references, and search tools at one's fingertips can help free up time for other tasks. Checking e-mails on the elevator or on the bus to work can give you the extra few minutes you may need to put the finishing touches on a presentation. The thing to remember is that there is a time and a place for everything. Pictures from friends do not belong on patient rounds, and electronic references won't likely be useful to you on a boat.

What I have found to be successful

Having the world at my fingertips with the accessibility of smartphones has definitely had an impact on my career. I'm able to respond to important e-mails faster and potentially avoid certain problems. Most handheld electronics have options to control e-mails and texts. I like to put my personal e-mail on hold while I'm at work, and turn off my work e-mail when I'm out with friends.

The most important thing to remember as a new leader who enjoys the quick communication with colleagues and friends provided by a smartphone is to be respectful of those around you. Whether it is your patient, your coworker, or your family, the person you are with should have your full attention. As a new leader, it's hard to gain trust with your patients and colleagues as a new leader if you constantly act like something else is more important. In order to build your relationships I would recommend the following:

- Leave your phone in your pocket when you're around patients. At the very least, make sure your ringer is turned off.
- Use your smartphone like you would expect your healthcare providers to use theirs. Don't allow yourself to focus on personal tasks when patient care is at stake.
- Some institutions and pharmacies are no longer permitting cell phones to be used in patient care areas. Be sure you know the rules about what is and is not allowed before you put your references on your smartphone.

It may be hard to realize that your authority may be diminished if you fail to show your professionalism while utilizing your handheld devices. All it takes is one unfortunate comment or picture to lose the respect of a coworker or patient. So, when in doubt, leave your smartphone out of sight.

Life as a resident

PRINCIPLE ■ Learning the difference between urgent and important deadlines

It is a month and a half into his first year of residency, and Tom is starting to get the hang of things. He has just finished his general orientation to the hospital, and more importantly, in the pharmacy. Tom now knows everyone by name, and if he doesn't know how to answer a question, at least he knows who can. This also means that everyone now knows Tom; he is the first resident to jump at any opportunity including projects, picking up shifts, or helping someone else. Tom knows that if he is to get everything he wants out of his residency, he needs to create his own opportunities and be sure to take advantage of the opportunities offered to him. Already this year, he has helped improve the utilization of the automatic dispensing cabinets, led a discussion with the clerkship students, and offered to help with a presentation for students interested in residencies. This is, of course, on top of his required staffing and developing his major project.

Now that Tom is about to get his first clinical rotation started, he begins thinking about what other opportunities this might provide him. First, he is really excited about being able to round with the ICU residents and attending physicians. He has already met one of the medical residents and knows that they are going to get along well since they bounce questions and suggestions for patient care off of each other all day. The medical resident has even suggested that Tom should give a presentation to the team on a new drug class each week.

During a meeting to plan his ICU rotation with his preceptor, Tom receives another list of opportunities. His preceptor is working on a medication use evaluation (MUE) to present to the pharmacy and therapeutics (P&T) committee. The results from the MUE might change the way the ICU physicians practice with regards to antibiotic use. Not only is this a practice change that the pharmacists would have to assess, but it might result in several teaching sessions for the physicians and residents. Later that week, Tom's program director asks him if he would be able to give a tour to a group of students interested in residencies. Tom's calendar is beginning to fill up faster than he had ever thought. He begins to wonder if he will even have time to round with the ICU team.

WHAT TOM MAY BE THINKING...

- What pharmacist doesn't have time to go on rounds?
- This is a great opportunity, but do I really have time for all of this?
- Rounds are not as important as all the publishing opportunities that this MUE might bring me!
- Don't patient care and pharmacy practice come first in the residency?

ON THE OTHER HAND, TOM MIGHT REASON...

- I have the best residency ever!
- Man I knew this was going to be a lot of work! I can't wait to get started!

- I just need to skip dinner tonight so I can keep working!
- Doesn't the director know how swamped I am?

MENTOR ADVICE

One of the best things about residency training is the variety of opportunities presented to the resident. Tom is being bombarded with great opportunities but sometimes too much of a good thing isn't so great. One of the most difficult things to do is to say no to a cool opportunity to decrease the risk of getting overwhelmed. Tom should connect his personal and professional goals with the various tasks he's working on. This will help him focus on the tasks or projects that actually align with his professional goals and thus help prioritize his work.

Tom needs to review his residency training goals and requirements and see if he can align the opportunities and tasks he's assumed responsibility for with these goals in order to clarify his thinking. For example, if he is interested in administration in the future he may want to take on the MUE to help with his experience in P&T considering it is an essential element of pharmacy management. Or if he wants to become a solid clinician, it would be great for him to leverage his time with the medical resident to challenge his clinical expertise. Is Tom considering a PGY2 in critical care? If so, he should focus on this opportunity to hone his critical care skills and ask himself what are his must-do versus his should-do tasks? Ultimately, it is his decision to determine which, if any, items on his list can be removed.

What I have found to be successful

As a new leader, you want to take advantage of opportunities but don't want to get trapped by saying yes to every cool idea that comes your way or you'll become overwhelmed.

- Review your project list and set deadlines for each task. Writing this down helps you visualize whether or not you have enough time to do it all. If you do not have the time, use your goal list to sort the must-do from the should-do tasks.
- Talk with your program director or boss. Share your project list to make sure they are aware of everything on it. They can help determine if you can say no to an opportunity or if you can reprioritize your list.

NEW LEADER ADVICE

Tom knew this was going to be a year full of projects, opportunities to expand himself (professionally and clinically), and plenty of late nights. Tom is on the right track, wanting to be involved and getting the most out of his residency. As with any new project, it is possible for Tom to adapt by improving his time management skills. One of the toughest lessons to learn is how to say no to projects, ideas, or opportunities that arise. Wanting to be involved in everything is exciting, but if it's not managed well, it will likely be a failure point for any leader and even more devastating for a new practitioner.

Tom should show his list of projects to both his program director and his mentor. They will both have different views of the prioritization and outcomes of his involvement in the different projects. Tom needs to take their advice and determine which projects will help him achieve his career goals. Additionally, as a resident, there are projects that will arise that Tom *must* complete. His program director can help him determine the best timelines for completing his projects and whether or not he will be able to fit additional opportunities into his schedule. Once he decides which projects are the best fit, Tom should learn as much as he can from the experiences he has chosen.

What I have found to be successful

One thing I struggled with as a new resident was my desire to be involved in every new activity or opportunity that was presented to me. It was the year to learn! I was being given opportunities I may never have again. Why would I want to say no? And then the time crunch hit. I had to learn that although these were all great opportunities for me, sometimes I just couldn't physically fit them into my day. When your sleep begins to suffer and it's next to impossible to crawl out of bed to complete your tasks, it may be a good time to re-evaluate the opportunities you're considering accepting.

My mentor asks what projects I'm currently working on during our meetings. She never hesitates to ask if I need help with anything. Although it's hard to admit to someone that you need help, having a mentor to help you evaluate and prioritize your opportunities may improve your outcomes. A mentor doesn't offer help when he or she is not able to help. But watch out, sometimes a mentor will continue to offer new opportunities to help you grow as a leader, and to learn what you can and can't handle on your own! As hard as it is, learning how to say no may be one of the most important things I learned during my residencies. It may have taken me over 14 months, but one day I said no. And my preceptor congratulated me on the accomplishment.

Another lesson I learned as a resident is that there are times when you just can't say no. If one of these times arises but you're not sure you can confidently say yes, try to find a compromise. Oftentimes the person asking for your assistance or involvement with a project would be more than happy to find a smaller piece of it for you to work on if you can't commit to the whole project. But be sure that before committing to a project, you think about whether you have the time and energy to participate. Don't commit and then back out—follow the project through to completion. And remember—you will surely get out of each opportunity what you put in!

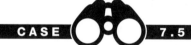

CASE 7.5

Balancing work, school, and life

PRINCIPLE ■ Evaluating the emotional challenges to time management

Rosalie can't believe her luck. In the middle of her first all-nighter of studying in pharmacy school, her 2-year-old son becomes sick. She spent all afternoon playing with him so she wouldn't feel like she was ignoring him and put off studying until he went to sleep. Now he is up, crying, coughing, and uncomfortable. Nothing she does for him seems to help. She finally wakes up her husband to help, but her son only wants to be held by her. Rosalie doesn't know what to do.

After starting her second year of pharmacy school, Rosalie decides that she needs to put some more effort into spending time with her family. Her son is growing up faster than she realizes, and her husband misses having her home for dinner. Their solution is for her to quit her part-time job as a pharmacy technician and live without some extravagant expenses until she is done with school. Additionally, in order to save on childcare bills, Rosalie comes home right after her last class and she doesn't study until she puts her son to bed.

For the first couple of months, the plan works great. Then Rosalie's exams began getting harder and more frequent. On top of that, her practice labs are taking more time this year and her involvement in the school pharmacy society is beginning to increase. The amount of time she has to sleep at night is getting shorter and shorter, her temper flares, and her relationship with her husband is being affected. As Rosalie realizes that her plan to spend all night studying may not be the best idea, she wonders how she can find time during the day to study. Her family time is important, but her grades are too.

WHAT ROSALIE MAY BE THINKING...

- Why can't my husband take care of my son when he gets sick in the middle of the night?
- If I don't get straight As, I'll never get the job I want!
- This wasn't supposed to be this hard! Maybe I should have waited to go back to school.
- Is there any way the pharmacy school can help accommodate my situation?

ON THE OTHER HAND, ROSALIE MIGHT REASON...

- Let the childcare bills pile up. I'll be able to pay them off in no time once I graduate!
- I'll graduate whether I get an A or a C. My son is more important to me!
- What about my pharmacy organization involvement too?

MENTOR ADVICE

Rosalie is in a difficult but not uncommon situation. What is the importance of achieving straight As? Is Rosalie planning to apply for a residency training program where grades are considered as part of the process? If not, she needs to consider the importance of a high GPA and how to balance that with her home situation. If she is planning to complete a residency, she should make sure she has a good understanding of the time commitment of a residency training program. With so many things on her plate, she may not have had a chance to think this through.

Few students are happy with Cs, so she needs to clarify her long-term goals and objectively look at her situation. Are there any areas of compromise that could buy her some time? Is there any time either before or between classes that could be scheduled as study time? Is there any flexibility in her husband's schedule? Could she put her son in daycare for a couple of afternoons per week? How about examining her options with her husband to gain his support? The bottom line is to understand that good time management includes taking care of herself as well as all of the other people and activities in her life.

What I have found to be successful

Finding the perfect balance between personal and professional life is a challenge, especially for new leaders like Rosalie. In fact, it is a life-long activity that shifts as one's priorities do but there are a few ways to tackle it:

- Objectively identify school/life balance issues. Prioritize these and assign time needed to complete each one. Eliminate low priority items to "buy" time for higher priority tasks.
- Ask for help. Faculty mentors can help identify strategies to set class schedules to build study time into your day.
- Bring ideas and possible solutions to your husband to demonstrate your commitment to finding ways to keep your family priorities.

NEW LEADER ADVICE

Balancing family and school life while completing graduate coursework can be a nightmare. I was always in awe of my classmates who were balancing three young children, a spouse, work, a social life, *and* school while I could barely balance school and work on some days. Rosalie is one of these amazing students and she has something special that allows her to complete the same amount of tasks and studying in about half the time that I did. Although it is a struggle, Rosalie should be proud of her skills and motivation. She is already developing skills to balance work, school, a social life, family, and other responsibilities. By choosing the activities each day or each week that are most important to each aspect of her life, it may be easier to find a balance between them.

High achievers often put their needs last. While new leaders in the same position as Rosalie may find it easier to put their needs above their families' needs, she has a responsibility to her son that must be her priority. She must give her family the same priority as exams and school activities by showing them they are as important to her; they will then become her biggest supporters throughout school and her career. Building strong relationships in her family life will reflect strongly in her relationships throughout her career.

What I have found to be successful

Don't let anyone else tell you what is most important to you. Missing an exam may set you back in school, but missing an important family event may set your emotions back even further. I had to take an exam in Europe one year in pharmacy school, because my family went to visit my sister. It was quite the compromise for my professor to allow me to take it out of the country, but being with my family was so important to me, we were able to make it work. Many times there is an alternate option to missing both events. I also had friends who had to take alternative exams due to family circumstances. While that short answer exam may be more intimidating than the multiple choice exam, being with family during tough times is worth it.

Sometimes it's necessary to take a break from work, school, family, and friends. Everyone has their own perfect, stress-free weekend. One of my most relaxing weekends during my residency was when I didn't talk to anyone, didn't do any work, and just worked out, cooked, and watched movies all weekend. That was what I really needed to recover from the stress in my life and rebalance myself and my priorities. Different people will have different ways to rebalance their lives. Try several different ways—a massage, a trip home, hiking, working out, or cooking—to find the way that works best for you.

Covey's circle of influence adaptation

PRINCIPLE ■ Being proactive and creating your own circle of influence

T's Pharmacy is a small, family-owned pharmacy in Sandy, a town on the outskirts of a large metropolitan area. Their daily prescription load has recently been increasing due to the addition of a new subdivision nearby. Victoria is excited about the increase in new patients that she can interact with. She has been a pharmacist at T's Pharmacy for almost 4 years and is very familiar with their regular customers. She can put a name on every face that walks through the door, and they love asking her expert opinion on the newest drugs available. Victoria is also in the midst of creating a new medication therapy management (MTM) program in conjunction with a local physicians' office, and she is beginning to feel like she can really make a difference in the health of her customers.

As the new customers slowly transfer their prescriptions to T's Pharmacy, Victoria becomes worried. The new customers are not as friendly as the current customers, nor do they want Victoria's advice regarding their medication regimens. "My doctor already told me how to take my medications," and "Why would I have any questions for you?" were common phrases spoken by her new patients. Victoria is beginning to wonder if they will appreciate her MTM program. If it isn't successful, she might not receive the funding she is expecting.

Soon it is autumn, and Victoria is getting ready to participate in the pharmacy's annual vaccination program. Her regular customers have been asking about it for months. The pharmacy has signs and flyers posted, and within a week all of the appointments have been filled. The vaccination program lasts a week and when it is done, Victoria feels accomplished. They have vaccinated more patients than any other year. Her feeling of success doesn't last long, however, when several of her new customers complain that they didn't know about or didn't have time to come to be vaccinated. Although Victoria had tried to reach all of the new customers, those that hadn't been vaccinated are not impressed by T's Pharmacy and threaten to transfer their prescriptions back to their old pharmacy. Victoria is more than upset. She was hoping the vaccination program would create an interest in the MTM program and draw more new customers to the store. Now, not only had that failed, but the pharmacy may be losing its new business as well.

WHAT VICTORIA MAY BE THINKING...

■ I have put so much energy into this project. It can't fail now!

■ I posted flyers and posters. What else do these people need?

■ What am I going to do if our pharmacy keeps losing patients? Are these complaints going to make us lose our regular customers too?

■ The new customers weren't friendly. I won't miss them at all!

ON THE OTHER HAND, VICTORIA MIGHT REASON...

■ At least the old customers were able to get vaccinated.

- My MTM program will still have some customers (my old customers)
- Hopefully, I can win over these new customers by killing them with kindness.
- I need to remember to get the word out earlier next time to attract more business!

MENTOR ADVICE

We choose how we deal with the issues in our lives. When we look outside of ourselves to assign blame for a project that didn't go as planned, we empower others to control us—a reactive approach that leaves us feeling victimized and powerless. A proactive approach is creating change from the inside out, where you maintain control of the changes you can impact. Victoria has focused a lot of energy on concerns that she has little influence over, for example, finding the new patients unfriendly and unwilling to hear her advice and complaining about the vaccination program. These issues are all outside her circle of influence as she cannot force changes in their behavior. She can, however, consider changes in her own behavior that might influence her relationship with the new customers. Victoria should try to be more patient, empathetic, and resourceful, thus causing the positive changes she is seeking.

Victoria considers the vaccination program to be a success with the regular customers. She has demonstrated her competence and empathy to these patients and has gained their trust and confidence, which places them in her circle of influence. Naturally, they would be the first to sign up for the vaccine program and come to her seeking her expertise. Victoria needs to do an honest self-assessment and look at how she has presented herself to the new customers. With the additional prescription load, time spent developing the MTM program, and the popular vaccination program, has Victoria inadvertently missed some of those subtle but important relationship-building cues from the new patients? This self-assessment will allow her to choose where to place her focus and energy in creating positive changes.

What I have found to be successful

As you gain leadership experience you'll find that building good relationships helps to get things accomplished, but you'll also find that you don't have relationships with everyone making decisions. There are a couple of things that you can do to be more effective:

- Focus on your circle of influence. Don't waste your time and energy on areas of concern where you have no control. Look inside yourself for opportunities to make positive changes that can drive the outcome you are seeking.
- Demonstrate your competence. Unfortunately, not all patients understand the role of the pharmacist. In order to build new relationships, patients need to trust the expertise of and be able to communicate effectively with their pharmacist. This takes time.

NEW LEADER ADVICE

Victoria needs to accept that she can't control customer behavior. As a retail pharmacy intern, I realized that I had to continue to do my best to share the information I had with the patients I was working with. When they came back the next month with the same problems, I tried to understand that it wasn't my fault (but I had to be careful not to blame them either). While it may be frustrating for Victoria to continue sharing the same information with the same people, talking to them and looking at their situation from a different angle may help her understand the best way to address their concerns.

Victoria should talk to her coworkers or mentors as it will help her analyze what went right and what to do in the future. Others can help her look at the positive things that happened and make suggestions for improving the vaccine program next year. Victoria could talk with her mentor about specific patient cases to evaluate alternate suggestions for improvement. Or Victoria and her coworkers could discuss how previous vaccine programs were similar or different to this one.

Chances are this won't be the last unsuccessful event Victoria has at T's Pharmacy, but it's important as a new leader to continue to put forth her best effort to care for her patients. She needs to continue working with the patients that appreciate her efforts and find ways to enhance their care. Eventually, she will find a way to expand her circle of influence to encompass the new patients as well.

What I have found to be successful

Victoria has committed one of the most common misunderstandings that new pharmacists often experience. We come into the pharmacy profession excited about the changes we can make in patients' lives and full of new ideas for how to produce these changes. But we often forget that patients are not always willing to make these changes themselves. For example, it's easy to think that I am going to be the pharmacist to convince my patient that taking her blood pressure medication is lifesaving and therefore improve her compliance. How many other pharmacists and physicians do you think she has encountered that have thought the same thing? Sometimes I have to remember that I can only provide the information and the rest is up to the patient. This essentially comes down to Victoria helping the patients that want to be helped.

It's important to remember that you can only change what you have influence over. Trying to change things outside of your circle of influence may be energy better spent elsewhere. For a fresh perspective on your circle of influence, ask a mentor or coworker to help you look at it from the outside, discuss the opportunities you have to impact it, and evaluate techniques to do so.

CASE 7.7

Setting and meeting deadlines

PRINCIPLE ■ Being organized and results driven

It is a typical Monday morning for Rob, a young pharmacist 1 month away from completing his PGY1 at an academic medical center. He is busy surfing the web and checking for updates in the news, sports, and music scenes. His patient list is slowly getting dirtied by the crumbs from his breakfast burrito falling onto it. He hears his e-mail "ding," alerting him to an update about a friend's weekend extravaganza—just in time for him to realize that rounds are starting in 5 minutes. Rob grabs his food-covered patient list, spills his coffee on it, and runs down the hall. Rounds go much quicker than usual, especially for a Monday. Rob wonders if this is because he hasn't taken a good look at his new patients.

Rob spends the afternoon catching up on the events of the weekend with his friends doing residencies across the country. His patient list never receives its full review, and he doesn't start his manuscript for his major project; however, he is now convinced that his friend has made the right decision by asking a girl for another date on Saturday night. Rob knows that his manuscript *has* to be completed before he finishes his residency, but he has to take care of patients, attend to rounds, finish a continuing education presentation, and present his last journal club next week. He knows that the manuscript is going to take several hours to complete, but these other projects kept coming up with shorter deadlines and smaller amounts of work needed for completion.

The weeks slowly pass by. Rob's journal club is his best yet. His preceptor finally catches on that he isn't always fully prepared for rounds, but Rob makes sure that never happens again. The continuing education presentation receives a few new slides every day, and finally, the day before he has to present it, Rob adds the finishing touches. The end-of-the-year resident picnic comes and goes, and Rob makes sure to spend lots of quality time with his coresidents before they all leave for their new jobs across the country.

Finally, the second to last day of the residency arrives, and Rob has run out of time. While the rest of his co-residents have finished their manuscripts and are out celebrating their last night together, Rob is sitting in an empty office, looking at a blank computer screen. How is he going to get this done by tomorrow?

WHAT ROB MAY BE THINKING...

- It shouldn't take too long. It's just a first draft, right?
- I don't actually have to have this done before tomorrow, right?
- Oh, that residency director! Why did you make the deadline the last day of the residency?

ON THE OTHER HAND, ROB MIGHT REASON...

- Why did I wait until now to start this? I'm going to be up all night!
- I can go out for a few hours with my coresidents tonight and finish this tomorrow morning.
- I know this will not be my best work product, but I am stuck with whatever I can pull together.

MENTOR ADVICE

Rob has gotten bogged down by the "trivial many" or lower-value activities while procrastinating on his most important project—an easy trap to fall into. But at this moment in time Rob needs to do what he can to complete his manuscript or negotiate an extension. If he had talked about this a few weeks ago with his mentor, they may have been able to break his projects into smaller chunks that could be worked on for even a few minutes each day. I've found that just completing one small part of the larger project creates a sense of completion and that positive energy propels me to accomplish more. Creating a project task list would allow Rob to accommodate other "vital few" projects into his schedule, which means that he could have continued to work on his manuscript while completing his other tasks.

Rob should revisit his professional goals and discuss how he plans to achieve them. What are his most important tasks and projects, and how is he spending his time? Completing residency training may be his top priority, but it seems like he has been spending more time social networking than working on residency projects. He needs to review his to-do list and due dates and then reorganize his list into a timeline that assures him success.

What I have found to be successful

I have been in this situation and it is not fun. It takes some discipline, but I've found some good techniques for getting the most important things done well and on time:

- Break down large projects into smaller, individual tasks. This allows you to get started and make progress toward your big goals.
- Apply the 80/20 rule to everything you do. Determine your top priority items (about 20% according to the Pareto Principle) and focus on completing these "vital few" projects before moving on to any of your "trivial many" (80%) projects.

NEW LEADER ADVICE

Deadlines sneak up on everyone. At this point, Rob is the only one who can produce the manuscript by tomorrow. By waiting this long, he has learned a valuable lesson—the downfall of poor prioritization and planning—and now understands the added stress it brings to an already tough situation.

So as to avoid this in the future, Rob needs to learn how to set his own deadlines. Applying the 80/20 rule to this situation may be a good suggestion. Rob should give himself the last 80% of his project time to complete the most important 20% of the project—editing, approvals, and so forth. By expecting to complete 80% of the basic tasks of his project during the first 20% of time allotted to the project, it's possible to start out feeling accomplished. And he mustn't let this discourage him when he's digging in to the last 20% of the project!

Another advantage of setting his own deadlines is that Rob will have more time to ask for help if he needs it. By setting up time to review his progress periodically throughout the manuscript-writing process with his preceptor, he may receive the much needed motivation to complete the paper.

What I have found to be successful

For some people, the only deadlines that mean something are the ones that are assigned to you, not the ones that you make yourself. This may be a downfall for some, but being able to identify that as a downfall might help you plan better in the long run. I am one of these people from time to time. When I find myself falling into this trap, I try to remember how many other people are affected by my decisions. This also helps when others offer to help: asking them to give me a deadline can help finish the project on time.

Focus on the "meat" of the project or paper that you're working on first. Complete the first 80% of the project in a small amount of time, so that the last 20% of the project can be detail-oriented and not impeded by time constraints. By assigning myself to write a minimum of one page per sitting, I was able to complete my manuscript in just a few days. This allowed me to be ahead of schedule and focus on the more social aspects of completing a residency.

A leader learns how to evaluate the importance and the volume of tasks needed to complete a larger project. Determining how these tasks need to be prioritized and divided up in order to best complete the project in a timely manner are skills that are learned—most often by spending late nights up working!

CASE 7.8

Asking for help: who, when, how

PRINCIPLE ■ Knowing your limits and learning to delegate

As a third-year pharmacy student, Sam is one of the most actively involved in her class. She is president of her school's student chapter of the American Society of Health-System Pharmacists (ASHP), the secretary in her school's student senate, and the recruitment chair in her pharmacy fraternity. She loves being involved in each activity and knows that not only is she setting herself up for improvement in her leadership skills and successes in her future pharmacy endeavors, but she is also setting herself up for failure as far as her grades are concerned. Her GPA has slowly slipped over the last year as she adds new student involvement activities to her calendar. She knows that this year, as president, she is going to have to work extra hard to get everything done.

Sam is currently balancing two big responsibilities in her leadership roles. Next week is the final week for recruitment for the pharmacy fraternity. This means Sam has to plan not only two social events, but also the final rush event for the new pledges. Sam has two other students on the membership committee who can help, but Sam knows the fraternity needs a solid group of new pledges to keep it going next year. On top of this, next week begins national pharmacist month, which Sam has to coordinate. The ASHP-ASP chapter started a new tradition last year, with a different celebration every day of the week. This includes dress-up days, class competitions, free food, and a visit from the school mascot. Sam is hoping that her social committee chair will step up and help, but so far Sam has done almost all of the planning herself. Finally, in class today Sam is reminded about the oncology therapeutics exam she has next Tuesday.

Sam knows she has to do well on this exam to keep her B average. Dropping down into the C range would mean that Sam might not get the residency she is aiming for after graduation. Although she likes oncology, she just can't manage to keep all the drugs straight. Brand names, generic names, adjuvant therapies—they all become jumbled in her head. As Sam is wondering how she is going to find time to study during the next week, she has a thought! What if one of the class competitions is related to the oncology drugs she is studying? Sam decides this is a great way to ensure she has time to study and continue with her plans for coordinating national pharmacist month. Now all she had to do is figure out how to gain another couple of days to study!

WHAT SAM MAY BE THINKING...

■ I don't know if I can trust my committee members to do the job I know I can do.

■ If I don't get a good grade on this test, I'm never going to pull my GPA up!

- Who cares about national pharmacist week anyway?
- Why aren't the committee members helping to finish these projects?
- What is more important? ASHP-ASP, the fraternity, or me?

ON THE OTHER HAND, SAM MIGHT REASON...

- Maybe I can design the class competitions and have the social committee put them together.
- Now I'm glad I have an internship! I've already been exposed to most of these medications!
- Learning how to prioritize and plan these activities now is only going to help me in the future.
- I need to delegate some responsibilities.

MENTOR ADVICE

Sam is on the right track. She has her to-do list, she understands the consequences of not completing the various projects, and she is thinking about ways to leverage her activities to meet multiple goals (e.g., structuring the class competition around the oncology drug test). She needs to take a look at some of her other responsibilities to see how she might accomplish all of them. First, she has two other students on the membership committee and three events to coordinate. Second, she has a social committee chair that can help her with National Pharmacist Week. And finally, she has to study for the oncology exam. Which of these activities can Sam only do? Which can someone else could do? And what are the consequences of not doing them? Clearly Sam is the only one who can study for the exam, but the other activities could be done by someone else, especially with Sam's support.

For example, Sam could meet with her membership committee and divide up the three events in a way that makes sense. With a bit of planning, she could come up with a list of tasks for the events, a timeline for each task, and assign each task to an individual. Next, she could meet with her social committee chair to discuss the events for National Pharmacist Week. Sam has a strong interest in planning the class competition so she can leverage her study time by planning an oncology drug competition, but the other activities do not require as much work. She has the experience from last year's events and with some planning and assistance, many of the other activities could be delegated to the social committee chair. This scenario is the best use of everyone's time. Since Sam has previous experience in these activities, she can perform the planning and oversight and her colleagues can build skills and gain expertise to provide leadership for next year's events. It also provides her with some much-needed study time.

What I have found to be successful

As much as leaders like to think we can do it all, it is just not possible. Learning how to effectively delegate is a skill that you should master now, early in your career.

- Delegate what can and should be delegated. It allows you to focus on activities that only you can do, and it gives colleagues the opportunity to build new skills.
- Consider the consequences of doing or not doing projects. Those activities that have positive long-term consequences for you should be your priority.

Sam should be applauded for being as involved as she is, for keeping on track with school, and for wanting to do more! Letting go of project pieces is hard to do. This is especially difficult when relinquishing tasks to someone whose work she may not have seen yet, but allowing herself to trust that others are competent enough to complete the tasks is a huge step in the process of learning how to delegate. Sam needs to remember that just because something isn't done to her specifications doesn't mean it will be a disaster. Other people have great ideas and twists on events or final work that can be just as creative and successful.

Sam should also remember that she still has control over the project. One way to prevent the fear of relinquishing control is setting up frequent meetings to check in on the progress. As someone who has both delegated and received delegated tasks, I have found that weekly or monthly meetings are the best way to do this. Checking in and making sure all parties are on the same track will ensure the process continues to unroll smoothly. The key is to know which tasks only she can complete and which tasks can be delegated to others.

What I have found to be successful

By creating a task list for a group project and checking off completed items, it becomes easier to juggle the number of tasks that are currently on your plate. What takes practice is being able to divide the tasks among the group to improve efficiency. Think about the strengths and weaknesses present in your group when delegating. It's important to avoid setting someone (or yourself) up for failure when assigning tasks.

One common mistake of a new leader is over delegating and appearing bossy. A piece of advice I received from a former employer is simple, easy to follow, and sure to be successful: never ask someone to complete a task you haven't done or wouldn't do yourself. When you appear to be "above" a task, delegating tends to appear more bossy than collaborative. If you notice that group members aren't actively volunteering to get involved, review the tasks that have been delegated. Are you successfully dividing up the work to provide the best outcome for the group or are you delegating the less exciting tasks? A successful leader is willing to take part of any task and motivate the group to work well together to create a positive outcome.

If you're struggling with task delegation, talking with your mentor about the project is a great way to evaluate the processes thus far. Another option is to find one or two other group members that you feel comfortable talking with—people who will provide you with honest feedback regarding the group dynamics and discuss as a team who would be the best member to complete the task. As you continue to delegate tasks, you will learn how to identify the team members with the skills needed to complete the task and ensure project success.

Summary

Effective leaders are individuals that can balance multiple people, projects, and priorities and still get things done. Working effectively requires you to develop a variety of skills in goal setting, time management, prioritization, organization, and focus while trying to maintain balance in your life. Unfortunately, nobody can do everything they might like to do so identifying those projects and tasks that align with your goals and have value (to you, to your organization) are the ones you should prioritize and focus on. Therefore, your first action item is to take time to set your professional goals. Consider them carefully, write them down, and post them where you can easily access them. These are your reference points for making many of your leadership decisions including time management issues.

With your list of goals as a foundation, you can begin to build your short- and long-term to-do lists. Prioritize your daily list to concentrate on activities that help you meet your goals. If a project is too large to complete in a day, break it into smaller chunks of work and focus some part of each day on completing that project. Ideally using 20% of your time to complete 80% of your project allows you the time you need to focus on the detailed work to finalize it. Aligning your to-do list to achieve those tasks that are most important to your long-term success helps you stay focused on achieving your professional goals.

Successful leaders understand the value of continuously developing their leadership skills to remain effective. One aspect of leadership development is taking advantage of specific opportunities that align with your professional goals to build your skills. Although continuous professional development is something to strive for, make sure the changes you make are planned, thoughtful, and do not overwhelm you or your coworkers. Additionally, there will be opportunities that you need to turn down because you simply do not have enough time to do it all. Learning to say no to certain opportunities or delegating tasks to someone else are two of the most important things you can learn. Luckily, your mentor can help you evaluate and prioritize opportunities that will meet your professional goals while attempting to maintain a healthy life balance. Why wait? Find that mentor and get started working effectively today!

• •

 Leadership Pearls

- Prioritize, prioritize, prioritize! Learn how to pick the hardest, largest, most intimidating task on your list and get started. Putting it off will not make it easier; in fact, putting it off may have a negative effect on *all* of your work!

- Take the time to think new processes through. It's great to try a new time management technique or implement new processes, but changing things too quickly may upset the balance in your workplace.

- Sometimes the highest priority you may have is yourself. Remember that school and work are important, but they may not always belong at the top of your list. Learn how to prioritize the different aspects of your life on a daily or weekly basis to ensure that all of your needs are being met.

- Big projects are easier to tackle when you break them into smaller tasks. Instead of waiting for a chunk of time to magically appear so you can get started, you can do smaller tasks that continually move your project forward.

Leadership Exercises

- Create a list of 10 goals you want to accomplish in the next year. Select the one goal that would have the most positive impact on your life and write it down. Determine a timeline and plan to achieve this goal. Then, take some action on your plan each day until you've achieved this goal. Practicing this behavior will make it a habit and keep you focused on achieving your goals.

- Perform a leadership skills inventory and make a list of areas you'd like to improve on or lack confidence in. Select and read books and articles in your areas of weakness. Attend professional meetings and seminars and participate fully in sessions focused on leadership areas. Download podcasts or audio programs that address these competencies. The more you know, the more your confidence grows.

- After discovering new techniques you'd like to try, write them down and keep them in a single place. Talk about how you would implement one of the techniques with your mentor. After trying the technique, be sure to evaluate the strengths and weaknesses you encountered and assess how you can improve the technique next time.

- Before your next meeting with your boss, take a moment to evaluate the projects you're currently working on. Think about how you have prioritized them. Would your boss put them in the same order? Talk with your mentor about looking at the list from your boss's view, your coworkers' view, your employees' view. How do each of these change the way you prioritize your projects?

- Based on what you've just read, develop a new time management habit. First, identify the new habit you want to cultivate. Second, practice the new habit again and again until it is automatic. Third, commit to locking the new habit into your personality (no backsliding!). You might be surprised how much efficiency you gain with just one change.

VETERAN MENTOR PROFILE

Cindi Brennan, PharmD, MHA, FASHP
(Ret.) Director of Clinical Excellence
UW Medicine Pharmacy Services
Clinical Professor
University of Washington School of Pharmacy
Seattle, Washington

Why did you decide on a career in leadership? I realized early on that my greatest impact in the profession would be coaching others to set up clinical programs. I love coaching others to become successful and to achieve their goals. I find it a real thrill to watch transformation in leaders and it feels good to know I helped to make a difference.

Where do you turn for advice when you are stressed? When I'm stressed, there are two places I always turn. First, I seek out my tremendously supportive network of colleagues in hospital and health-system pharmacy. Second, I look to my mentors, who always seem to be there at the right time.

What is your favorite leadership book? *Synchronicity: The Inner Path of Leadership* by Joe Jaworski. This book reminds me that my primary job is to foster relationships, discuss strategy and vision and, when the moment is right, connect people who have similar visions in order to get things done.

From your perspective, what is the most important issue facing pharmacy leadership today? Our biggest issue is continued demonstration of the value that health-system pharmacists bring to patient care. Our front-line clinicians need to take responsibility for the entire medication use process and our pharmacy leaders need to align our pharmacy departments with the goals of the organization.

Looking back over your vast experience in pharmacy, what one to two things do you know now that you wish you would have known as a student and new practitioner?

1. Change is hard. Things that may seem simple to you are not always perceived in the same way by your colleagues. Hang in there!
2. Networking is paramount to our professional success and fulfillment. It takes a village to nurture ourselves and our profession, to support each other through the lean times, and to celebrate our successes.

What is your best advice for a new pharmacist today? Nuture your vision. Don't let tradition and mediocrity stop you from doing the right thing.

How do you envision this publication assisting student and new practitioner leaders? I thought it was fun. The case-based approach is a great way to dig through the issues. Hopefully the reference will inspire new leaders to continue down the right path with the right set of tools.

NEW PRACTITIONER PROFILE

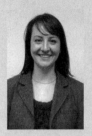

Katherine A. Miller, PharmD
Pharmacy Operations Manager
United Hospital
St. Paul, Minnesota

Why pharmacy: Growing up I was interested in math and science. Some of my family members were healthcare professionals but being a doctor didn't really appeal to me. My uncle was a pharmacist and pharmacy seemed to fit my interests.

Advice to readers: To students: get involved nationally as early as possible. Attend meetings because it is time and money well spent because you begin to build your professional network. My biggest learning since graduation has been that I will never feel totally comfortable as every patient is different. I also have learned to trust myself and the education I received, however I also realized I will never quit learning. In starting your career, be open to advice from people, seek out uncomfortable experiences and seize opportunities. Seek out precepting and teaching opportunities because you will never stop learning and obtaining new ideas from students. Remember others did it for you and I find you gain satisfaction from "paying it forward." As a new practitioner, get involved in professional organizations because they provide you an overall perspective of what is happening and the more deadlines you have the more you will perfect your time management skills thus becoming more efficient.

Tips for work-life balance: My advice is to consciously schedule your personal time especially time with friends, otherwise it may be less likely to happen.

Personal career: I had worked in retail and wanted to make more clinical decisions versus just handling products so my best career decision has been to do a general PGY-1 residency to experience all the various practice options in health-system pharmacy and then a PGY-2 Administration residency. So far the major value of my residencies is the opportunities and networking connections that I have received, such as contributing to this book. My residencies have allowed me to try out various roles and thus determine what the best fit is for me. Residencies have also provided me background, perspective and context for various practice areas. At this point in time my career goal is to get the most out of every experience I have. I am not in a hurry to "move up quickly" with leadership titles as I want to enjoy increasing responsibilities as I go through my career. I define my career success as more responsibility as time goes on and being happy with my accomplishments. My major success so far has been completing the residencies I wanted and knowing my parents are proud of me.

Why leadership: Growing up I was told I would make a good teacher because I influenced others. I was introduced to leadership roles in my PGY-1 residency by my mentor and discovered I enjoyed leadership as it played to my strengths. My favorite leadership books are Tracy's *Eat the Frog*, Komisarjevsky's *Peanut Butter and Jelly Management*, and Roth's *Strengths Finders 2.0*.

Recommended change for pharmacy: I would like to empower pharmacists to make stronger clinical decisions and have every pharmacist be willing to make suggestions for possible solutions to our profession's challenges.

Using this book: I think this book will suggest ways to improve the readers' career and life. My hope is that the cases enable readers to realize they are not alone when they encounter new situations.

References

1. Tracy B. *Eat That Frog!* 2nd ed. San Francisco, CA: Berrett-Koehler Publishers; 2007:28-32.

2. Covey SR. *The 7 Habits of Highly Effective People.* New York, NY: Simon and Schuster Publishers; 2004:81-88.

Suggested Additional Readings

Bell CR. *Managers as Mentors.* 2nd ed. San Francisco, CA: Berrett-Koehler Publishers; 2002.

Covey SR. *The 8th Habit: From Effectiveness to Greatness.* New York, NY: Simon and Schuster Publishers; 2004.

Hammond JS, Keeney RL, Raiffa H. *Smart Choices.* Boston, MA: Harvard Business School Press; 1999.

Kouzes JM, Posner BZ. *The Leadership Challenge.* 4th ed. San Francisco, CA: Jossey-Bass Publishers; 2008.

Additional Materials

Working Efficiently Checklist

(* those you need to work more on implementing)

_____I have documented my highest value activities.

_____I start each day with my most challenging task.

_____I minimize distractions.

_____I know what only I can do that will make a real difference.

_____I always ask myself what is the most valuable use of my time right now.

_____I employ the 80/20 rule.

_____I use technology wisely

_____I manage my cell phone versus it managing me.

_____I set and meet deadlines and if needed negotiate them with my superior to avoid being overwhelmed and missing deadlines.

_____I am able to say NO when appropriate and not feel guilty.

_____I am able to balance my work/school with my personal life.

_____I focus on my circle of influence and not my circle of concern.

_____I ask for assistance when I need to such as from a mentor.

_____I continue to learn new efficiency techniques.

 *Read "Success Skills" article 4.*

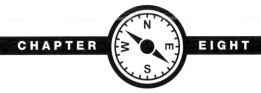

Leading Yourself

Philip W. Brummond, PharmD, MS; Toby Clark, RPh, MS, FASHP

Introduction

As a pharmacist you have the ability to be part of something bigger. You have the opportunity to positively affect the lives of the patients you serve. Your pharmacy education has provided you with the foundation and knowledge and you should be ready to practice those skills in the real world. When the time comes to do so, will you be ready to lead? In order to lead you will have to look inward and discover your inner strengths and weaknesses. In order to lead practice you will have to start the process of introspection and self-evaluation. This chapter will focus on the importance of leading yourself to achieve the success you desire.

The ever-changing healthcare environment is providing pharmacists with the opportunity to challenge the norms of the past and come up with new and exciting ways to care for our patients in the future. Our profession's ability to move forward is on the shoulders of new practitioners and seasoned professionals alike. As you look at your abilities and visualize how you will influence change in the profession, you must understand what skills you possess and how you can use them to move change forward.

Every pharmacist has the opportunity to make a difference and you possess the foundation needed to be successful. As you reflect on your abilities while reading through this chapter, identify areas where you feel can be a catalyst for change in the profession. Leadership is not about being out in front of others; it is however, about knowing yourself in a way that will help you make a difference in the lives of the patients that you serve. Will you be up for the challenge when it is knocking at your door?

What are the things that can make you successful in both your personnel and professional life? Looking through the glass with a positive attitude is a trait that can help you overcome whatever is placed in front of you (Case 8.1). It is important as you take the initial steps to becoming a leader. If you think you can, then you are more likely to be successful in accomplishing your goals or tasks. Some of the most effective leaders across the country make others believe through their actions that the future contains hope. The hope that our patients deserve better and that you will deliver on your ability to rise to the challenges needed to overcome the barriers that prevent this from occurring. As you lay the foundation for success with a positive attitude you should consider a few other traits that will separate you from your peers in your quest to achieve your goals. Personal confidence, accepting responsibility, and following through with action are important first steps to leading yourself.

Confidence, or more aptly self-confidence, is an important trait that should be toward the top of your list of abilities that must be self-evaluated. To trust one's ability to assess a situation adequately, make decisions about the situation, and then to act on those decisions to produce the desired outcome is an important task. As with most skills the more this is done with the desired results the easier it is to feel good about the process.

Accepting responsibility is another important trait to possess, which can result in having the capability of making rational decisions on one's own as well as holding one accountable for those decisions. Maturity and responsibility go hand in hand. Responsibility to one's self must be modeled when making process decisions. It makes no difference what the process is, whether it is furnishing medications to a patient or obtaining your certification as a board-certified pharmacotherapy specialist.

Follow-through with action is important and should be done in a way where a thought is trailed by an action and accomplished in a timely manner. Follow-through is a deliberate activity that must be in the mind of all professional persons as they think about the next steps. Also it is a person's thoughts about the sequence of steps that will bring them accomplishment.

The trait of having an inner drive and subsequent passion about oneself can come from a variety of stimuli. Frequently for healthcare professionals it comes from purpose. A purpose to help others by using the knowledge, ability, attitude, and skills attained through professional education and training is an important force to many (Case 8.2). How is drive created in those that have this characteristic? For many, drive is established by wanting to do things correctly and to the fullest potential. For others, especially achievers, they need to be first in whatever they do so they excel in their professional activities. And some others feel a burning desire to be recognized. Sometimes the passion for accomplishment is derived from wanting to give back to others and to help them. Very frequently drive and passion complements the already known concept that people are good at some skills and they wish to make them better and more complete.

Documentation is a unique expression of thought. When you move a concept from the human brain to paper (or computer screen) you do so with deliberation and thoughtfulness. Sometimes one will think is this what I want to express? So after it is read and reread it will be altered in a way that is in fact what you really want to express. By putting thoughts in writing, one will also move them out of his or her thought processes and be ready for new ones to come into the thinking pattern. Meeting challenges and being creative are traits that are very useful in personal and professional situations.

A 360-degree evaluation is a method of evaluation where everyone around you will assess you. The term *360* comes from a circle where you are in the middle. This evaluative feedback comes from your supervisor, peers, your subordinates, others who work with you, and yourself. The scope of the evaluation can include how you get along with others, your cooperation skills, what is your level of initiative, your level of dependability, and your understanding of the quality and quantity of work you produce. The aforementioned factors deal with your performance generally related to your working relationships. But many of the same factors can be applied to the personal side of your life. It is believed by many that an individual's personal life and work or professional lives are strongly related. The results from 360-degree feedback are often used by the person receiving the feedback to plan their development and improvement.

Another important part of leading yourself is establishing a life plan, which is the start to making your life more goal oriented and successful. Without it aspirations and dreams may only be thoughts in the mind. A life plan will help you create reality from your dreams and aspirations (Case 8.3). This works because the plan gives you not just a destination but also a way to get there. A life plan does not have to be complicated, as it should answer two basic questions. First, what is my destination? And second, how will I get there? You need to find your destination as a beginning step in life planning. You need to dream big. A famous architect, Daniel Burnham, many years ago said "Make no small plans." Dream big. If you dream small you will not move past mediocrity. Along the way to your destination you need to have some milestones. Look at these as goals to help you stay on the right pathway. As you move toward your destination you will need some guiding principles to keep distractions from blocking your path. You can use your values as guiding principles to keep you focused on your pathway.

Establishing a life that contains self-reflection and work-life balance is necessary to lead and influence. Reflection is the process of personal evaluation of experiences, memories, values and opinions in relation to a specific issue or topic. Reflection develops a deeper understanding of one's culture, personal and cultural biases, experiences, and beliefs as these may influence future actions, purpose and learning. Self-reflection is a process of looking at oneself that can be used to maximize personal satisfaction and strengthen commitment.

Work-life balance is the achievement of equality between time spent working and one's personal life. At the core of an effective work-life balance are two key concepts that are relevant: achievement and enjoyment. These simple concepts have real meaning as life planning is thought about. Achievement and enjoyment are the front and back of the coin of life. You cannot have one without the other, no more than you can have a one sided coin.

When we focus on people who have made a huge historical impact we think of presidents, visionary artists, great spiritual leaders; however, we sometimes forget that we too are making history. It can be said that we as professionals have an obligation to leave the world in a better place than when we found it. Thus we too are influencing the future with the way we live our lives.

It is good to ask ourselves, what will our legacy will be? (See Case 8.4.) We have all heard stories about family members we may or may not have known; sometimes it is their humor that shines through in others' memories, their contagious positive energy, or their skill in managing the family assets. People outside our immediate family may have changed the course of our lives. They could have encouraged and inspired us. For example, maybe a neighbor helped us in a time of need or a stranger came to our aid in a difficult situation. When we remember these people, we realize that however small our daily lives seem they are actually very important. How we treat people in each moment with each interaction can have a major impact. Professionally we can have a great impact in the lives of our patients. We should never forget that.

It helps to begin our days with an acknowledgement, taking a moment to consider how we want to be in the world and how powerful we really are. We must remember that our lives are not meaningless, quite the opposite actually. Every day we have an opportunity to "make history" and influence the future for the better and for the betterment of those we have chosen to serve.

The term *role model* has come into general use to mean any person who serves as an example, whose behavior is emulated by others. It has been hypothesized that individuals compare themselves with other people or groups of people who occupy the social role to which the individual aspires (Case 8.5). It becomes the individual's frame of reference and source for ordering his or her experiences, perceptions, cognition, and ideas of self. It is important for determining a person's self-identity, attitudes, and social ties. It becomes the basis of reference in making comparisons or contrasts and in evaluating one's appearance and performance. True role models are those who possess the qualities that we would like to have and those who affect us in a way that makes us want to be better a better person. Role models help us advocate for our goals and ourselves and take leadership on the issues that we believe in.

Critical thinking is purposeful and reflective judgment about what to believe or what to do in response to observations, experience, arguments, or expressions. Critical thinking may involve determining the meaning and significance of what is observed or expressed and determining whether there is adequate justification to accept the conclusion as true. An important aspect of personal and professional growth and development is the realization of the need to observe and be mindful of the behaviors of others that have caused them to be successful. Some of these behaviors have been gained by positive experiences and some unfortunately by negative situations. However, whatever the situation the observer can benefit from the experiences of others. It is important to remember that one does not always need to reinvent the wheel.

Everything begins with a decision—that is to decide to be in charge of others' perception of you (Case 8.6). Many factors influence the way in which we perceive the world and the people in it. Our cultural competency, life experiences, and personal values all affect our interactions and relationships with others. Our personalities, social skills, dress, mannerisms and our styles of dealing with people and problems also affect our relationships with others. In school or the workplace, especially as professionals, we need to learn the skills that enable us to understand and manage other people's perceptions of us. This is not as difficult as you may think, although it does require a good deal of thought, motivation, self-awareness, and practice. Once you have the skills, you will find it easier to communicate with people and to motivate and lead them. You will be judged not only on what you do but also on how you do it—so other people's perceptions and evaluations of you play an important role in your career. People with the skills to influence others' perceptions have a far better chance of controlling their own destiny. Perception management is the ability to create an impression through conscious activities and awareness of other people and how you are able to impact them through your behavior. Impressions that others form of you are a result of both your journey and your destination. Do you behave ethically and are you service focused? People are watching, even when you think they are not. Throughout your career, awareness and management of the perceptions you create are essential.

When we think of teamwork we should be thinking about collaboration, cooperation, synergy, and leadership as we think of a group of pharmacists who do similar functions with the same end point related to serving patients. Teamwork in many cases is not an easy activity to achieve, but with effort on the part of the leader and each participant it can be achieved (Case 8.7). Team members need to feel they are part of the team. Building this team spirit and attitude is one of the roles of the team leader. Team members in turn need to actively participate in performing tasks that contribute to the overall effort of the team. If each person does 110% of their effort then the cooperation and synergy will happen and the team will rapidly come together and be strong.

Jumping to conclusions without having all the facts is a common trap that many novice leaders fall into. What they don't do is ask questions to gain a better understanding and listen to the answers of others. They sometimes will also not go to their superior to ask questions for clarification of issues. The reason teams are supposed to meet on a regular basis is that they will share the information they have with one another to help each other in reaching the team's common goal.

Team leaders, team members, and coworkers of any definition need to show compassion for one another. This is part of being a good team member. Compassion and understanding others situations is absolutely necessary when groups of people work together. Without compassion we don't have an understanding of the other person's situation, which is necessary for cooperation.

CASE 8.1

Approach opportunities with a "can-do" attitude

PRINCIPLE ■ Overcoming obstacles through self-reflection and motivation

Jordan is a 25-year-old pharmacy student who is completing his PharmD degree from a new school of pharmacy. He graduated with an undergraduate degree from a competitive university at the top of his class with a BS in molecular biology. Grades have always come easy for Jordan throughout high school and college. He decided to go into pharmacy school because his undergraduate advisor told him that the medical profession was growing and that pharmacists made a great salary and did not have to work nights and weekends.

Throughout his undergraduate schooling, Jordan worked for an independent pharmacy filling prescriptions for patients within his community. His pharmacy school career started out like many others, with high expectations. Jordan attended his first day of orientation where the school of pharmacy faculty discussed the different roles that pharmacists play in the healthcare field. Jordan decided that he would not have to pay attention since he was going to go back and work for the independent pharmacy he worked at during his undergraduate schooling. He started classes and sailed through the first year without becoming involved in pharmacy organizations because he wanted to be the best student in his class. His memorization skills were superb and he knew that he was going to graduate being a member of Rho Chi with a very high GPA. During his third year he was going through the selection process for student rotations and decided to choose them based on what upperclassmen had recommended for someone of his caliber.

Upon entering his fourth year, things were different. His first rotation did not go as smoothly as he had planned, receiving his first unsatisfactory grade within his academic career. His preceptors felt that he lacked initiative in clinical practice and did not follow through on the goals and objectives discussed during the first day of the rotation. Rotation after rotation Jordan heard similar feedback and was questioning whether he was fit for the pharmacy profession. Jordan's final rotation was in critical care, which would require him to be thoroughly engaged and truth be told his engagement had declined significantly after receiving rotational evaluations. On Jordan's second day of critical care his preceptor overheard him telling another student that he "just wants to finish this rotation and start making the big bucks."

Jordan's preceptor sat him down shortly after hearing him vent and told him that if he did not change his negative perspective that he would not pass this rotation. Jordan drove home that night and reflected on what his preceptor had told him and reminisced of that first day in pharmacy school where he felt unstoppable and ready to take his pharmacy career by the horns.

WHAT JORDAN MAY BE THINKING...

- I'm scared that I may not be good enough to practice pharmacy.
- Did I choose the right career path for me?
- Was there something I could have done in pharmacy school to better prepare me for my fourth-year rotations?
- Should I have been more open minded about the pharmacy profession and been involved in things outside of just school?

ON THE OTHER HAND, JORDAN MIGHT REASON...

- What do my preceptors know? They are just out to get me!
- I just want to finish this rotation and take the boards.
- If pharmacy school had better prepared me, I would not be in this situation.
- What did I do wrong? I am a straight-A student.
- If I could only start over and show them how smart I am.

- -

MENTOR ADVICE

Jordan is in a complicated but repairable dilemma. He needs to ask himself: What is my purpose? What are my responsibilities to me, my preceptors, and my patients? What do I expect to learn about patient care? Am I being open-minded about how I can contribute? Jordan needs to self-evaluate to see what his strengths really are. And last but not least, he needs to question where his strong level of confidence has gone. Does he have a negative attitude and does he see that he has become his own barrier? These are difficult but important questions that need to be addressed for his future. Jordan needs to honestly assess his own skills to determine what his strengths are. The skill-assessment process includes having a mentor who will reflect back to him and perhaps tell him sometimes what he doesn't want to hear but needs to hear. A mentor of this caliber is hard to find, but Jordan should search until he finds such a mentor.

Jordan should also try to develop a positive attitude in every situation and turn those difficult situations into opportunities to help other people. Remembering his purpose can also help keep a positive attitude. In order to be a more positive and responsible person, he needs to view new situations as opportunities to learn and expand his knowledge, skills, and abilities. Becoming less risky while being responsible and accountable in his behaviors will add to his ability to learn at any age.

What I have found to be successful

It has been my experience that when in confounding situations like this, I need to honestly ask myself "What am I doing wrong?" or "What did I misinterpret as what is going on?" I have coupled this type of questioning and thinking with advice from others I know who know me. Before asking the questions, I write them down and then when I have gotten some of the answers either from myself or others, I continue to reduce to writing the answers. By writing the questions and answers, I am able to reflect and make the determinations I need for myself.

NEW LEADER ADVICE

Many individuals enter into pharmacy school with high expectations and falling short of those expectations can be a real dilemma. Jordan may not have gone into pharmacy with an open mind; however, Jordan has been presented with multiple opportunities to change his perspective throughout his education. Now that Jordan is in his fourth year of school and stuck in a situation, he must take responsibility for his actions and will have to work very hard to change his preceptor's perception. Jordan must face his challenge with confidence—the same confidence he entered pharmacy school with. He was able to be successful before, now he must face his fears and enter his final rotation with the same drive and motivation that got him into pharmacy school.

Jordan must take responsibility for his patients and should be ready to learn new things along the way. He has struggled with being accountable for his actions throughout his rotations. Jordan needs to branch out of his comfort zone and rely on others to help him along the way. If he can finish his rotations on a high note, he will not only impress his preceptor, he will also start laying the foundation for success.

What I have found to be successful

Life always presents obstacles. Whether it is not passing an exam, a personal loss, or overcoming a unique challenge, everyone must take responsibility and accountability for their actions. The obstacles themselves do not lead to success or failure; it's how one responds to them. Jordan has had many obstacles, and he has failed to act in a manner that would lead to success. There have been times in my career where it would have been easier to react to an obstacle that presented itself instead of overcoming it and taking accountability for my actions. As you begin your career, it is important to remember that whatever obstacle may lie in front of you, you can overcome it.

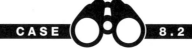

CASE 8.2

Begin with the end in mind

PRINCIPLE ■ Importance of setting goals and seeking out challenging experiences

Sally is a new practitioner who in the upcoming months will be completing her second year specialty residency in pediatrics from one of the most prestigious academic institutions in the country. She has started preparing for an interview in a large academic medical center as a pediatric clinical specialist. She sat down to write her cover letter and reflected on her past to help her articulate why she was the right person for the job.

While Sally was growing up her family was instrumental in shaping who she is today. Sally has always been dedicated to the tasks that have been handed to her, putting forth 110% in everything she does. When Sally was 19, her younger sister was diagnosed with non-Hodgkin's lymphoma. Up until this point in her life she was unclear as to what she wanted to do when she "grew up." When her sister was diagnosed, the stress that was put on their family was overwhelming. Sally dropped out of school for the semester to spend time with her sister in the hospital. Many different physicians and nurses cared for her sister throughout her hospitalization.

One evening while sitting at her sister's bedside a pharmacist walked in and discussed the chemotherapy treatment plan that was going to start the next morning. Up until this point, Sally had never seen a pharmacist in the hospital before, let alone one who walked into a patient's room to discuss medications with family members. The pharmacist discussed in detail the pros and cons of the treatment and what to expect over the months ahead. Sally questioned the pharmacist about the different medications that were being administered to her sister. She was amazed at how calm she felt when talking to the pharmacist. The next morning on rounds she realized that the pharmacist had been caring for her sister throughout her entire stay.

That following spring she went back to school with one goal in mind, to be a pediatric pharmacist just like the one she had met at her sister's bedside. She started shadowing pharmacists and became involved in pharmacy organizations in her state. One of the pharmacists that she shadowed asked her to write out her personal and career goals, which would later become the platform for her growth and development. At the time, Sally questioned the importance of writing out her goals and had been told by others that writing out her goals would be a waste of her time.

While writing the final paragraph of her cover letter, it clicked; she had come this far not by chance, but by having set goals that continually challenge her. Sally knew that because she had the skills, the drive, and the passion there was no stopping her in the quest for the perfect job.

WHAT SALLY MAY BE THINKING...

- Why is it necessary to write down my goals?
- How did I go so long without assessing my goals and writing them down?
- What types of characteristics would make me a successful pharmacist?
- Why should I seek out challenging experiences?
- Does drive and passion make that big of a difference in my career?

ON THE OTHER HAND, SALLY MIGHT REASON...

- Life experiences have shaped who I am today.
- When the going gets tough, it may be easier to go the other way!
- I do not need to write out my goals because I know they will change over time.
- Where will my motivation and long-term goals take me?

MENTOR ADVICE

Writing personal and professional goals is a different way of thinking for most people but this clearly is what Sally needs to do. It is hard to do but extremely important because it forces us to think ahead and set a vision of what we want in the future. By thinking first and then writing we have a documented record of what it is we want to achieve and why we were thinking that way in the first place. It is like a mental compass that helps us to keep on the track we desire. It also helps us to not react to a whim of something we desire just for the moment.

Sally should review her goals every 6–12 months so she can self-evaluate and ask herself if she's on track. A quick review of her already established goals will help her get out of that quagmire/mental funk and build her confidence and self-esteem. Successful leaders plan, self-evaluate, and take action to achieve their goals. At the same time it is ok to change her goals after careful deliberation. Successful people do not leave to chance their life work and career outcomes. Successful leaders also look for ways to expand their knowledge and experience to learn more and to have new skills. They also have the attitude to seek out and make the best of whatever opportunity or situation is before them. In many cases leaders seek the hardest or the most complex opportunity to challenge themselves and others that may be working with them.

Some would call this challenging effort a part of the drive and passion that causes one to move ahead and do more. It is also important in this regard for Sally to do more than what is required. She needs to establish a sense of personal pride and accomplishment for things she likes to do as well as things she doesn't like to do. How will she come across these situations in the first place? Well, she must experience many different situations and then judge these situations to be either good or bad, but she should view them as opportunities to learn.

What I have found to be successful

You shape what you are by your beliefs, attitude, and actions—you are in control. Above all else, you must always have a positive mental attitude. Even in the face of the strongest adversity you must be a positive force for yourself. A constant positive attitude requires work to be maintained, but the payoffs are enormous in the long run. Remember the age-old adage that "attitude is everything."

Success is based on a roadmap or a plan. Plans need to have a vision for the preferred future and this is where your goals come in to the picture. Your plans need to be written and kept in a spot where they can be reviewed from time to time. On days when you think things are not going well, whatever that may be, it is reasonable to look in mirror and give yourself a little pep talk. If you think that you can do something, then most likely you *can*.

- -

NEW LEADER ADVICE

Up to this point in Sally's career, drive and passion have been established through life experiences and they have molded her into who she is today. Sally should strive to be the best and should continue to do so with the hopes of providing better care for her patients. As Sally looks for a new job, she should understand how important it is to establish goals and put them into writing. She must push herself both personally and professionally to reflect back on the goals that she has written down and modify them as needed. It is also very important that Sally seek out challenging experiences that will fulfill her thirst for knowledge and wisdom. This next chapter in her career is a critical step that will continually challenge her to strive for excellence. With Sally's goals set high, she should be confident that she can handle any situation that may lie ahead in her path.

What I have found to be successful

I have been blessed to have many mentors throughout my career who have taken an active role in assuring that I am headed in the right direction. One of my mentors spent the better part of 6 months with me discussing what my career and personal goals were and helping me put them into writing. This exercise was very useful and helped lay the foundation for my career decisions. Without having done this, it would have been much more difficult to know where I wanted to go. As you start putting your goals into writing it is important that you aim high and not limit yourself. Your goals should be concise, objective, and measurable. It will be important to continually reflect on your goals and make changes over time to adapt to your current and future state environments.

CASE 8.3

What's your life plan?

PRINCIPLE ■ Living your life to the fullest and planning for the future

David is a 26-year-old pharmacy resident who is struggling with deciding what exactly he wants to do with his pharmacy career. David has done rotations in general medicine, neurology, and critical care. The ASHP Midyear Clinical Meeting is on the horizon and David wants to make sure he is able to secure the job of his dreams. Up to this point in his residency he has had multiple evaluations from both his superiors and subordinates. His residency program recently implemented a 360-evaluation program to help coach and develop the residents. As part of this process the residency program brought in weekly speakers to discuss important pharmacy topics ranging from clinical practice to administrative leadership.

One week in November, David attended a resident seminar where the speaker discussed the importance of a life plan. The speaker also detailed out the importance of self-reflection and philosophical development. David became intrigued by the speaker's message and discovered that this could be the missing link in his quest for deciding what he wanted to do in his career. All the way through school and residency the plan had always been to get done and get out, make money, and be happy. He was almost done with one foot out the door and the money tree was starting to grow, but he was unsure what would make him happy. Following the presentation David went back to his office and thought long and hard about what had been discussed, then he started typing.

David realized that he had been living his life in the past and not in the future. Everything up to this point in his career was about work. The presentation opened his mind to a new way of thinking. He picked what he felt were the five most important elements in his life and included them in a short and concise plan. In going through this process, David realized that his career was only one element of his plan and that in his quest for the perfect job and happiness, he had forgotten the other very important things that will make his life whole. David realized it was about having a balanced life plan that would bring him success both at the ASHP Midyear Clinical Meeting and into his future.

WHAT DAVID MAY BE THINKING...

■ What makes a life plan so much different than just setting goals?
■ How much weight will my career play in my life?
■ Should I explain to potential employers my general life plan?
■ How do I decide what should go into my life plan?
■ How can I be successful as I move into an uncertain future?

ON THE OTHER HAND, DAVID MIGHT REASON...

- I know that it is important to have plans; I just don't have time to write them down.
- I don't need to know where I am going with my future; it will just happen and I have little control over it.
- I haven't done anything yet, how would "the writing" of a life plan be worth my while?
- Can't I just get a job, make money, and figure out my life plan later?
- Why should I focus on other things when all that is important is my residency?

- -

MENTOR ADVICE

David is on the right track after he realized that a life plan and balance in life would help him establish thoughts about success in his life. He needs to start the process of learning and thinking about what his values and beliefs are by reducing these thoughts to writing. By writing down his values he can better go back in a few days and see if he still feels the same way now about his thinking. This process will help him in his reflection and subsequent self-evaluation. His construction of a balanced life plan now will stimulate his thinking that in his residency he is more focused on learning new knowledge, skills, abilities, and attitudes at the present time. While he needs to do this his entire professional career he is doing it now with a greater intensity. He needs to think that this intensity of learning will decrease a little after residency. In other words his current state of uncertainty will decrease as he moves into his professional career.

In addition to writing his life plan David needs to seek the counsel of a mentor who can help reflect on this thoughts. A mentor should not tell David what to do, but rather stimulate his thinking on what is best for David based on David's dreams, goals and aspirations. David does need to be careful about his thinking that money is going to bring him a level of happiness and success. While he can have a nice income from his profession he needs to think about how his chosen profession can assist him in finding the satisfaction and subsequent achievement he deserves.

What I have found to be successful

Learn to evaluate yourself in personal and professional matters. Learn to ask yourself questions and then listen to your answers. Take time to ask yourself did I do the right thing? You can learn to apply self-evaluation in both your personal life as well as your professional life. Think about what you did in the past and how it will apply to the future, both short- and long-term.

The concept of thinking about planning for life balance is extremely important and cannot be understated. But what is more important is to actually prepare the written life plan. While life planning is a personal and confidential process it is important each of us have someone that serves as a reflector to our thoughts. We all need someone to bounce ideas to and from. So find a mentor who will be a confidant.

NEW LEADER ADVICE

David needs to realize the importance of a life plan and how the 360-evaluation process can be the springboard for this plan. David has learned so much about himself throughout the residency program. As he writes his life plan he should use what he knows about himself and establish guiding principles that will lay the foundation for his plan. As David set his sights high, he should establish a relationship with someone who will be there to bounce ideas off of. He can use this individual as a mentor and confidant to help guide him in the right direction.

Establishing a rewarding career is important both personally and professionally. David's patients will benefit if he likes what he is doing. David should try his hardest to push himself professionally by also striving to be happy personally. As he moves throughout his career, he should continually reflect on what is going on day to day as well as apply what he is doing to help accomplish his life goals. Having a plan in place will give him the opportunity to lead his life toward a purpose; a purpose that he has planned and articulated for himself.

What I have found to be successful

Work-life balance is important for many finishing pharmacy school these days. Completing a residency can be difficult and establishing work-life balance is nearly impossible during that time of your life. If you take the opportunity to complete a residency, I would recommend writing your life plan during the final month of residency. By doing it at that time, you will have received feedback throughout your residency and you will have had ample opportunity for self-reflection. You will likely have identified a mentor and will be ready to start articulating what you want in your career and personal life.

Working through the elements of a life plan will assist you in identifying the important things in your life that you will derive success from. I have established a life plan and put it into writing about 2 years ago. I have reviewed it once or twice since then and the themes are still relevant. It is broad enough to encompass many areas of my life. If you have not done so already, put to writing a life plan to assist you with identifying what is important in your life. You will not regret it.

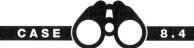

CASE 8.4

What will be your legacy?

PRINCIPLE ■ Developing relationships and making an impact on patient care

George is a pharmacist, 5 years removed from pharmacy school, who recently moved to a rural community to start his own pharmaceutical care practice. Upon his arrival, members of his community had been familiar with traditional pharmacy services—medication dispensing, drive-through windows, and a building full of knick-knacks. George joined the community with the hopes of offering new services that would improve the community's health through the management of drug therapy. His goal was to offer medication therapy management services to patients in his small community.

When George first started building his practice, he struggled in getting it up and running. People did not see the value in the services that he was offering. He spent a significant amount of time developing relationships with many members of the community. George joined local community organizations and started speaking at the senior center. After about a year he established a collaborative practice agreement with a local provider, which opened doors. Patients started scheduling appointments with George and were discovering what type of impact that he could have on their lives. George was saving his patients hundreds of dollars a month and was able to improve medication therapy use and compliance.

A year later local business organizations started to realize the impact his services were having on their employees. Businesses started contracting directly with George for the services he provided to their employees. His practice began growing exponentially over night, which required him to hire new pharmacy practitioners and bring them into the area.

WHAT GEORGE MAY BE THINKING...

- How can I have an impact on the patients I am serving?
- Why did I move to a rural community to offer new services?
- How can I change the attitude of the community toward pharmacy?
- Does taking a risk really pay off in the long run?
- Can I as a pharmacist leave a footprint on the community in which I serve?

ON THE OTHER HAND, GEORGE MIGHT REASON...

- Just for being a pharmacist, people should worship the ground I walk on.
- Why do I need to develop relationships? They don't really matter!
- Perceptions are just perceptions. Who cares what people think?
- Now I have the "big" money employers in my pocket and I can ignore the other patients.

- -

MENTOR ADVICE

George has a dream and he aimed high to change the perception of the role of pharmacists in his community. He made a strong impact on the health of his community and took a risk, and others in addition to him are the winners. His level of professional satisfaction must be very high and that surely gives a great feeling of accomplishment. George had a plan and worked his plan.

George should continue to keep his mission, vision, values, and purpose. He should make sure he is training his new pharmacy practitioners in his philosophy of doing what is best for patients. He should make sure that he has quality measurement activities so that the safety and quality of his pharmacy practice is upheld no matter who is providing the professional practice activity. George should also lead his professional team of pharmacists and technicians in reading the literature and keeping current with the latest drug therapy and technology aids to continue to serve patients. George should not forget how he got where he is today and continue to strengthen his relationships with patients and care providers with whom he has established the collaborative practice agreements.

What I have found to be successful

I have found that making plans must be done with a distinct purpose in mind. That purpose must be greater than to serve one's self. Making plans for the future necessitates preparing bold and big plans that stir the hearts and minds of others, not just yourself. It has been my experience that when making bold plans, others will want to participate with you as you prepare to change the future if they see what is in it for them.

In my experience the personal trait of persistence is one of the most important human interaction characteristics. One must have the personal philosophy of being persistent in everything. If you are going to be an effective person in helping others as well as being a professional pharmacist you must be ready to face bumps in the road and obstacles to success.

- -

NEW LEADER ADVICE

Throughout George's career, he has lived his life in a manner that portrays his values and beliefs. He walked into a small town and did not know what to expect. It was important to aim high and dream big. Though he faced some adversity young in his career, the persistency of knowing that he could provide better care for his patients helped establish his drive.

What George found that helped him achieve his full potential was to develop relationships with everyone throughout the community. This task was not easy nor should it be. Establishing the trust of others should not be taken lightly. Relationships must continually be worked on to maintain the level that is needed to influence change. George has made the choice to put others first and the rest just fell into place. He knows that he can have an impact on others and be part of their history. George should continue to make decisions and influence outcomes that will put his patients first. By doing this, there is little that can come between who George is and how he cares for his patients.

What I have found to be successful

I believe it is important to approach situations with the possibility of leaving it better than when you started. I have tried to practice the philosophy of leaving a footprint in each place you cross that represents you. George did not go into his community and think "What will my legacy be?" Instead he started doing the little things that make a difference. Those things that make a difference will form his legacy over time. Surrounding yourself with people who are successful and trying to emulate the characteristics that make them successful is important. I have learned that if you can approach situations with an open mind and put importance on developing and strengthening personal relationships, it will be easy to accomplish your goals. If the foundation of those relationships is trust, you will have a higher likelihood of success.

Importance of a role model (both good and bad)

PRINCIPLE ■ Understanding oneself through mentorship and relationships

Robert is an associate dean at a university school of pharmacy. He has been involved in many different activities throughout the course of his career and has been in his current role for the past 10 years. He has practiced in a variety of settings including clinical hospital practice, pharmacy administration, research, managed care, and ambulatory practice. His resume is filled with numerous publications and presentations both on the national and international level. Many in the pharmacy profession would consider Robert a seasoned practitioner with attributes of a leader written all over him. On the weekends, Robert loves to hang out with his students and socialize—whether it is at the bar, tailgating, or just hosting poker night at the house. Robert's professional and personal lives do not always overlap—one minute he is all business and the next a social butterfly.

One day Robert is preparing to leave the office and notices that one of his students, Ken, is standing at his doorstep. Robert invites Ken in and asks him to sit down. He can tell that something is on Ken's mind since he has come to visit him at the end of the day. Ken asks Robert if is willing to sit down and talk through things with him as he prepares to seek out a residency in the next couple of years. Robert would always mention to students on the first day of orientation that individuals could seek him out if they needed someone to talk to. Very few students actually took him up on the offer; however, today it appeared that the student in his office is serious.

Ken explains to Robert that is interested in learning from someone who has experiences in many different areas of pharmacy. He also wants someone to provide him with critical, open and honest feedback both personally and professionally. Lastly, Ken is hoping to develop a professional relationship with Robert. Robert welcomes Ken's honesty and asks him to set up regular meetings with him over the course of the next few months, with some meetings at the beginning of the day and some later in the afternoon. Ken questions the need for specific meeting times, and Robert replies that they can have some of the discussions in a fun environment outside of school where the real learning occurs. Ken agrees and then sets up some meetings with Robert's secretary the next day. Over the course of the next several months, Robert challenges Ken to think differently than he has done in the past. Robert shares his life experiences and helps Ken expand his horizons. The development of the relationship also occurs over time and both Robert and Ken appreciate their meetings.

One fall afternoon at their team's tailgate, Ken sees Robert and walks up to greet him. Robert has been having a little too much fun throughout the course of the afternoon and is not representing himself in a professional manner. Ken decides it would be best to walk away. The next day Ken reflects on how he had seen Robert at the tailgate. Ken is concerned with how his role model had portrayed himself and wonders if things could ever be the same again after seeing Robert in a different light.

WHAT KEN MAY BE THINKING...

- I feel disappointed and embarrassed by Robert's behavior in public.
- Do professionals really act this way?
- Does this change the way I interact with Robert in the future?
- Should I begin to seek out another person as a role model?

ON THE OTHER HAND, KEN MIGHT REASON...

- Everyone makes mistakes including myself.
- Should I share with Robert how his behavior made me feel?
- Doesn't Robert deserve to have a little fun too?
- What can I learn from this experience?

MENTOR ADVICE

Robert has a lot to learn about relationships with himself, his students, and his peers. Too much fun in the form of overindulgence of alcohol and/or foolish behavior shows little respect for himself and those around him. By virtue of his position with the university as well as a professional person, he should know he is a role model for others to emulate and look up to. Robert has an outstanding professional record of accomplishments—for that he should be praised and others should aspire to be so accomplished. However, his personal behavior needs to reflect his professional accomplishment. Robert needs to realize others are constantly viewing him as a model of behavior.

Ken clearly has some soul-searching to do to decide if he can trust and rely on Robert for advice and counsel. Yes, all of us make errors in judgment, but repeated errors as evidenced by Robert's behavior do show great cause for concern on the student's part. Ken should give careful consideration to finding another person from whom advice is sought. It is important for Ken to think through this "tailgating experience" the next day. This shows a real sense of maturity on the part of Ken to question Robert's behavior.

What I have found to be successful

The relationship between the mentee and mentor, student and teacher, and advisee and advisor is a precious affiliation. Both parties should regard this situation as a privilege as well as a responsibility. Students should relate to role models that don't tell them what to do, but rather role models that help students broaden their horizons and act as a sounding board for reflective thinking. Role models come in all shapes and sizes, and students will come across role models that they do not wish to emulate.

NEW LEADER ADVICE

Ken should be concerned with how Robert is acting in public. Ken should think long and hard whether or not he should continue to foster his relationship with Robert. As a professional, Robert is well-accomplished and has taught Ken much over the time he has spent with him. Robert's behavior should make Ken critically think about the consequences that could come about with associating himself with someone like Robert. His sphere of influence is impressive; however, his social habits may be overshadowing his positive traits.

Ken should consider seeking out another role model. It is highly unlikely that Robert would change his behavior if Ken brought his behavior up to him. Robert clearly has prioritized what is important to him and socializing is a big part of it. Ken can learn from this experience and know that through the relationship that he established, Ken was able to discover himself and know what he does not want to emulate in his future. Another option Ken could take is continue to use Robert as a professional role model and not a personal one. It can often be difficult to separate the two; subsequently, the risk may be worth the benefit. Ken must continually use what he has learned up to this point to make the right decision.

What I have found to be successful

Having a mentor who is dedicated to your success is important and should be sought after. I have found that there will be times when the person you look up to does not hold up their end of the deal. Ken finds himself in this type of situation with Robert. When situations such as these are presented to me, I try to spend time understanding what can be learned from the situation. Ultimately having a negative experience can lead to further self-reflection and helps me not make the same mistake. You may find that you can learn much about what not to do in these types of situations, and knowing what not to do can be extremely valuable.

CASE 8.6

How to influence others' perception of you and why you should want to

PRINCIPLE ■ Becoming the pharmacist you want to be

Robyn, a third-year pharmacy student, is standing in front of her colleagues as the ballots are being counted for the student pharmacy society presidential election. Things have not always fallen into place for Robyn. Throughout her early years of college, she was known as a quiet loner that did not get involved in activities outside of studying. Throughout her first year Robyn spent most of her time with her nose in the books and little time socializing. She did not see much value in wasting her educational dollars on fun and games. One evening as she was leaving school, Robyn saw a group of her classmates laughing and socializing in the student lounge. As she walked home she reflected on that moment and realized that there might be more to pharmacy school then just studying.

When Robyn began her second year she decided to become involved in activities such as Operation Diabetes and Katy's Kids (community service activities). With these opportunities she was able to portray to others some of her core values and beliefs. She also decided to take on more and more responsibility within organizations and school functions. Robyn began viewing herself as someone who was providing value to others and contributing to the better part of the profession.

One afternoon, during a student society meeting, a problem arose that required a tremendous amount of resources to pull everything together. The school had decided to cut funding for their student organization because of state budget cuts. The student group was going to have to cancel some of their events, including their spring social if funding could not be obtained. People were in shock of the news and when asked for ideas, the group did not come up with anything substantial. At this point in time, Robyn had just started attending the meetings. She felt as though she was part of the team and offered an idea to the group. She stated that it might be wise to have a grass roots campaign to solicit funding from past members and graduates of the school. As part of the donation, the past members could attend their spring social event, network with pharmacy students, and be recognized for their contributions.

After unanimous approval, Robyn led a team of individuals to call, e-mail, and write letters to past graduate members of the student organization. Her efforts and the efforts of her team did not go unnoticed by the school and her classmates. She raised over $10,000 in 2 months. The spring social ended the year with a bang, and at the same time members of the student society approached Robyn to run for president the following year. As Robyn stands in front of her classmates and the votes are being counted, she hopes what she has done in the past is enough.

WHAT ROBYN MAY BE THINKING...

- I am scared about what other people think of me.
- Am I really experienced enough to be the president?
- I hope that I changed others' perceptions enough to become elected.
- I think that I have shown others through my actions what I am capable of.
- I have done all I can to leave an imprint in the lives of those I have interacted with.

ON THE OTHER HAND, ROBYN MIGHT REASON...

- I have tried my best and it really doesn't matter what people think of me.
- I am right for the job.
- If I don't win the election, I am going to go back to my comfort zone and never do this again. Besides I am here to learn in the classroom.
- People should know that I have changed from my first year of school and should vote for me just because of that reason alone.

- -

MENTOR ADVICE

Robyn should care about what others think of her and needs to demonstrate her best skills and a positive attitude. Robyn made the decision to become involved in activities and make life more than just about her. She also used some creative thinking as she proposed an idea to solve a problem. Having one's ideas accepted starts to promote an idea of leadership from the group. This is what happened to Robyn as she led a successful team effort in fundraising. The members viewed her as a potential leader when they approached her to run for president.

Her ideals and ethics play a big part in how she creates her image. At the same time she needs to be respectful of others and their thinking by being a good team player. Being a good team member is an important quality to exhibit because team members share and trust one another.

Emotional intelligence also cannot be overlooked. It describes the ability, capacity, and skill (or self-perceived ability) to identify, assess, and manage one's emotions. Robyn seems to have good emotional intelligence. She was focused during her first year in school and was not balanced, but she realized balance was missing and did something about it.

What I have found to be successful

Be proactive in your thinking and raise your hand to volunteer if you want to be involved. If you decide to be part of the solution rather than part of the problem, let others know of your desire in a way that is likeable but not bossy. Don't use the term *I*, but rather mention to others that you have a suggestion. For example, say "perhaps this idea has merit" and then explain the thought leaving out the word *I* and using the term *we* or *our*.

I have found that I need to be prepared to be proactive in my thinking and then active when entering the conversation. I try to offer suggestions—not direct dictates. At the same time be flexible in language and thinking, using such terms as perhaps and maybe. This works well when I support the thoughts of others and don't cut them off in discussions. It is important to make sure others have their say in the matter. Always remember that the term team has no *I* in it. Speak with others in their terms and framework. In other words, try to have conversations about them and what they are doing. Focus on them—not yourself. This will have a definite influence on others' perceptions of you. However, don't live your life trying to always please other people and be liked. I have found that I must find a balance between being a team player that contributes and being myself.

- -

NEW LEADER ADVICE

Robyn has changed the perception of her peers, and she is still learning what is and what is not appropriate. She wants to be liked by those around her; however, she still wants to be herself. As Robyn became involved in activities outside of her comfort zone, she realized that there is more to life than just her. She found a way to not only fit in but to stand out. She is not sure if she will be elected president, but she does know that she has done everything she can to change the first impression that others have of her. Robyn has strived to show that she is a team player and is willing to take action when necessary.

Robyn should never give up! This experience has helped her realize how important it is to show others who she is through her actions. Robyn could go back to her comfort zone and be a loner, but then again she's not so sure that being a loner *is* who she really is. Robyn has developed herself as someone who has strong morals and is respected by many.

What I have found to be successful

First impressions are important and are very hard to overcome if the impression is negative. I learned this at a young age when I had overheard a group of faculty members taking about my appearance. The experience made me wonder why we live in a society that puts so much emphasis on conforming to social norms. I spent a lot of time reflecting on this and concluded that it is not necessarily me they are judging but rather how I portray myself. This experience made me stronger as a person and ultimately showed me the importance of how first impressions can make or break you. Once people have formed an opinion of you, it can be difficult to change that perception because their perception is their reality and changing that perception requires deliberate actions. Everyone wants to be recognized for the good that they bring to situations. So strive to form good first impressions and work to change negative perceptions that others may have of you.

Don't play the blame game or be the victim

PRINCIPLE ■ Working with a team to achieve success and overcome failure

Becky is a 29-year-old pharmacist who has been practicing as a clinical specialist in anticoagulation for the past 4 years. She has spent the better part of the last year intimately involved in leading an initiative aimed at showing the impact of a pharmacist-led anticoagulation service. As part of the project Becky measured the impact that pharmacists had on medication error reduction. After 6 months into the initiative, she thinks individual pharmacists who have a higher incidence of errors are causing patient harm. Becky is shocked by these conclusions and begins to think that certain individuals on the team are attempting to sabotage the initiative.

Over the course of the following weeks, Becky spends time trying to build up evidence to support her theory with the hopes of proving that certain pharmacists are at fault for the negative outcomes. Her ambition to hang some of her colleagues out to dry is consuming her work life and has started to impact how the initiative is being led. Instead of working to correct the problems and trying to positively influence the outcomes, she is badmouthing pharmacists on her team. Word spreads quickly that Becky is not supportive of anyone not working on the anticoagulation service. She is coming in on her days off to work side-by-side along other pharmacists to prevent what she thinks is the inevitable failure of the initiative.

The director of pharmacy asks Becky to put together a presentation for their monthly staff meeting highlighting the outcomes of the initiative. With quite a bit of hesitation, Becky agrees to put together the presentation. Later that month, Becky presents the preliminary results of the project and sarcastically bashes the other pharmacist members on the team. She realizes halfway through the presentation that members of the department are chatting with each other and raising eyebrows at her comments. Becky portrays their lack of interest in her presentation as disrespectful.

The next day Becky calls a team meeting to further discuss the outcomes of the anticoagulation service. There is a mix-up and the team members meet in a different location than where Becky is waiting. They are disgusted with her absence at the meeting as well as her recent attitude and behavior. They discuss Becky's findings, determine that her analysis of their work was done incorrectly, and proceed to tell the director of pharmacy. The director reviews the results and agrees that Becky's analysis was bogus and that her behavior at the staff meeting was inappropriate.

Later that week, the director meets with Becky in his office. His plan is to remove Becky from the project and promote another team member to lead the initiative. Once Becky discovers that she was going to be overthrown as the project leader, she decides it is best to bring in other healthcare professionals to meet with the director to tell him how good of a job she is doing.

WHAT BECKY MAY BE THINKING...

■ I feel like I am in the right and that my team members should not accuse me of wrongdoing.

- What could I have done differently to gain the respect of my colleagues?
- Did I make a mistake by assuming people made errors that harmed patients?
- Should I begin looking for a new job where people will respect me?

ON THE OTHER HAND, BECKY MIGHT REASON...

- I did nothing wrong, and people should understand that this is my initiative and it is important to me.
- My director will support me once he finds out the real story.
- My team should all be removed from the initiative and then I will pick people that can do the job well.

MENTOR ADVICE

Becky needs to think about what has happened and why it happened. The team has fallen apart and feels betrayed by its leader. It happened because Becky was more interested in herself than in the team and the team's results. Becky started to blame others when she did not have the facts. She needs to understand that she did not build a team who would work together for the common goal. Becky clearly needs to assess her attitude and reflect on how she can relate better to the team. Becky should have been continuously evaluating the team's results as a group from the start of the initiative and not waited 6 months to see results. Clearly, Becky should not have made any conclusions without reviewing the information with the team members early in the project. As her director of pharmacy provides Becky with critical feedback, she needs to be open to criticism without being defensive.

What I have found to be successful

In my experience when project teams come together, the leader of the team and the team members need to understand how the project results will be reviewed and by whom. Team leaders and others at any level of authority need to be told, in no uncertain terms, that blame or blaming others is unacceptable behavior. I have made sure the project sponsor or other high level leader not on the project team sets ground rules of behavior that excludes the "blame game." Project evaluation methods should be written and well-understood by the team members; however, project team meetings can take valuable time that is often hard to come by so short, stand-up meetings between shifts can help keep the meetings brief and to the point. Project team reports should be posted or e-mailed for all to see before team meetings. This keeps the team informed and up-to-date. Make sure to send one clear message to update the entire team and ask them to bring feedback to the meeting. This is not over communication, but rather a mechanism to facilitate team communication. People like to be kept informed!

NEW LEADER ADVICE

As a new practitioner, Becky should practice her leadership skills including project management and team leadership. She has not made all of the right decisions up to this point, and it will be very hard to re-establish the trust and respect of the team and her director. Becky has not been true to herself or to her team members. She has lost the compassion she once had and needs to find the spark to reignite it. Becky is not sure what will lie in store for her in the near future, but one thing Becky knows is that she has made mistakes and hopes to learn from them as she moves forward.

As Becky attempts to break down the barriers that she has put up for herself, she must remember that things are not always as they seem. If given another opportunity, Becky should take the feedback that is given to her seriously, with the hopes of being able to renew broken relationships and move toward one common team goal. This experience has been challenging, yet Becky will look back and know that this event changed her outlook on how she deals with individuals on a day-to-day basis.

What I have found to be successful

Making mistakes can sometimes be one of the best ways to learn. It can be difficult to experience a mistake; however, the learning potential is great. I have made mistakes in my career, and my philosophy is that if I learn from the mistake and do not let it happen again it was worth it. Put yourself in situations that foster creativity and push yourself to the limit. By putting yourself through these types of situations you will have ample opportunity to learn. If you make a mistake, you will be able to reflect on what worked and what did not. Self-reflection should be done to minimize the chances of putting yourself in a similar situation.

Summary

Leading yourself is an important first step to influencing others. As you embark on your journey, remember to approach opportunities with a "can-do" attitude and begin with the end in mind. Write down your plans, spend time reviewing them with your mentor, and establish your legacy as you become the pharmacist that you want to be. It is important to recognize that mastering the skills described throughout this chapter can take a lifetime. Take things one step at a time. Now that you have the tools to lead in the ever-changing healthcare environment, it is time for you to use them through practice and repetition.

 Leadership Pearls

- Assess your skills to determine what your strong strengths are and develop a positive attitude in every situation.
- See new situations as opportunities to learn and expand your knowledge, skills, and abilities.
- Always remember the age-old adage that "attitude is everything."
- Making plans for the future must be done with a purpose in mind.
- Seek mentors who assist in understanding different points of view.

Leadership Exercises

■ Set aside 30 minutes and write the answers to the following questions:

1. What are my strengths?

2. What are my weaknesses?

3. What opportunities do I need to make my strengths even stronger?

4. What can I do to improve my areas of weakness?

5. What do I like to do in my personal time and pharmacy practice related time?

- Assess your attitude. Is your glass half-full or half-empty?

- Think about and then construct your own life purpose statement.

- Attend leadership/management skills workshops available through your organization, local colleges, or professional organizations.

- Volunteer to be a committee member of your local, state, or national professional society.

- Using your developed career and life plan, periodically assess your progress on meeting your goals and targets. Remember you only hit the targets you aim at.

VETERAN MENTOR PROFILE

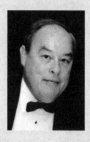

Toby Clark, RPh, MS, FASHP
(Ret.) Director of Pharmacy and Adjunct
  Professor of Pharmacy
University of Illinois at Chicago Medical
  Center
Chicago, Illinois
Lead Surveyor, Accreditation Services
American Society of Health-System
  Pharmacists
Bethesda, Maryland

Why did you decide on a career in leadership? It was a natural career path for me because my dad owned the only pharmacy in a small Indiana farm town and he had a big influence on my career path. I remember him taking me to professional meetings and teaching me that professional people have a leadership obligation because you get from the community so you have to give back to the community. There was always an expectation to go into leadership.

Where do you turn for advice when you are stressed? I turn first to my wife and second to mentors and colleagues in the pharmacy profession. I ask them for help—it's not complicated. I find it helpful to partner with people in similar positions and to lean on colleagues for advice from time to time.

What is your favorite leadership book? I have favorite authors, not necessarily favorite books. I like Peter Drucker, John Kotter, and John Maxwell. In 1972 I was given a Drucker book to read and discuss. It sparked a thirst for reading in management topics.

From your perspective, what is the most important issue facing pharmacy leadership today? The biggest issue is the lack of pharmacy leaders building people to be supervisors because you can't be a good leader without being a good supervisor. Since 2002 this issue has been phenomenally addressed by Sara White to expand the number of leaders with residency experience and through other leadership programs.

Looking back over your vast experience in pharmacy, what one to two things do you know now that you wish you would have known as a student and new practitioner? I wish I would have known as a student and new practitioner when to keep my mouth shut. It's important to think things through and listen before you speak, which is a topic that relates to situational planning. It is important to develop a vision for yourself. In essence, this is an amplified life plan.

What is your best advice for a new pharmacist today? Establish a preferred vision for your future and work with a mentor to help see that vision come true.

How do you envision this publication assisting student and new practitioner leaders? The use may be different for students than for new practitioners. Students can use the cases for group discussions in classes or as a self-learning guide. New practitioner learners can apply the cases to their individual practice settings although they will need to apply their own motivation to get the most out of the book.

NEW PRACTITIONER PROFILE

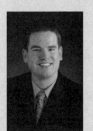

Philip W. Brummond, PharmD, MS
Pharmacy Manager
Department of Pharmacy Services
University of Michigan
Ann Arbor, Michigan

Why pharmacy: I was introduced to healthcare as a growing field by my mother who was a nursing director. I later shadowed a pharmacist and was able to see the impact pharmacists could have on their patients.

Advice to readers: In pharmacy school I would suggest becoming more involved in community service activities in addition to being involved in pharmacy organizations. By doing so, you can start developing relationships within the communities where you are being trained. Get involved in professional organizations because it will foster new ideas and expand your network. For the time you devote to professional organizations, there is an opportunity to gain ten-fold back in value. Seek out mentors who can assist you with personal and professional decisions that lie on the horizon. Do not restrict your thinking to what the current practice of pharmacy is today, but see and seize opportunities to do things differently that will ultimately improve the care we provide our patients.

Tips for work-life balance: Expect the balancing to always be a bit of a struggle. Surround yourself with people who are also trying to have a reasonable work-life balance (i.e., consider as you select a job). View your personal life as equally important as your professional life.

Personal career: The best career decision I have made thus far is completing an MS Administrative Pharmacy Residency because it challenged me to think differently and provided me with the tools to start my career. In my residency I learned that I could handle anything that was thrown my way. My career goal is to continually strive to advance the practice of pharmacy and improve the care that is provided to our patients.

Why leadership: My mentors sparked my interest in leadership through their dialog and passion for what is needed in the profession and how I could be part of influencing change. My favorite leadership book is Maxwell's *25 Ways to Win with People*.

Recommended change for pharmacy: We need to take bigger risks with regards to what we as pharmacists can do to care for our patients. These risks should be calculated as to how we organize and process our work. We must challenge one another to ask the question: Is what I am doing today providing value for patients?

Using this book: My hope is that this book will provide exposure to new thoughts and ideas, which will stimulate readers to think differently about their ability to influence change.

Suggested Additional Readings

Cottrell D. *Monday Morning Choices: 12 Powerful Ways to Go From Everyday to Extraordinary.* New York, NY: HarperCollins Publishers; 2007.

Cottrell D. *Monday Morning Mentoring: Ten Lessons to Guide You Up the Ladder.* New York, NY: HarperCollins Publishers; 2006.

Drucker PF. Managing Oneself. *Harv Bus Rev.* 2005;93(1):100-109.

Holliday M. *Coaching, Mentoring and Managing: A Coach Guidebook.* Franklin Lakes, NJ: Career Press; 2001.

Johnson R, Eaton J. *Coaching Successfully.* New York, NY: Dorling Kendersley Limited; 2000.

Maxwell JC. *25 Ways to Win with People.* Nashville, TN: Thomas Nelson; 2005.

Maxwell JC. *The 21 Irrefutable Laws of Leadership.* Nashville, TN: Thomas Nelson; 1998.

Maxwell JC. *The Right to Lead.* Nashville, TN: J. Countryman; 2001.

Additional Materials

Self-assessment

PART A

Complete the following questions with an open and honest mind.

Do I set high expectations for myself?

———— 1 ——————————— 2 ——————— 3 ————— 4 —————————— 5 ————

Strongly Disagree   Disagree   Neutral   Agree   Strongly Agree

Are my personal and professional goals established?

———— 1 ——————————— 2 ——————— 3 ————— 4 —————————— 5 ————

Strongly Disagree   Disagree   Neutral   Agree   Strongly Agree

Are my professional goals compatible with my personal goals?

———— 1 ——————————— 2 ——————— 3 ————— 4 —————————— 5 ————

Strongly Disagree   Disagree   Neutral   Agree   Strongly Agree

Do I have a plan and use it for professional development?

———— 1 ——————————— 2 ——————— 3 ————— 4 —————————— 5 ————

Strongly Disagree   Disagree   Neutral   Agree   Strongly Agree

Am I a contributing member of a pharmacy professional association?

———— 1 ——————————— 2 ——————— 3 ————— 4 —————————— 5 ————

Strongly Disagree   Disagree   Neutral   Agree   Strongly Agree

I ask others to give me feedback on my self-performance?

———— 1 ——————————— 2 ——————— 3 ————— 4 —————————— 5 ————

Strongly Disagree   Disagree   Neutral   Agree   Strongly Agree

Am I a likable person?

———— 1 ——————————— 2 ——————— 3 ————— 4 —————————— 5 ————

Strongly Disagree   Disagree   Neutral   Agree   Strongly Agree

Am I respectful to all those around me?

———— 1 ——————————— 2 ——————— 3 ————— 4 —————————— 5 ————

Strongly Disagree   Disagree   Neutral   Agree   Strongly Agree

Do I regularly perform a self-evaluation?

——— 1 ————————— 2 ————————— 3 ————— 4 ————————— 5 ———
Strongly Disagree   Disagree   Neutral   Agree   Strongly Agree

Am I a team player in my professional and personal activities?

——— 1 ————————— 2 ————————— 3 ————— 4 ————————— 5 ———
Strongly Disagree   Disagree   Neutral   Agree   Strongly Agree

PART B

After completing Part A, brainstorm and write a plan that will help you address some of the areas you have identified as opportunities for improvement.

PART C

Reassess the plan 6–12 months later to determine if you are moving in the right direction and make changes in areas you feel need more action. Review your progress with a mentor and develop strategies to overcome the gaps you may have. Also consider gaining experience in areas where you may be deficient.

Read "Success Skills" articles 7, 8, and 10.

CHAPTER NINE

Marketing Yourself in Pharmacy

Samaneh T. Wilkinson, MS, PharmD; Harold N. Godwin, MS, RPh, FASHP, FAPhA

Introduction

Exceptional leaders connect with people. They have an understanding that people are the greatest asset to a team, department, and company. These leaders take the necessary time to build rapport, establish credibility, and show a genuine interest in getting to know others. Leaders possess strong social skills with a purpose: build relationships and network "up and down" the organization. Relationship building begins by winning others over. Although it may be a time-consuming process, it is accomplished through consistency, competence, expertise, and trustworthiness.

Many different relationships will be established throughout your career: classmate, coresident, other healthcare colleague, superior, employee, and a multitude of others. However, one must never forget that the most important relationship will be with our patients. Successful leaders always keep this relationship at the forefront of all actions.

Implementing cutting-edge practice models and expanding pharmacy services, new rounding teams, new software and programs, and medication therapy management are not possible without sound leadership skills. The relationships previously mentioned quickly become your network. When a solid network is in place, it's easy to be successful and collaborate with peers when the time for action is necessary. The principles that we will be discussing in this chapter will assist you in the art of relationship building and establish opportunities to market the profession and your role as a leader. Although there is no set marketing strategy as a pharmacist or pharmacy leader, we have identified five key elements: professionalism and role modeling; a positive attitude; self-awareness; persuasion and winning others over; and last but not least, motivation (Figure 9.1).

The single most important aspect to marketing yourself as a professional and a leader is role modeling—always maintain a high professional standard and put the care of the patient first. Cultivate the philosophy of professionalism amongst others on your team and let this be the tone and expectation as their leader. Professionalism and role modeling are important as all pharmacy employees are ambassadors of the profession and anything less than exemplary behavior and exceptional care for patients is unacceptable. This can be a difficult lesson for leaders but one that is crucial to success.

A positive and friendly attitude creates an environment that will attract others to you, and this is element number two. Positivity does not imply that you must always be in a good mood but rather dictates the manner in which you react to situations. Humor and a positive attitude is contagious and encourages teamwork and job satisfaction. As a leader, you should be generous with praise and always quick to smile. This positive demeanor will add to the ability to influence the behaviors and attitudes of others along the way. This simple concept is an extremely powerful tool.

Element number three requires an understanding of self-awareness (who you are). Self-awareness is the ability to recognize and understand your moods, emotions, and drives as well as their effect on others. Successful self-awareness requires an honest self-assessment and evaluation of your self-confidence level. This is critical when marketing yourself because having a deeper understanding of your strengths, weaknesses, and drives will determine how you perform on certain tasks and in certain roles. It is important that you find a position that is the right fit for *you*, so that you can leverage your strengths appropriately. Developing goals and focusing on situations that play into your strengths and

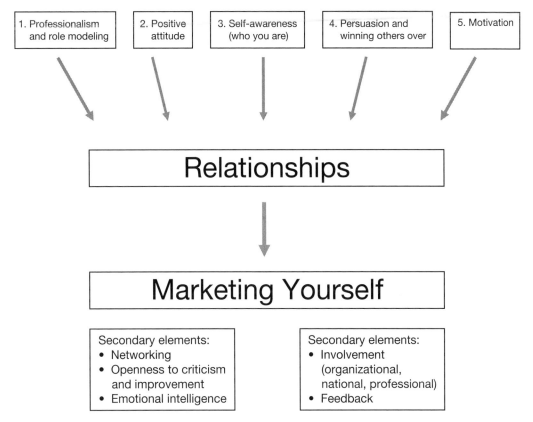

Figure 9.1: 5 Elements leading to successful marketing within the profession.

then applying them to create win-win solutions is a great marketing strategy. This concept is very difficult as many people are not keenly self-attuned; however, as a leader, matching the right person for the right job or task is extremely important. Mastering this element comes with experience and true internal evaluation. Failure of even one team member could cause the entire group to fail the organizational mission or project goal.

The fourth element in marketing yourself involves the art of persuasion. Persuasion should be tailored to appeal to specific audiences and specific outcomes. This element is supported by the professional credibility established when you have proven to be a competent expert. Your credibility should support the persuasion without creating a situation that may appear to lack authenticity. When developing new projects and procedures, it's important to bring lots of energy and passion to encourage others to follow your lead.

The fifth and final element is motivation. Motivation is defined as "a passion to work for reasons that go beyond money or status" and "a propensity to pursue goals with energy and persistence." Although this element fits into many chapters of this book, motivation and marketing go hand in hand. When leaders have a passion for their work, it is evident. These leaders do not accept the status quo; they seek out challenges and investigate appropriate solutions. They are persistent with their goals and are always looking to improve situations and explore all options. They are restless and have a strong commitment to and a connection with the mission of the department and organization.

The five elements that we have discussed directly and indirectly support a place to start when marketing yourself as a leader within the profession. There are many other components that one should consider while evaluating self-marketing strategies. Some of these include participation in committees both organizationally and nationally, accepting challenging projects and situations, openness to feedback and criticism, patience, and persistence. To that end, volunteering for committees, projects, and presentations as well as attending national and local meetings is essential. Take the time to meet new faces and introduce yourself to names that may sound familiar. An easy goal for every opportunity should be to meet and connect with two to three people. Remember that authenticity during networking is extremely important. The elements discussed play a key role in aiding in the development of strong and meaningful relationships with colleagues within and outside of the profession. Solid relationships are the foundation to marketing yourself within the profession.

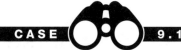

CASE 9.1

Representation is key

PRINCIPLES ■ Professionalism and role modeling ■ Customer service

Suzie is a recent graduate of a 2-year Residency-MS program. She is thrilled to start her new job at Washington Memorial Hospital, a 600-bed academic medical center. She recently finished her orientation to the organization and department. One part of the orientation process that she did not complete was spending time in the cardiology satellite, due to a summer staffing shortage. She was unable to meet with nursing leadership for the cardiovascular operating room (CVOR) due to other commitments. However, she was able to spend some time with the clinical pharmacists. This is great since she will be managing the cardiology pharmacists (teams) in her new role.

The cardiology teams support not only rounding cardiology services but also a CVOR. Suzie is also in charge of the pharmacy satellite that supports the CVOR. Although the satellite is relatively small, there is a dedicated CVOR pharmacist primarily responsible for providing medications to the six to eight cases being performed daily. Medications provided include anesthesia medications, pain medications, anti-emetics, and vasoactive agents as necessary.

A few weeks after starting, Suzie gets a call in her office from Betty, the CVOR nurse manager. Betty is pretty upset and immediately starts asking Suzie who she is and why she was transferred to her office when she clearly asked for the CVOR pharmacy manager. Since Betty had previous commitments during Suzie's orientation, she was unable to meet her; however, once Suzie gets Betty to realize she is the new CVOR pharmacy manager, she receives some very disturbing news.

It appears that the pharmacist staffing in the satellite on this day has refused to dispense medications for a case that was originally scheduled for the main operating room but was rescheduled to the CVOR due to high patient volumes. The pharmacist has never been involved in this type of patient case before and due to personal religious beliefs is having a problem caring for this patient. Betty and the surgeons are furious, as clearly the case cannot continue without these medications. The patient has been prepped for surgery and is on the operating room bed waiting for the procedure to continue.

WHAT SUZIE MAY BE THINKING...

- That pharmacist is so fired!
- What did I get myself into?
- How am I supposed to help this situation? I can't dispense medications from my office.
- Why can't Betty and the surgeons just be more empathic to my pharmacist's religious beliefs?
- Why is Betty so demanding?

ON THE OTHER HAND, SUZIE MIGHT REASON...

- I've got to get this patient the necessary medications immediately.
- I'm sure this is all a misunderstanding.
- That pharmacist must not know the entire story.
- The CVOR must be really busy today. I wonder if they are short-staffed.

MENTOR ADVICE

Susie certainly has hit the ground running. It is unfortunate that she did not meet the CVOR nurse manager during her orientation. However, in the healthcare practice world there are often new players in the organization that might not be aware of the pharmacy service or its leadership team. A good leadership style is to lead by example, which allows a more personalized approach to management. Had Susie known the CVOR nurse manager, I am sure that the conversation, while critical, would not have been so confrontational. Suzie's focus should be to calm the nurse manager down through an effective conversation that is empathic to her feelings. As soon as Suzie is clear about the issue, she should not hesitate to act responsively to her staff in the satellite.

The critical issue at hand is assessing the situation and taking prompt action, aimed at taking care of the patient immediately. In this case, as long as the medications needed are appropriate for the patient and are in the appropriate doses, the needed medications should be provided immediately.

Next, the critical discussion must take place with the pharmacist who refused to dispense needed medication to a patient on the basis of personal religious beliefs. While Susie must respect her staff member's right for conscientious objection, this staff member must be made aware that the patient's needs come first. Suzie should have this conversation in private and work on an alternative plan should this situation present itself again. Suzie should also focus on her expectations for the pharmacist and review the unacceptable behaviors to avoid any further confusion. If there seems to be no resolution or an agreement is not possible, the patient's needs must become a priority over beliefs and Suzie may consider rescheduling this pharmacist to another pharmacy area, thereby removing any future barriers or by having another pharmacist on call to accept the responsibility to the patient.

The most important issue here is to realize all individuals represent the pharmacy department and patient care must always come first. Suzie has made her expectations clear by stepping in and providing the necessary medications and acting in a calm, assertive, and professional manner.

What I have found to be successful

New managers should always begin their tenure in a department by meeting as many staff members outside the department as possible. They should study the hospital's organizational chart so they understand who's who in other departments and when the situation presents itself, quickly introduce themselves as new managers representing the pharmacy. Always strive to be an ambassador for the department and a role model for the profession.

Pharmacy has a unique responsibility within the hospital of being responsible for drug distribution in a timely manner and managing drug therapy as a clinical service. Since this is the responsibility of the department, the staff member also has that broad responsibility. Always remember, however, that the patient comes first. Once a patient care issue is resolved appropriately, the incident should be immediately discussed with the staff or pharmacist involved to develop a plan to avoid this incident again.

NEW LEADER ADVICE

It's unlucky that Suzie got placed in such a difficult situation so quickly into her new role. Unfortunately, this is common in every practice setting (hospital, community, leadership) and, if not addressed appropriately, may set the tone for future relationships. Suzie is being pulled in three very different directions: one by her staff pharmacist, one by the patient, and one by nursing and physician leadership. Suzie should address the patient's needs immediately before addressing any other issue. As previously mentioned, there should be a conversation with the staff pharmacist. Although everyone is entitled to their beliefs, the patient's needs must be a priority. It's important for Suzie to understand the underlying issues so that this can be avoided in the future through the development of a system or process where both the pharmacist's beliefs and the patient's needs can be accommodated. This collaboration allows the pharmacist to be an active part of the solution and demonstrates that Suzie is empathic as a manager and leader.

Diversity is a very important aspect and one that should be respected and accepted in the workplace. Once this situation is resolved, Suzie needs to take the time to formally introduce herself to the nurse manager, apologize, be prepared to ask a lot of questions, and listen. It's probably not going to be a pleasant meeting, but it must be done. Suzie should have no expectations for that meeting except to make sure that she begins a collaborative relationship with the nurse manager. Suzie must assure her that she takes responsibility for providing a system that makes the patient's needs a priority. If a face-to-face meeting is not possible immediately following the incident, Suzie could contact the nurse manager via e-mail as soon as possible. This should be a very carefully composed e-mail with some personalization as well as a plan for addressing the current issue. Immediate attention also allows the situation to be addressed and future processes to be developed. A request for a followup meeting would also be a very good idea. Although this is a very uneasy situation, it can be a win-win situation. Resolution of this issue can put Suzie in a positive light as a manager and help establish credibility with nursing leadership and the pharmacist. It's a great opportunity to show that she is onboard and willing to do whatever it may take to care for her patients and listen to her pharmacist at the same time.

What I have found to be successful

When faced with difficult situations, I have found being empathic to the other person's needs and situations tends to create a less hostile environment. This can be accomplished by listening closely, asking lots of questions, and apologizing when necessary—especially if I have violated that person's trust. Although apologizing may be a difficult thing to do, it's a very important step that is often overlooked. Apologizing doesn't mean having to take fault or blame for the situation—it can simply be that you are sorry for the outcome or the unpleasant feeling experienced through that situation. I'd encourage more people to apologize as well as say thank you. It's a small thing that can make a huge difference. It's easy to be defensive or suggest your solution to the problem; however, you should consider not saying much and listening to the other people involved, both the pharmacist and the nurse manager in this case. Enter a situation with some thoughts on a potential resolution and work toward that goal. In this case, it would be to establish a collaborative relationship between myself, the pharmacist, and nurse manager. This goal would not take place if the issue wasn't discussed or addressed. Although the conversation will not be an easy one, it is one that will make a difference now and in the future.

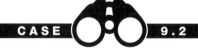

CASE 9.2

Remain positive and optimistic; seize every opportunity

PRINCIPLES ■ Positive attitude ■ Friendly demeanor

Molly, a new practitioner and a "millennial," started working in an outpatient pharmacy about 1 ½ years ago. The pharmacy has seen an increase of 25% in their prescription sales as well as taking on a recent expansion role in the local hospital clinics focusing on discharge counseling for high-risk patients (greater than 10 medications and/or on high-risk medications). Unfortunately, the pharmacy department has not been able to obtain approval for increased resources. In addition to her new patient care responsibilities and increasing workload, the pharmacy department has just added a community practice residency program and increased the number of pharmacy students completing rotations at the practice site due to college expansions. Molly just has no way of meeting all of her job requirements as well as educating the resident and students. Molly is extremely dedicated to her patient care responsibilities and so she has no choice but to ignore the resident and students that are on rotation with her throughout the year.

It's August 1st and on the first day of her rotation, Molly starts off with 5-minute introduction to the resident and students where she shows everyone the restrooms, the department, and her office. "Let me know if you have any questions. Just jump right in and help fill some prescriptions or help with the window. If you have any questions, we'll discuss tomorrow." Since Molly didn't bother to ask any questions, she is unaware that the students and resident are new to the organization and have no idea how to navigate the computer system. All the while, the students and the resident try their best to help fill prescriptions. The resident even took the initiative and answered a request from a physician to assist with discharge counseling. Excited about his accomplishment, the resident looks for Molly, but she is nowhere to be found. She never takes the time to wrap up their day and offers no feedback. The following day, Molly asks them to take care of a new patient recently discharged from the hospital on Tikosyn®. While the resident is entering the prescription, the computer system indicates a severe interaction with one of the patient's current home medications (hydrochlorothiazide). Unsure how to proceed, he asks Molly for help and she types in her override code, paying no attention to the issue or the fact that these two drugs are contraindicated. Assuming that all is well, the resident fills the prescription and proceeds to counsel the patient on Tikosyn. The following week, Molly is informed that the patient has returned to the outpatient clinic with changes evident on an EKG. The doctor is extremely frustrated that the pharmacist didn't prevent the interaction and immediately calls the outpatient pharmacy manager to discuss the situation. When Molly is called into her manager's office for a fact-finding discussion, she says "There is just no way that I can precept students and the resident. I am entirely way too busy and simply have no time, energy, or desire to dedicate to them. It's not my responsibility to teach them—that is why they went to pharmacy school. Anyway, what's in it for me? Precepting is all give, give, give."

WHAT MOLLY MAY BE THINKING...

- Why in the world do I have to be nice to the resident and the students? I'm never going to see them again.
- I am already working 10 hours a day and it's an 8-hour shift.
- If the resident or students really want to know what it's like, they should just jump in the deep end and get the job done. They stand around so much!
- I should just go work somewhere where there aren't students and residents.
- What in the world is in it for me? My preceptors were horrible and I turned out fine.

ON THE OTHER HAND, MOLLY MIGHT REASON...

- It's important to have a positive attitude and have a friendly demeanor.
- Precepting is a core responsibility for my position.
- I owe this to my profession.
- Precepting is rewarding because I learn a lot from the students and residents as well as contribute to their education.
- Engaging the resident and students may help me meet all of my job responsibilites.

- -

MENTOR ADVICE

Molly appears to be frustrated by having more and more responsibility without additional resources. She has not had any orientation to her educator role nor has she had any discussion on the value of this new role. The workload appears to be increasing. The supervisor and the staff should be addressing methods together for improving operational efficiency and time management in order to cope with the increasing workload. This is an important step regardless of the increasing educational responsibility.

During the time of the responsibility change, it is important to provide for a planned transition into her new role and responsibility. The manager should have frequent discussions with Molly to prepare her for her new educator role and monitor the transition to her responsibility change. Time should be provided for this transition. Perhaps a sample student and resident orientation template and packet should be given to Molly for her use for the resident and students. The manager should engage her thoughts in this process so that she has "buy in" to the orientation and can champion her own thoughts and ideas. Molly's manager also needs to explain how the resident and students, once orientated, can assist Molly in her own clinical responsibilities thus creating the win-win situation.

Molly should be told that by serving as a good role model for the resident and students, the likelihood of being able to hire one of these well-trained students will increase. This should take the pressure off the workload if eventually all new hires are well-trained.

What I have found to be successful

Position responsibility changes require significant explanation and description, detailed expectations, orientation, and guidance. However, this role change process may take considerable time and a well-planned process depending on the complexity of the role change. Certainly, in this case, the new educational role is a major shift or addition of responsibility for Molly.

Always remember that challenges and difficulties can provide an opportunity for personal development and a positive growth experience. Look at the big picture for not only improving the individual employee but also for improving the department or unit. The department of pharmacy team is made up of a mixture of generational types each with their own strengths. The key is to place employees in a position in which they can have success in their strengths.

Lastly, remember to discuss the originating issue (the patient drug interaction) and the patient care problem. As discussed in the first case, the patient *must* be the first priority. This case illustrates two problems facing our profession today: the essential need for staff orientation and the continued requirement to provide quality patient care.

- -

NEW LEADER ADVICE

It's easy to relate to the situation that Molly is in. Increasing responsibilities without increasing resources is a situation that everyone (students, residents, technicians, pharmacists, and leaders) faces in our profession. New healthcare reform expectations will only continue to bring light to this issue and we will be expected to do more with less. Although Molly is extremely busy, education is a fundamental responsibility that should not be taken lightly. With the number of residency positions available across the nation and double the applicants, most likely Molly will be precepting residents throughout her career.

It's unfortunate that Molly has such a poor attitude and even more unfortunate that many of us have experienced a situation like this either as a student or preceptor. It is a horrible feeling to know that your preceptor doesn't care, doesn't want you around, and doesn't have the time to dedicate to teaching and precepting. I am extremely empathic to Molly's situation. Though I would like to give Molly the benefit of the doubt, her overall attitude is unacceptable. When faced with difficult and challenging situations related to time commitments, it's important that one maintains a positive attitude. A "glass half-full" attitude will get you much further than a "glass always empty" attitude. A positive attitude is energizing and magnetic and one that attracts other people and their support. It's important to note that Molly is also modeling this poor attitude to our future leaders, which is particularly alarming.

Like many preceptors in our profession, Molly needs some guidance on how to accomplish all of the tasks in her busy day. She also needs support in identifying her priorities and learning how she can better delegate some of her patient care activities to others, including the resident and students. Regardless of her precepting skills, her attitude should also be addressed immediately. It's easy to dismiss her "what's in it for me" attitude as a generational issue—millennials have been praised for their ability to multitask, and they have been identified as a sociable generation that enjoys variety and opportunities.[1]

Molly needs to set up a meeting with her manager to discuss expectations and to revisit the benefits of precepting. She should also ask for some guidance in the other areas that she is struggling. If Molly doesn't feel comfortable doing this with her manager, then she could find a mentor in her department or the profession that has experienced similar day-to-day challenges. One thing for sure, Molly must address the errors that have occurred because she is responsible for making sure that this never happens again. Most new practitioners struggle with fitting precepting responsibilities in their day. Time management skills are essential for success and Molly would benefit from some direction. A great place to start would be with the residency program director. What support is in place for development? Is there a teaching certificate program? Can Molly be a part of this? Although the residency program should focus on precepting development, some of the ownership is also Molly's. She should take some personal measures to improve, such as reading articles or attending a national preceptors' conference. Molly has the opportunity to use her knowledge of department operations to engage the residents in helpful department activities, which may help alleviate some of the tension related to the recent growth until a more permanent solution is found. Molly has numerous opportunities to be part of the solution rather than part of the problem. Maintaining a positive attitude and implementing some coping strategies will allow her to become an approachable voice of reason.

What I have found to be successful

It seems like everyday, I'm being asked to do more with fewer resources. As our profession continues to be challenged with shortages, a positive attitude and working environment continues to be important in job satisfaction. I have found that work friendships help maintain my positive attitude even during the most difficult situations. Numerous studies have shown that friendships at work predict performance (12 elements) and it's important to have someone to confide in. I am extremely lucky in that I have numerous colleagues and mentors that I can rely on at my organization. Finding someone to confide in when frustrated is one of the best things that you can do for yourself. Find someone that will openly listen without passing judgment. A relationship like this will be essential to your success as a leader. Remaining positive also requires some work-life balance skills. It's essential to identify means to manage stress and prevent burnout. There are lots of activities that can allow you to do this. Burnout leads to lower performance and a lack of motivation. Maintaining a solid work-life balance and coping mechanisms will eliminate this burnout and continue to support your positive attitude. As a leader, you should always strive to be "part of the solution." It's easy to complain about processes and changes; however, it's difficult and takes initiative to be part of the improvement. Do that as much as possible!

Know your strengths

PRINCIPLE ■ Self-awareness (who you are)

Pete, a new practitioner, has been working as a clinical pharmacist at a local community hospital in Juno, Iowa. Although the hospital census is nothing in comparison to the large university hospital 25 miles away, Pete sees the impact that clinical pharmacy can make. In his short time at the hospital, he has been able to make significant improvements as a pediatric clinical pharmacist. Pete actually worked as a clinical pharmacy intern at the university hospital and has been able to use his experience to implement numerous clinical protocols for his area since he was hired. Due to his initiative and ongoing clinical improvements, Pete has been recently promoted to clinical coordinator and is in the process of training his replacement, David.

David's path to the community hospital is very different then that of Pete's. David is a new graduate with no hospital experience except his minimal time during rotations in pharmacy school. On those rotations, he was often overheard saying "Why do I need to know that? I'm never going to work in a hospital, and I already have a job so why are you making me do this?" David's work experience outside of his required rotations has also only been in the retail independent practice setting. His career goal was to purchase the retail store where he worked but due to the recent economy, he was unable to secure a loan and couldn't purchase the store. The only job left in Juno was this pediatric clinical pharmacist and because of his financial situation, David had no choice but to accept the offer.

Pete has been training David for 2 weeks. Before his arrival, Pete gave him a pediatric pharmacist guide that included all of the policies and procedures as well as the protocols recently developed. Doing his best to cover all of his bases, he spends every minute with David during his training. Much to Pete's disappointment, David does not ask any questions or need any clarification on the training. David seems extremely disengaged and unmotivated. Although he doesn't have any background experience or training, he acts as a know-it-all. He also seems to have a chip on his shoulder and his arms are always crossed when Pete is discussing something with him. His overall attitude is really getting Pete down and he is starting to wonder if David is the right fit for the position.

WHAT PETE MAY BE THINKING...
- What have I done?
- How did I get talked into this? I should have gone with my gut.
- Why did we ever hire him?
- He's going to blow it. I just know it.
- How can I make him see that this is a great job with lots of potential?

ON THE OTHER HAND, PETE MIGHT REASON...
- If I just work a little harder, he will get it.

- Maybe I can cover his patients for a while during this transition period.
- If I were Pete, what else might I be thinking?
- I need to figure out how to motivate David.

MENTOR ADVICE

Pete is in a difficult position. Perhaps he should have realized that the fit of this pharmacist, David, in this clinical practice area might have not been the best choice. The focus of this case is on the development of the pharmacist in a clinical role but actually Pete himself is also learning a new role or position being a new clinical coordinator. He now must develop leadership skills of managing through others rather than being an "independent" clinical pharmacist.

Pete should seek counsel from his superior in order to gain additional insight on how to train and develop David. The question could also be raised on how much effort and planning has been devoted to developing Pete as a manager. Since Pete is in a relatively new role or position, he must also realize that he is continuing to develop his own leadership and management abilities. He should not only seek advice from his supervisor for how to coach new employees but also how to properly orientate and develop them for their new positions.

Orientation to a new position takes time—certainly longer than 2 weeks. Since Pete had this position previously, I would have David shadow his practice as a part of the orientation and then gradually transfer the responsibility over to David completely. This should give David confidence and perhaps would demonstrate that he does not "know it all" but needs growth and development. If after a reasonable period of time, David's attitude and performance is not at the proper level, it may come to having a "heart-to-heart" with him relative to the position. Perhaps there is an ambulatory care position within the department that he would be better suited for, which would allow him to continue his interest in this area. Otherwise he may feel trapped by this position and would probably continue to create issues or leave as soon as a position is available elsewhere. Since pediatrics is a very unique and specialized clinical service, the pharmacist replacement choice should probably have been someone who had at least some general medicine clinical experience. Perhaps one of the current clinical staff should have been moved into this position and David hired for a general clinical position first.

What I have found to be successful

It is critical to always choose the correct person for the position. Determine this attribute as best as possible during the interview process. Remember that there is a significant investment in training new pharmacists for a new position or role. It is essential that your choice be the best person for the job considering all factors such as qualifications, personality, interest, and fit.

Communicate, communicate, and communicate. Always seek help or ask advice when you need it and likewise do not assume that new employees do not have any questions or are not having any difficulties in adapting to a new position. Assess and not assume. Remember, you are striving for your own leadership development when you are developing and managing others.

NEW LEADER ADVICE

Based on the case, there are two people struggling in this situation—both for different reasons, but mostly because they are new to their respective positions. Although Pete is doing the best that he can based on the situation, he should have requested some time to develop his own leadership skills before offering to mentor and train a new hire. Remember that Pete has only been practicing for a year! Ideally, he would have done this prior to the arrival of David. Since this was not the case, Pete should investigate leadership courses and development programs within the organization or nearby institutions immediately. Some dedicated time to key leadership elements such as communication, time management, and team building may assist with the current state. Pete should also find a mentor that will help him develop his own leadership style and assist in preventing this from happening again.

Once Pete has participated in these classes, he may be able to sit down with David and evaluate his motivations for this position. If Pete is going to be David's mentor and trainer, it is important for him to know David as a person as well as a pharmacist. Getting to know David's strengths, weaknesses, and priorities will help direct and mentor Pete into the appropriate way to deal with David. There are some difficult questions that Pete will have to address with David such as "Is this the right position for you?", "Are you happy?", and "How does this job make you feel when you wake up in the morning?" It's important to discuss this openly as David's future may rely on this particular conversation with Pete. Pete needs to understand David's point of view and his motivations, or lack thereof, before any changes or solutions can be proposed. Pete should also not pass any judgment on David. Just because he loved being a pediatric clinical pharmacist doesn't mean that David will. Results of this conversation should enable Pete to either change the orientation plan based on David's personal style (including his learning style) or should direct Pete to finding an alternative placement for David if possible. Listening to others is a very important skill that Pete will need to utilize often in his new role as a leader within the department and this is a great opportunity to utilize these skills.

Since this is a learning opportunity for David as well, David needs to do some serious soul searching. It's clear that this was not David's first choice for a position upon graduation; however, he needs to realize that his actions are not going to solve anything. Not only is the position in a completely different practice setting, but it is also a specialized practice setting (pediatrics). Since he has been orienting to the position and now has some idea on the responsibilities and daily duties, David will need to assess whether or not he is the right fit for this position. He can do this by spending some time evaluating his strengths, weaknesses, and priorities. Often new practitioners spend time trying to fix their weaknesses and don't spend enough time cultivating their strengths. Once David understands his strengths, he should then focus on goal development. Goals can keep you on track and help you prioritize and evaluate your career both personally and professionally. Goal setting is a very important tool in marketing yourself. If David is honest with himself (who he is), he may see that there are other opportunities within the organization or department that may not have been presented to him at the time of hire.

In addition to the coaching and mentoring that Pete can provide to David, Pete should take the time to inform the department manager of the issues at hand in person. Solid examples, objective information, and even data (if applicable) will be key for the manager to begin to assess David's performance. David may not want to move on, but he may have to move on if his goals and motivations are not in line with the department and organization. I would also recommend that Pete engage the manager at this point in the current orientation plan for David so that if changes need to occur, the manager is aware and onboard. Pete, as a new leader himself, may also want to invest in identifying his strengths and focus on cultivating these as a rising leader within the department. Identifying each person's strengths will assist the manager in developing a well-rounded team and help him focus on areas of improvement. Knowing who you are is a fundamental element of how to market yourself. Focusing on the strengths that you have to offer teams, projects, and departments will create personal success.

What I have found to be successful

Identifying my strengths early in my career has assisted me in finessing the responsibilities of my position within the department. I often find myself volunteering for projects and improvements that force me to work with others, internally and externally. Knowing that I am a "people person" and extrovert has helped me realize that those collaborations create happiness and success for me. In addition to focusing on my strengths, I often evaluate goals on a quarterly basis. It is something that I have found to be extremely valuable as a leader. Goals (short- and long-term) should be developed based on your different roles (mother, wife, daughter, manager, friend, residency coordinator, etc.). It's important to include all of your roles so that the balance doesn't tip one way or another. Once solid goals are established and strengths are evaluated, developing a mission statement is also a great exercise. Strengths, goals, and a mission statement help keep you on the right track. Review these often (ideally monthly) to assess your progress. Always have a self-development goal in place to improve skills throughout your career.

Utilizing components from *Good to Great* by Jim Collins, I have found that it's extremely important to address personnel management issues immediately. Allowing employees to continue in a position that makes them unhappy or doesn't utilize their natural strengths is usually an equation for failure. Although the performance conversation is never enjoyable, the moment that you sense that you are working harder at someone's success, you may need to reassess that position or project. As a manager, it's hard to admit when you have selected the wrong person for the job or task, but your success as a leader depends on addressing the situation as soon as possible. Allowing the wrong people to continue in their role kills morale and is detrimental to all the right people; great vision without great people is impossible to deliver.

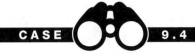

CASE 9.4

The art of persuasion

PRINCIPLES ■ Persuasion ■ Selling a plan/idea

Tyler, a recent pharmacy school graduate, is working on the surgical intensive care unit (SICU). He has just overheard the attendings discussing the expansion of more beds on the SICU and the addition of a second trauma rounding service. Tyler is very anxious about this news; he is already monitoring over 20 intensive care patients and knows that this is above the national average. He lets his supervisor, Kathy, know that there is no way that he can take on the new service patients and it's time to add a critical care pharmacist.

Kathy takes her conversation with Tyler to heart. She remembers that at the last hospitalwide leadership meeting, the CFO mentioned how well the organization was doing financially and how nursing is recruiting double the number of positions from last year. Kathy starts to think that maybe it is time to start the request process for an additional pharmacist FTE. She immediately starts thinking of how she will accomplish this task. She also thinks that this is a great opportunity to get Tyler involved, so she sets out to work on this together. First, Kathy decides that she should contact the attendings and gather the facts. When will this take place? Have they hired new physicians? How many patients will be on service? She also asks Tyler to contact some of his fellow critical care pharmacists across the nation to gather benchmarking information. How many patients do they follow? Is there a pharmacist assigned to every rounding team? What are some of the policies and protocols that are in place for critical care pharmacists?

With this data and written support from the physicians, the proposal is finalized. In addition to the critical care specific data, Kathy decides to include additional workload data to show how increasingly busy the department has become over the last few years. This has also caused some decreases in nursing satisfaction. Now, Kathy is waiting to set up a time to meet with the hospital vice president (VP). Once she determines who will be at that meeting, she alters her executive summary to include only the key information that the VP will be interested in: quality, cost, and outcomes. She deletes all of the additional information she had included when presenting the proposal to her department director. She recalls that the last time she asked for a pharmacist it was a disaster. One thing that she has done differently with this proposal is that she has taken the time to discuss with all of the key stakeholders that this is a necessary addition for patient care. Numerous meetings with physician leadership, nursing leadership, and benchmarking data have resulted in a solid proposal. One of the attending physicians even said, "I won't round without my clinical pharmacists. They are just too valuable. If you want me to come to that meeting with you, I will." What a change from previous attitudes regarding pharmacists and rounds! She knows that the relationship that Tyler has with this group has made a large impact on this support for additional pharmacists. As she is walking to the VP's office, she is a bundle of nerves.

WHAT KATHY MAY BE THINKING...

- There is no way that anyone can get additional resources during this economic downturn.
- What is included in the proposal that will provide the picture for how busy the department is?
- The VP doesn't care about pharmacy.

ON THE OTHER HAND, KATHY MIGHT REASON...

- This is really the best time to ask for support.
- I have all of my ducks in a row and know what I am doing.
- This should work out well.
- I talked to everyone that I should have. This is not just me asking for additional resources—this is a team proposal.

MENTOR ADVICE

Kathy is to be commended for being attentive to the issue that Tyler brought forth. It is important he felt comfortable raising this issue with her because he appreciated the pharmacy department's mission. Likewise, it is good that Kathy recognized the value of Tyler's contribution and appropriately used his enthusiasm to collect some of the data for creating the business case.

The timing appears to be excellent—the hospital is doing well financially, the new service rounding team is developing, pharmacy has current experience on this service, and nursing has recently gained resources to help their workload. The time is very opportune for action. While Kathy has the support from physicians, she needs to gain more support from nursing. In addition, nursing satisfaction scores for the pharmacy are down. Kathy must use this data to put them on her side.

While Kathy is nervous about her presentation, it might be advantageous to take Tyler, a representative of the new SICU team and a RN supporter, with her to meet with administration. She could lead the discussion but would be able to demonstrate her allies in nursing and medicine. In addition Tyler would be available to answer specific questions about the role or function of the pharmacist on this service as well as time or workload issues for the service. This also provides excellent recognition for Tyler's work and dedication.

What I have found to be successful

Always analyze the situation by gathering data, obtaining peer data, and including internal support for your business case or proposal. Always provide the business case in written form with an executive summary. However, present your proposal verbally if at all possible so that you are able to answer any questions or clarify any misconceptions.

Always anticipate your nonsupporters in advance and analyze what issues that they may raise. Be prepared to counter in a professional, nonthreatening manner to any issues that are raised. Do not "bluff." Be well-prepared but always listen to comments and questions as well. If you do not know the answer or have not encountered the issue, promise to follow up with that information. And remember to respond back to all members who were in attendance at the presentation. Opportunities knock—you must react swiftly with action.

NEW LEADER ADVICE

An element in asking for additional resources (people, time, funding, and equipment) is timing; it's crucial to realize the difference that timing can make on a situation. A leader who pursues the wrong action at the wrong time is sure to suffer negative repercussions. Kathy is very lucky to have been proactive about the additional pharmacist as well as to be working at an organization that is doing so well financially. When the right leader and the right timing come together, incredible things happen. Another key component when asking for additional pharmacist resources is persuasion. Kathy has done a great job connecting her ideas (proposal) to people. Her persuasion has lead to endorsements from key physicians and this is something that she can be extremely proud of. Persuasion also requires a lot of energy. Again, Kathy has done this well as she is succeeding at promoting her new positions. By evaluating benchmarking data, Kathy is giving hospital leadership incentives to say yes.

One thing Kathy needs to do is to engage Tyler in the process more. It's crucial for staff members to understand the process for future situations when everything may not be in Kathy's favor. Kathy should also share all triumphs and pitfalls with her staff so that they are aware and understand the process. This transparency will ensure her continued credibility.

What I have found to be successful

Pitching proposals (clinical service expansions, changes in services, and staff scheduling changes) can be a very intimidating experience for anyone. Regardless of the audience, it's always a situation that could go very bad. I have found a few things to be successful as a new leader. The first is to make sure that the key stakeholders internally and externally are aware (similar to Kathy's approach). It's easy to overlook the internal stakeholders in proposals so never forget to discuss your thoughts with others before pursuing them. They may not always be on board with the solution or overall change, but they always need to be aware of what is going on. Can you imagine if two pharmacy leaders asked for resources a day apart without knowing! The next thing is be aware of the audience of your proposal. Again, Kathy did this well in the case, but you want to make sure that you are selling your idea to an individual and you will need to tailor your information to that individual. Presenting proposals or any type of information should be altered to fit that person's preferences as well as professional background. Also, make the presentation memorable. There are numerous ways that this can be done. Tell a story and put your heart into it, bring props for visuals, and offer supporting documents (e-mails, letters, etc.). All of these tools enable you to grab your audiences' attention and may be the deciding factor when proposals are being evaluated.

Finally, throughout the entire proposal process make sure to communicate back to the key stakeholders as well as to the department staff. As previously mentioned, it's important for staff members to understand and address new programs, protocols, and staffing additions. This "loop back" keeps them involved, engaged, and supported.

CASE 9.5

Stay motivated and keep your vision

PRINCIPLE ■ Motivation

Jim is the lead pharmacist covering services for an emergency department (ED) at a community hospital in the outskirts of Lincoln, Texas. Since there are no other hospitals or clinics in the area, the ED usually has about 190 visits a month and half of those visits result in hospital admissions. The number of visits has increased since Jim started 2 years ago and he's thrilled that the pharmacy director was able to leverage for a new pharmacist to help in the ED. This will put the total number of pharmacist full-time equivalents (FTEs) available to support the ED at 3.0. Although there are numerous other opportunities for clinical expansion, the primary responsibility of the ED pharmacist is to gather a full medication history on patients being admitted to the hospital.

As soon as Jim is notified that they will be hiring an additional pharmacist, he calls a team meeting with his other team member, Julie. Jim wants to discuss how they will expand services to cover additional hours in order to capture more admissions. Before Jim can even get to the first thing on his agenda, Julie bounces into the room and yells, "Guess what, I'm pregnant! I wanted to wait to tell you until I was half-way along and I'm due in 5 months. I'm planning on taking a 12-week maternity leave so we need to make sure that we have that covered." Jim immediately thinks that there is no way they are ever going to expand if Julie leaves. How will they capture all of these admits and meet The Joint Commission expectations on medication reconciliation?

Rather than focus on the disappointment that he feels, Jim starts discussing the possibility of how they will accomplish what they need to with the upcoming staffing changes. Although hesitant because the potential new pharmacist coverage schedules won't be ideal for her work-life balance, Julie suggests changing the times of their shifts since they won't be able to fully expand in the coming months. As a team, they decide that it's not necessary to be in the ED early in the mornings as there aren't many admissions during that time. They decide to move one of the shifts back and have an overlapping time during the early evening in order to help capture more admissions. They also discuss the possibility of having the pharmacy administrators train in the ED and familiarize themselves with the medication history process so they can assist in extremely busy situations. Jim and Julie put together a staffing plan to submit to their pharmacy director for approval prior to the start of their new hire.

WHAT JIM MAY BE THINKING...

- It's not the pharmacists' responsibility to come up with an alternative when staffing situations come up. That is management's responsibility.
- Administration will just have to hire another pharmacist.
- I'm a pushover.

ON THE OTHER HAND, JIM MIGHT REASON...

- This is an opportunity for me to set the service and coverage up exactly the way I want.
- Maybe through this process I will learn some leadership skills and they will be noticed by the department administration.
- This new staffing model may save the department crucial resources (time, money, pharmacist hours).

- -

MENTOR ADVICE

Jim has done a good job of leading new emergency department pharmacy services. Apparently this service has been successful in the 2 years in which it has been established. It must have been recognized as very desirable and very successful in that the pharmacy director has justified another pharmacist in order to expand services to 3.0 FTE for the service. Leadership is required not only for establishing new programs or services but also for maintaining the service and resolving problems as they develop.

Certainly, Jim must have mixed emotions when he hears from Julie that she is pregnant. This means that the expansion of 3.0 FTE will probably be delayed and this may place the addition of the FTE in jeopardy. On the other hand, Julie is certainly happy with her new news and she has the right to take FMLA for the 12 weeks allotted for her absence. On the other hand, this provides Jim with an unexpected challenge that he was not expecting. This challenge can be a good test for his leadership abilities.

Julie should be applauded for her dedication to the department and to the service that she and Jim have developed. She has a good attitude and with Jim's leadership together they will start planning on how they can reduce the blow to the program. They have done a good job of thinking outside the box in using data of ER visits to formulate their staffing schedule so that they can handle the maximum number of patients for the resources provided. This illustrates the value of such data that has been collected even though they probably never anticipated that they would need this data for this particular reason.

In looking at the schedule, they should be mindful to hire the new pharmacist prior to Julie's pregnancy leave to allow adequate time for orientation and training. In addition, with the patient workflow data they have collected, they may be able to have the new pharmacist staff a lighter portion of the workload initially until he or she becomes accustomed to the service. Thinking out of the box might also prompt consideration of other resources that may be available. There has been a suggestion of having the pharmacy administrators assist during Julie's maternity leave. They may also consider some staffing by any pharmacists that are currently trained and functioning as medication reconciliation pharmacists on the inpatient units or even using pharmacy residents if they are available to cover during these shifts. This would be an interesting experience for any of these pharmacists.

It is important to develop a best proposal (but feasible) to solve this problem in order to present the proposal to the director. They may not be able to staff the 3.0 FTE during the maternity leave, but if they have adjusted the schedule to maximize the number of patients they can cover, there may still be a gain in the service provided from the current coverage. In addition, such a challenge may provide an educational opportunity for current staff and/or residents. This may even provide future back-up staff to cover vacations and holidays later in the program.

Jim and Julie should demonstrate their leadership and planning by presenting these proposals to the director of pharmacy. A well-organized plan with possible solutions to maintain the current service, preserve pharmacy creditability, and increase the pharmacy service even with limited resources should go far in resolving the dilemma. When faced with a difficult situation, leaders will present their supervisor with a solution rather than a problem. Julie should also be complimented for her dedication to the department. Hopefully, this will result in a "win-win" situation for all.

What I have found to be successful

Encourage the development of a team approach. A dedicated team can usually come up with solutions much better than one person. On the other hand, it usually takes a leader to serve as a catalyst for this process. Take responsibility for your professional practice and career. When faced with problems or challenges always attempt to present resolutions as solutions rather than problems for someone else to resolve. Always do your best to sustain services through creative solutions versus to delete the services or temporarily stop them. The department worked hard to develop progressive services and to meet a patient care need. Sustain them any way you can.

NEW LEADER ADVICE

As the team leader in his clinical area, Jim is extremely dedicated to medication reconciliation and providing the multidisciplinary team support when admitting patients. It's clear that his professionalism and role modeling enables him to motivate his team during some difficult times. It seems as soon as the department becomes fully staffed, there is an alternative situation that arises. How the situation is dealt with is extremely important, and Jim's attitude is a good one. He's committed to accomplishing this goal and is open to alternative suggestions while keeping the end result in mind. His vision on medication reconciliation hasn't changed, and he's open on how to get to the final outcome, which is a great approach. Once he assesses the situation, he should develop a staffing plan for himself and the new hire and then immediately share those recommendations with the ED services manager. In that staffing plan, he should review the changes with nursing and physician leadership in the ED. Changing coverage without having input from those groups may be difficult down the road. Jim could also consider finding an ED department that may have similar issues in another town so that he could set up a site visit and find out what other organizations are doing when faced with the same challenges. Finally, when meeting with the director Jim should ask what other resources are available. Pharmacy interns, technicians, externs, and residents may be appropriate alternatives during staffing situations so it never hurts to ask!

What I have found to be successful

Adaptability is a skill that I have had to rely on heavily as a new leader. Walking into a situation open to only your ideas or solutions will not always gain the respect and credibility needed to complete the task at hand. Remaining open and flexible while maintaining the end result in mind has allowed me to complete a lot of project-related goals. It's not always how you get to the final result as long as you get there. I've found that remaining motivated and adaptable has helped when I have issues that require immediate attention and have a need for a quick solution. These skills have also been helpful when working on a long-term project or goal. It's easy to lose sight of the end result, but remaining motivated to complete the task or project is critical for success. I would encourage new leaders to work on their adaptability skills to make the most out of all circumstances and create the best win-win situation for all those involved.

Summary

There are many different aspects to marketing strategies; however, relationship building is one of the key components that we have elaborated on. Identifying your strengths and goals will further enable you to focus on establishing solid relationships with a variety of people, including colleagues, mentors, students, subordinates, and other team members. Relationships, collaboration, and teamwork should be a goal of all leaders. Utilizing the key elements discussed in this chapter are a starting point in facilitating relationships. Creating relationships will in return result in professional and personal marketing opportunities within the great profession of pharmacy.

Leadership Pearls

- Be a role model for the department and pharmacy profession at all times.
- Remain positive and approachable in challenging situations.
- Be prepared to challenge yourself outside of your comfort zone, and know your strengths and use them!
- Ideas cannot be implemented without support from others.
- Remain motivated and never lose sight of the end goal and be open to alternative paths.

Leadership Exercises

- Take the time to introduce yourself to someone that you may not know. Take a few moments to establish a relationship with that person. It could be professional, personal, or that person could simply be an acquaintance. Whatever the case, make it out of your comfort zone.

- Next time there is an issue that leads to a disagreement, make sure to address it and have a conversation with the parties involved in order to resolve it.

- Volunteer to be a representative for your class, department, school, or other organization. When appropriate, practice representing the organization and marketing your role within that organization.

- The next time you are in a group or team working on getting something completed and have some people that are less than interested, take the time to ask them some questions about their interests and skills rather than make assumptions based on their performance.

- Develop a proposal for additional resources you feel is lacking in a particular area of your life (school, home, work). What data points will you include in the proposal and how will you deliver the proposal?

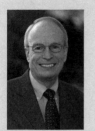

Harold N. Godwin, MS, RPh, FASHP, FAPhA
Professor of Pharmacy Practice and Associate Dean
University of Kansas School of Pharmacy for
   Clinical and Medical Center Affairs
Overland Park, Kansas

Why did you decide on a career in leadership? I chose a career in leadership to help others and to contribute. As a young kid I had an assignment to interview a town leader and I chose a pharmacist. He took the time to show me their compounding practice and script filling. This began my career in pharmacy and interest in leadership. People usually start leadership at a young age—it's just who you are.

Where do you turn for advice when you are stressed? I turn to my network and to my mentors (mentors can be within or outside of pharmacy). Having a network is one of the blessings in pharmacy because you can turn to your colleagues for advice when you need it, and then return the favor when they call you.

What is your favorite leadership book? *Strengths Finder 2.0* by Tom Rath demonstrates that every person has strengths that can be capitalized on. Individuals who make up a team need a variety of strengths in order to be dynamic, and when selected appropriately, the different strengths can lead to synergy and creativity in a team.

From your perspective, what is the most important issue facing pharmacy leadership today? Health-system pharmacy is a recognized clinical profession by other providers in the community. It is important to have a chief pharmacy officer (CPO) at the table for the decision-making process. The CPO is not a title but a position. Other important issues include having strong leadership both in health-system and community practice to create comprehensive pharmacy practices and having a clear vision for the whole profession.

Looking back over your vast experience in pharmacy, what one to two things do you know now that you wish you would have known as a student and new practitioner?

1. Patience and persistence. Learn your environment and be patient. Patience is very important because while you have a vision, it's all about timing if you are to gain the necessary support. To get a vision across you need the endorsements from others to show a collaborative effort. Timing is critical.
2. Concentrate on your victories, not your defeats.

What is your best advice for a new pharmacist today?

- Know, work with, and thank your mentors. Remember, you need to have a mentor(s) for life.
- Find your mentor(s). Develop your professional network.

- Reflect on your vision but be patient and persistent in achieving it.
- Recognize that you don't achieve success by yourself—you need collaboration and a team.

How do you envision this publication assisting student and new practitioner leaders? The approach used by this book for leadership learning is unique in that it blends the experience of new practitioners with that of experienced leaders and shows collaboration of thought. The material in the book applies at all levels of an organization and will be helpful to new leaders in any pharmacy practice setting.

NEW PRACTITIONER PROFILE

Samaneh T. Wilkinson, MS, PharmD
Clinical Manager, Inpatient Clinical Services
PGY1-Residency Director and HSPA PGY-2 Residency Coordinator
Department of Pharmacy
The University of Kansas Hospital
Kansas City, Kansas

Why pharmacy: I was interested in the medical field so I started out in biology and had friends who were in pharmacy. I knew that I wanted to take care of patients and felt pharmacy would be great profession to do so. The profession was also appealing to me as a female with the option to work part-time and have a family.

Advice to readers: In school my only true perspective on pharmacist positions was independent practice. My advice to pharmacy students is to explore as many practice settings as possible. I've learned throughout my career that there are a vast number of opportunities. I was able to find a hospital job in the middle of my pharmacy schooling. But looking back I would have liked to have had more experience prior to residency. My biggest learning since graduation is to trust my own judgment in making decisions even after I gather everyone else's opinions. Having served as president of my local professional organization and on committees at the national level, I realize that this involvement is also vital to my success as a leader. Getting involved professionally has allowed me to create relationships beyond my workplace, and through those I learn what others are doing so that I can bring best practices back to my organization and continually improve practice models and services. When starting out as a new leader, be patient. It takes time to get a career started so be realistic in your expectations and goals. It also takes time to establish rapport and credibility with internal and external peers, thus sudden major changes will make it difficult to partner in the future. Don't ever forget the little wins! There will always be an insignificant thing that makes a major difference for others. Don't be dismissive and work toward getting resources needed for people to do their jobs well. Ask and listen to advice from others. If resources aren't readily available to you, find a mentor. Become a mentor. Seek teaching opportunities and create difficult situations for yourself. Constantly utilize your strengths and strive to personally move to the next level. Always take the time to introduce yourself and allow others to put a name with a face. Be friendly and smile often!

Tips for work-life balance: Set up a support system. I am fortunate that both grandparents live close and are willing to assist with child care. When I am evaluating work-life balance, I look at it as a long-term balance rather than a daily balance. Consider evaluating on a month-by-month or week-by-week basis. There will be times when you will have to devote more time to work. Evaluating work-life balance on a daily basis is frustrating and difficult to achieve. Leadership positions often allow for flexible schedules as long as they are not interfering with daily responsibilities. Discuss options with your administrative team and try and arrange a flexible schedule if possible. Some organizations may allow work from home days or alternative hours as long as they are planned in advance. Sometimes I work on Sunday to get days off during the week, and I use those days off to plan time with my daughter. Dropping her off at school is a big deal for her, so I try to fit it in when possible and move meetings into later hours. It is a balancing act and prioritizing your daily responsibilities is essential. Research services such as cleaning services or Super Suppers (prepared meals that can be frozen and just heated up each night). Whatever it is, always have a plan!

Personal career: My best career decision has been doing a Hospital Administration residency because of the leadership opportunities and experience. It's incredible how much you learn about yourself and your abilities in a 2-year period. I also learned to use mentors and build a network early on. My residency allowed me to become part of a family—a leadership community that continues to provide me with opportunities and support. As a manager at an academic medical center, I've had the opportunity to work on a variety of projects, such as starting a PGY-1 residency program and expanding key clinical services (cardiology, solid-organ transplant ICU, internal medicine, and others). I've also had the opportunity to be involved organizationally in key quality programs, and I am a pharmacy representative on a large number of external committees. My ultimate career goal is to lead inpatient clinical services at an academic center.

Why leadership: My introduction to leadership was in my elective health-system course. Since I was interested in clinical practice and knew that the University of Kansas residency program offered a variety of clinical rotations, I decided to interview for one of the residency positions here. When I started, the first question I asked my residency director was, "Do I really have to complete all of these management rotations?" He laughed and told me that I signed up for a management residency and, yes, I would need to complete those to successfully graduate. One of those required rotations was with the assistant director of clinical services at the time. During my rotation, she happened to start her maternity leave the same month. I was given the opportunity to cover some of her responsibilities, and that is when I realized that through a leadership position I could affect many patients, not just the ones I intervened with during daily rounds. I also knew at that point that I wanted to be heavily involved in personnel development. Creating and supporting other leaders is a passion of mine. I enjoy identifying strengths in people that they may not realize they had and placing them in positions or projects that are successful. Becoming a residency coordinator and director was something that was very important to me. Although I have a number of leadership books that I often reference, some of my favorites are John Maxwell's *The 21 Irrefutable Laws of Leadership: Follow Them and People Will Follow You* and Tom Rath's *Strengths Finder 2.0*.

Recommended change for pharmacy: I would like to see a practice model that enables consistency and has key elements for all organizations to adhere to when developing or expanding pharmacy services. Additional improvements for the profession include more residency positions and fewer pharmacy school admissions. Metrics to evaluate the value of pharmacists in hospital and healthcare systems is also something that would be extremely helpful for pharmacy leadership.

Using this book: This book is a means for students, residents, new practitioners, and clinical leaders to know what opportunities exist within the profession and how to seize every moment in their career so that they can continually improve and strive to be the best pharmacist and leader possible.

Reference

1. Howe N, Strauss W. The next 20 years: how customer and workforce attitudes will evolve. *Harv Bus Rev.* 2007;85:41-52, 191.

Suggested Additional Readings

Collins J. *Good to Great: Why Some Companies Make the Leap... and Others Don't.* New York, NY: HarperBusiness; 2001:20, 46, 96, 124.

Patterson K, Grenny J, McMillan R, et al. *Crucial Conversations: Tools for Talking When Stakes are High.* New York, NY: McGraw-Hill; 2002:21.

Goleman D. What makes a leader? *Harv Bus Rev.* 1998;76(6):93-102.

Maxwell JC. *The 21 Irrefutable Laws of Leadership: Follow Them and People Will Follow You.* Nashville, TN: Thomas Nelson; 1998:109-115.

Shell GR, Moussa M. *The Art of Woo: Using Strategic Persuasion to Sell Your Ideas.* New York, NY: Portfolio–Penguin USA; 2007.

Additional Materials

Complete the strengthsfinder.com profile and learn about your unique talents and strengths—and of those you manage. Read *Now, Discover Your Strengths* by Marcus Buckingham and Donald Clifton, PhD.

Complete *The 7 Habits of Highly Effective People Personal Workbook* by Stephen R. Covey and focus on goal development and completing a mission statement. Evaluate and include your strengths and personal and professional goals.

 *Read "Success Skills" article 15.*

Index